Death, Religion and Law

This practical guide summarizes the principles of working with dying patients and their families as influenced by the commoner world religions and secular philosophies. It also outlines the main legal requirements to be followed by those who care for the dying following the death of the patient.

The first part of the book provides a reflective introduction to the general influences of world religions on matters to do with dying, death and grief. It considers the sometimes conflicting relationships between ethics, religion, culture and personal philosophies, and how these differences impact on individual cases of dying, death and loss. The second part describes the general customs and beliefs of the major religions that are encountered in hospitals, hospices, care homes and home care settings. It also includes discussion of non-religious spirituality, humanism, agnosticism and atheism. The final part outlines key socio-legal aspects of death across the UK.

Death, Religion and Law provides key knowledge, discussion and reflection for dealing with the diversity of the everyday care of dying and death in different religious, secular and cultural contexts. It is an important reference for practitioners working with dying patients, their families and the bereaved.

Peter Hutton was Professor of Anaesthesia at Birmingham University, an Honorary Consultant at University Hospital Birmingham and a Medical Examiner. He is now a non-Executive Director of the Royal Brompton and Harefield Hospitals.

Ravi Mahajan is Professor of Anaesthesia and Intensive Care at Nottingham University, UK.

Allan Kellehear is 50th Anniversary Professor (End of Life Care), Faculty of Health Studies, University of Bradford, UK.

Death, Religion and Law

A Guide for Clinicians

**Peter Hutton, Ravi Mahajan and
Allan Kellehear**

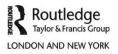 Routledge
Taylor & Francis Group

LONDON AND NEW YORK

First published 2020
by Routledge
2 Park Square, Milton Park, Abingdon, Oxon OX14 4RN

and by Routledge
52 Vanderbilt Avenue, New York, NY 10017

Routledge is an imprint of the Taylor & Francis Group, an informa business

British Library Cataloguing-in-Publication Data
A catalogue record for this book is available from the British Library

Library of Congress Cataloging-in-Publication Data
Names: Hutton, Peter, PhD, author. | Mahajan, Ravi P., author. | Kellehear, Allan, 1955- author.
Title: Religion, Law and Death : A Guide For Clinicians / Authors, Peter Hutton, Ravi Mahajan & Allan Kellehear.
Description: Abingdon, Oxon ; New York, NY : Routledge, 2019.
Identifiers: LCCN 2018057798| ISBN 9781138592889 (hardback) | ISBN 9781138592896 (pbk.) | ISBN 9780429489730 (e-book)
Subjects: | MESH: Attitude to Death | Religion and Medicine | Terminal Care—ethics | Jurisprudence | United Kingdom
Classification: LCC BF789.D4 H86 2019 | NLM BF 789.D4 | DDC 155.9/37—dc23
LC record available at https://lccn.loc.gov/2018057798

ISBN: 978-1-138-59288-9 (hbk)
ISBN: 978-1-138-59289-6 (pbk)
ISBN: 978-0-429-48973-0 (ebk)

Typeset in Sabon
by Swales & Willis Ltd, Exeter, Devon, UK
Printed and bound by CPI Group (UK) Ltd, Croydon CR0 4YY

Contents

List of figures   *viii*
List of tables   *x*
Foreword   *xi*
Preface   *xiii*
Acknowledgements   *xvi*

PART I
Belief systems in society and human history:
interpretations of the mysteries of life and death   **1**

1   Introduction to death and religion in society   2

2   Faith, why people believe and the need for tolerance   5

3   The characteristics of a religion or belief system   15

4   The range of belief paradigms   26

5   What happens when we die?   32

6   The soul: what is it; where is it; and does it exist?   49

7   What does death mean to patients and their relatives?   61

8   Near-death experiences, deathbed visions and
    visions of the bereaved   65

9   The entanglement of religion, ethics and societal
    development   69

10 The uses and abuses of religion   80

PART II
Managing death in different faiths and doctrines   89

11 An introduction to religions and belief systems   90

12 The landscape of religions worldwide and in the UK   97

13 The Baha'i faith   103

14 Buddhism   107

15 Chinese religions   117

16 Christianity   124

17 Hinduism   136

18 Islam   144

19 Jainism   155

20 Judaism   161

21 Rastafarianism   171

22 Secular philosophies and other belief systems   175

23 Shintoism   186

24 Sikhism   193

25 Zoroastrianism   201

PART III
Legal aspects of death in the UK   205

26 Life and death as biological and legal constructs   206

27 Medico-legal issues at the end of life   221

28 The responses of professionals and relatives around death   237

29 Medical certification of the cause of death (MCCD)   245

30 The registration of death   253

31 Coroners and autopsies   260

32 The body after death   271

33 Disposal of the body   278

34 Life support, brain death and transplantation   283

35 Performing last offices   291

36 Less common circumstances   293

37 Deaths in Northern Ireland and Scotland   297

38 Future changes in England and Wales   311

Index   *316*

Figures

11.1   Chinese and Japanese beliefs   92
11.2   Religions originating in the Indian subcontinent   93
11.3   An outline of Zoroastrianism   93
11.4   Abrahamic and related faiths   94
11.5   Secular ethics and new faiths   95
14.1   Mahāyāna Buddhism in Asia. Reproduced under license
       from Keown D (2013): *Buddhism: A Very Short
       Introduction*, Oxford University Press, p. XVI. The hatched
       area shows where the Buddha taught and lived.   111
14.2   Theravāda Buddhism in Asia. Reproduced under license
       from Keown D (2013): *Buddhism: A Very Short
       Introduction*, Oxford University Press, p. XV. The hatched
       area shows where the Buddha taught and lived.   112
15.1   The *taijitu* symbol of yin and yang: yin is associated
       with darkness, water and the female, yang with light,
       activity, air and the male   120
16.1   An outline of the history of the Christian faith   126
18.1   The main divisions of Islam   148
18.2   The rise and spread of Islam. Reproduced under licence
       from Ruthven M (1997): *Islam: A Very Short
       Introduction*, Oxford University Press, p. XIII   149
20.1   The main branches of Judaism   166
24.1   Map of Punjab, showing the undivided Punjab before
       1947, its division between the new state of Pakistan
       and the sub-division of India's post-partition state of
       Punjab in 1966. Reproduced under license from
       Nesbitt E (2016): *Sikhism: A Very Short Introduction*,
       Oxford University Press, p. 10   194

26.1 A single-celled organism, the amoeba 208
26.2 Schematic diagram of a higher mammal 210
26.3 The three sets of criteria for diagnosing death 217
29.1 The front side of an MCCD 248
29.2 The back side of an MCCD 249
30.1 A completed death certificate 256
34.1 Judith in the tent of Holofernes. Reproduced under licence
from National Gallery Picture Library, London 284
34.2 Detail of neck with spurting arteries 285
37.1 A sample Northern Ireland handwritten MCCD form.
Please note that each MCCD has a retained counterfoil
section similar to the English MCCD shown in Figure 29.1 299
37.2 A sample electronic Northern Ireland MCCD form.
The doctor works through a series of screens, the first of
which is shown in Figure 37.2a on p.300. After this is
complete, a paper record of the necessary information for
registration is printed out in hard copy as shown here
(Figure 37.2b) 300
37.3 A Scottish MCCD form: it has four pages, as shown 304

Tables

10.1	Life expectancy and social class	80
10.2	Charitable income raised by faith groups	81
12.1	The percentage distribution of a faith's adherents in the six major regions of the world	99
12.2	The projected percentage growth among different religious groups by 2060	101
12.3	Distribution of faiths in England and Wales in 2011	101
18.1	The current distribution of Muslims across the world	144
26.1	The essential criteria for diagnosing circulatory death	218
32.1	A list of notifiable diseases	274
37.1	International comparisons in autopsy rates	298

Foreword

Dame Joan Bakewell

Death is a mystery. It remains a mystery even for all those who deal with it professionally: priests, doctors, nurses, social workers. Most of us don't think about it at all until someone we love dies and the shock hits us directly. However, care professionals are confronted regularly with the realities of what dying means for different people. It falls to them to understand and treat with sympathy the many different ways people make sense of the world. . . especially when they're leaving it.

This is where science and religion meet, and it is a brave book that sets out to explain and understand what happens when they do. This is such a book.

We in the West live in a multi-cultural society, enjoying the benefits of cultural differences in the arts and in domestic life – cooking, holidays and such. But what we often find difficult to understand is the totally different worldview that other belief systems follow. More isolated parts of the world have a more unified culture, unaware of the variety of beliefs the world holds, but no area of the inhabited planet is so remote as not, on occasion, to overlap with other values. People travel widely, people take up work in far-away places; the need to have a tolerant understanding of other beliefs is paramount in our all getting along together.

I present a BBC Radio 4 series, *We Need to Talk about Death*. It covers a wide range of topics ranging from different forms of burial to the consideration of grieving. What this work brings home to me is the variety and intricacy of people's faiths and the important detail of observance and behaviour. This, observed in their lives, is intensified when someone is ill and dying. It is then, more than ever, when people of and without faith are looking directly into the unknown that an informed knowledge about their beliefs will be so important to those who care for them.

Carers, for their part, have their own philosophies and religious beliefs. Their work will reflect those beliefs and need to be considered in their treatment of others. We are living in times different from any other; we are more globally connected one with another; we are more sensitive to cultural hurt and insult. We have recognised that to live together we must understand what is of value in people's lives. People entrusted with the care of others have a particularly sensitive role. It is part of their calling to understand that. This book has successfully set out to make managing the process of death easier for patients, relatives and professionals and will be of value across many cultures and outlooks, including our own.

Preface

Everybody will die; there are no escapees. This book has been written because the authors, from their own professional experiences, feel that there is a need to improve the information related to, and the teaching of, the process of managing death. It is intended for doctors, ward and community nurses and social workers or any others who manage the dying and their relatives.

The book is meant to assist all those working in our multi-cultural, multi-ethnic society to better understand and care for those outside their own immediate cultural circle. It is hoped that two groups will benefit:

- those being cared for because their religious and psychological needs will be better understood and provided for, and
- those doing the caring by increasing their knowledge and confidence and reducing their anxiety about what should be done for the best.

The text tries to give support in the round by proportionately encompassing medical, cultural, religious, philosophical and legal aspects of death. In modern British hospitals, GP practices, care homes and within the social services, the cultural, religious and ethnic mixes in both the carers and those cared for is such that it is common for patients or relatives to be attended by a professional from outside their own culture and religion. There remain large sections of professional groups and the public who are unfamiliar with any belief system other than that within which they were raised. Whilst it is unreasonable to expect the patient and their relatives to anticipate and understand the attitudes and norms of their attendant, in contrast, it is absolutely incumbent upon the attendant to both understand and meet the specific needs of the patient or relative.

Nowhere is this need for knowledge more important than in looking after the person who is approaching death. A 'good death' for the patient and their relatives and friends should not be left to chance. A 'bad death' can linger corrosively and significantly delay healing in the bereaved. It remains a sad fact that a 'bad death' hangs on in the minds of the survivors for a long time; it does not evaporate with the disposal of the body. Furthermore, it can raise anxiety levels about their own dying, and how they will be treated at the end. Hence, there is an imperative to 'get it right' on every possible occasion.

Compassion does cross cultures, usually successfully, but additionally, managing a death requires some knowledge of the beliefs by which the dying person has lived, how they are likely to approach death, what they think is important and what they think will happen after life is extinct. It is also essential to be completely clear about the legal aspects of death and particularly to know what is mandatory and where discretion can be applied. The text tries to address what the authors perceive as the knowledge base a professional needs if they are likely to meet with the dying and their relatives in the UK. The content has been arrived at empirically – it has evolved from experience of what has been observed, and what, if it had been present in both knowledge and behavior, would have made things better.

The book is divided into three parts. These are as follows.

Part I Belief systems in society and human history: interpretations of the mysteries of life and death

Part II Managing death in different faiths and doctrines

Part III Legal aspects of death in the UK

Part I looks at the basis for faith and belief, including secular beliefs, from the dawn of man to the present. It describes the constant inter-twining of belief systems with cultural changes. It has been included because much of what it contains is absent from modern curricula, yet is essential to understanding the landscape of care.

Part II describes how the major religions originated and developed together with the important issues in managing the deaths of believers and non-believers. All the major religions are covered. Some small faith groups are missed, but it was necessary to apply a limit since there are hundreds of different sub-divisions each with their own individual characteristics. The text necessarily assumes that a carer of any affiliation could be dealing with a patient of any affiliation. Furthermore, the wider family group may encompass several beliefs, which may or may not align with the wishes of the recently dead. The intention is that the carer(s) will have a reference source to quickly establish what is important as death approaches and what will be important after death has occurred.

Part III reviews the legal aspects of death in the UK. Over recent years there have been changes to the Coroners Acts in England and Wales and a new Medical Examiner system is being introduced. Scotland, which has a different legal system, has also had modifications to its registration system, as has Northern Ireland. Overseas staff coming to the UK may have little knowledge of the legalities of death registration here, because they will come with experience of their own country's system.

In conclusion, it is hoped that this book, in presenting the information as it does, will be timely, interesting and of practical use. Above all, we hope that it will ultimately benefit those who are dying and those who grieve.

It should be noted that there is no consideration of abortion, stillbirths and childhood and maternal deaths, which are specialist areas.

Acknowledgements

In particular, the authors would like to acknowledge the time and valuable assistance given by Professor Jack Crane, former State Pathologist for Northern Ireland, and Dr James Grieve, former Senior Lecturer in Forensic Pathology at the University of Aberdeen, in the composition of Chapter 37.

We are also grateful to the following friends and colleagues who have contributed through conversations, commenting on drafts and suggesting modifications: Chrissie and David Ashton, Julian Bion, David Bogod, Tom Bowden, Brian Cooper, Paul Dias, John Hillborn, Karrar Khan, Meriel and Christopher Hutton, Brian and Nina Johnson, Bertie Leigh, Charlie Ralston, Andy Reddy, Denis and Margaret O'Riordan, Maria Rollin, Susan and Michael Orlik, and Johannes Niederhauser.

The responsibility for what is written rests with the authors.

Part I

Belief systems in society and human history

Interpretations of the mysteries of life and death

Chapter 1

Introduction to death and religion in society

Doctors, nurses, physiotherapists, social workers and all other health and social care staff follow undergraduate and postgraduate training that is predominantly designed to give them the professional tools to practise safely. This is as it should be because the application of specialized skills to meet agreed standards is the cornerstone of quality care.

During training there will be some teaching on the wider issues of management such as ethics, withdrawal of care and legal issues surrounding death. It is however generally only in advanced practice, several years after professional qualification, that practitioners look at the patient in a truly holistic manner and consider their beliefs and societal context when deciding with them and their relatives the best course of action. Yet when patients are approaching the ends of their lives and when they actually die, at key moments such as breaking bad news or confirmation of death it is often those who are only recently qualified that are the ones present to speak to patients, manage events and have discussions with relatives.

The management of the final days is so important for the patient and their loved ones. Also, after death, how these events evolved and the manner of their happening are crucial factors for relatives or close friends in determining poor or positive bereavement outcomes. This is even more so when death is sudden or tragic. Clinical staff do their best at handling death and its consequences, but good will, although vital, needs to be underpinned with a knowledge and appreciation of how major life events are interpreted, shaped and dealt with by persons who, both socially and in their belief systems, are unlike themselves.

The majority of healthcare staff do think about life and death but it is inevitably against a background of their own social and religious beliefs. These various beliefs (both explicit and implicit) are ingrained into all societies and have been so for millennia. There is normally an appreciation of the variations of the attitudes and beliefs of others in a modern multi-cultural society, but this may simply be formed and bounded by the lottery of life's experiences. Albert Camus in his novel *L'Étranger*[1] and Henrik Ibsen in his play *An Enemy of the People*[2] focused on the importance of the membership of one's 'tribe' in society and the penalties and alienation that result when an individual declines to conform to social norms. Such tribalism inhibits spontaneous assimilation of other people's lifestyles. A special effort and an appreciation of 'where the other person is coming from' has to be made by a healthcare worker to properly engage and interact at a meaningful level with a member of 'another tribe'.

As will be seen in Part II of this book, religion and belief systems are another visceral component of a person's constitution, whether they necessarily appreciate it or not. In approximately 700 BCE Homer declared that:

all men have need of the gods[3]

and over 2,000 years later Voltaire in one of his epistles wrote:

If God did not exist, it would be necessary to invent him.
Let the wise man announce him and kings fear him.
Kings, if you oppress me, if your eminencies disdain
The tears of the innocent that you cause to flow,
My avenger is in the heavens: learn to tremble.
Such, at least, is the fruit of a useful creed.[4]

Today things are just the same, even if the players are different. Religions are living, ever changing mediums into which people are born. Faiths consider the metaphysical nature of being and the hereafter, care for the psyche and provide social structures with their own behavioural norms. They are constantly morphing as time passes. Some grow, others contract and different belief systems cope well or not so well with the modern world.

The possible combinations of social tribes, religious beliefs (or otherwise), metaphysical ideologies, ethnicities and legal structures that surround dying, death and the disposal of bodies are limitless. There is a vast literature available covering all these aspects, but they are dispersed and not always easy to source. In short, it is difficult for a busy healthcare professional to easily access a succinct review of what matters to different people in life and death so as to be able 'to put themselves in their shoes'. In this book we attempt to provide an overview of this landscape. The drivers for faith, tolerance and intolerance, the characteristics of religions, the possibilities of a soul and an afterlife, what death means to different people, the entanglement of religion, ethics and societal development and the uses and abuses of religion are all discussed.

To demonstrate the breadth of approaches, which those who have tried to tackle these issues of human existence have used, examples are drawn from the past and present, countries across the world, religious and secular texts, poetry, plays, musicals and scientific papers. Our hope is that this text will provide a conveniently accessible, unbiased and readable source for those who want the knowledge but who, in the jargon, 'are not time rich'. Although they will probably find more questions than answers, knowing what others think and believe is fundamental to compassionate practice.

Notes

1 Camus A (2013 [1942]): *The Outsider (L'Étranger)*, translated by Smith S, Penguin Modern Classics.
2 Ibsen HJ (2018 [1882]): *An Enemy of the People*, translated by Marx E, CreateSpace Independent Publishing Platform.
3 Homer (2003 [*c.*700 BCE]): *The Odyssey*, translated by Rieu EV, Penguin Classics, book 3, lines 45–50.
4 Voltaire (1877–1885 [1768]): *Epître à l'auteur du livre des Trois imposteurs (Oeuvres complètes de Voltaire*, edited by Louis Moland, Garnier, tome 10, pp. 402–405), available at: www.whitman.edu (search for The Voltaire Society of America).

Chapter 2

Faith, why people believe and the need for tolerance

Although there are anthropological views suggesting that some cultures believed in an afterlife whilst others did not, from the time it was possible to chip thoughts into stone and paint images on walls, generations of humans have conjectured on the purpose of existence and the possibilities of life after death.

These questions are not new, but their resolution and the belief systems created to explain them depend upon a contemporaneous interpretation of society and scientific knowledge. Since these change, so too do perceptions of reality and belief. Proposed paths to understanding commonly, but not always, result in the postulation of one or more great powers or gods, or a Creator, or a single divine being or God who is eternal. As time passes, following the traditional ordained creed can set a group apart as it observes its stipulated rules and tries to maintain them within a wider social or pluralistic national setting.

Fundamentalists adhere to what they assert to be the original beliefs and prescribed behaviours set out when a religion was created, but many others would argue that to do so is illogical because the personal, local and world situation is constantly changing. Each generation gains new insights into their sacred texts through the lens of their current times and culture. This is the sociological meaning of the term 'revelation', which should not be confused with the religious meaning of 'revelation' that describes a divine or supernatural communication to a man or prophet from a god. Re-interpretation and/or modification to original tenets create branches and divisions within the founding faith: this phenomenon is present throughout all the major world religions. Hence for many, religion is a living paradigm within which there is a need to respond and to modify one's beliefs and practices as time progresses, knowledge accumulates and society changes.

Consequential links between religious belief and practice and social development were analysed by Weber in his classic *The Sociology of Religion* where he introduced the term 'theodicy'. The theodicy of fortune (privilege) and misfortune (disprivilege) is the theory of how different social classes adopt different belief systems to help explain their social situation. These distinctions can be applied not only to class structure within a society but also to denominational and ethnic segregation within religions. In relation to ancient Eastern religions he writes:

> Wherever a developing priestly ethic met a theodicy of disprivilege half-way, the theodicy became a component of congregational religion, as happened with the pious Hindu and the Asiatic Buddhist. That these religions lack virtually any kind of socio-revolutionary ethics can be explained by reference to their theodicy of rebirth, according to which the caste system is eternal and absolutely just. The virtues or sins of a former life determine birth into a particular caste, and one's behaviour in the present life determines one's chances of improvement in the next rebirth.[1]

This process of never-ending and repetitive life cycles called 'Samsara' is of course entirely different to the concept of the Abrahamic religions where a person gets only one shot at life, and everything that follows might depend upon it forever – hence the construct of belief and the organization of society are fundamentally different in these contrasting faith systems.

In 1998, the late Ninian Smart, an authority on the world's religions, was interviewed and commented on the modification of religions and the ways they change, especially when they start to interface with different faiths. He said:

> What happens when Religion A meets Religion B? Well, A becomes a little B-ified, and B becomes a little A-ified. Then people in A don't like the B-ification, so they become AA types. And the same goes for B. So there is always that dynamic going on when religions meet.[2]

Interpersonal frictions and local and international wars have often been the result of not accommodating the beliefs and lifestyles of others. This unhappiness continues today and there are many examples across the continents. On an interpersonal level contraception and homosexuality are still unacceptable in some faiths; in local societies, faith schools and the wearing of religious icons offend some citizens; and internationally, corrosive inter-religious conflict continues in many places such as the Middle East, Nigeria and Myanmar.

Dissensions of this nature are not new. The need for an understanding of another person's deeply held beliefs and what they consider to be the proper way of conducting their life was recognized in the writings of the ancient

Greek historian and traveller Herodotus (484–425 BCE) who related a social experiment performed by the Persian king, Darius (550–486 BCE):

> When Darius was king, he summoned the Greeks who were with him and asked them what price would persuade them to eat their fathers' dead bodies. They answered that there was no price for which they would do it. Then he summoned those Indians who are called Callatiae,[3] who eat their parents, and asked them (the Greeks being present and understanding by interpretation what was said), what would make them willing to burn their fathers at death. The Indians cried aloud, that he should not speak of so horrid an act. So firmly rooted are these beliefs; and it is I think, rightly said . . . that custom is king of all.[4]

Underpinning this social experiment are the conflicting Persian belief that fire is a god deserving reverence and the Callatiae's respect for inherited spirits. The latter's custom in a different part of the world continued into the 20th century in the Fore people of Papua New Guinea which allowed the discovery that prions (mutant or 'rogue' intercellular proteins postulated as the cause of diseases such as scrapie and bovine spongiform encephalopathy, also known as mad cow disease) were transmitted from one generation to the next by the consumption of the deceased's cooked body and brain.

Difficulties over the management of dying and death continue to this day. Jews and Muslims want quick burials with no interference with the body; Hindus want the body to be cremated; traditional Zoroastrians wish to have it eaten by carrion; and Christians allow a choice. Difficulties can arise when the death is deemed suspicious or unnatural and the legal system over-rides religious choice, introducing obligatory examination of the remains and delays to disposal.

Ideological[5] or religious belief, maintained by custom and social reinforcement, is a major driver that determines how people think and behave. This was a theme developed by Hume in the 18th century in his *Treatise of Human Nature*. He argued that 'all our reasonings concerning causes and effects are deriv'd from nothing but custom'[6] and that 'belief is an act of the mind arising from custom'.[7] He famously asserted that 'generally speaking, the errors in religion are dangerous, those in philosophy only ridiculous'.[8]

Hume's conclusion was that religious belief had no logical justification and that a further illogical or emotional step of believing was necessary for faith. He emphasized that belief was often resistant to change and that

> All those opinions and notions of things, to which we have been accustom'd from infancy, take such deep root, 'tis impossible for us, by all the powers of reason and experience, to eradicate them.[9]

This was also a view held by the Jesuit Order in their commonly quoted aphorism:

Give Me a Child Until He Is Seven, and I Will Give You the Man.[10]

In more modern times the importance of belief, and the receptiveness of the young mind, was illustrated in the novel *Whistle Down the Wind* which was turned into a musical in 1998. In this, an escaped killer is mistaken by children as Jesus in a Second Coming, and rather than turn him in, they secretly hide and feed him, despite the warnings of their parents about the dangerous convict. This resulted in the now well known hit single by Boyzone of which the refrain is:

No matter what they tell us
No matter what they do
No matter what they teach us
What we believe is true.[11]

Furthermore, it is an accident of birth as to which religious denomination a person starts out with in life – just like the language and social customs they learn. Although there is a trend towards secularization there are very few proselytes who convert through analysis of the available faiths, so the majority of devotees die in the faith they were born into.

Whilst examining the justifications for different beliefs and the content of religious texts, if we fast-forward via the modernism and post-modernism of the 19th and 20th centuries, we terminate at the confusion of 'relativism' which has been, in its various guises, both one of the most popular and also one of the most reviled philosophical doctrines of our time.[12] Whilst relativism has several sub-divisions, what it means here is the concept that experience is personal and its interpretation and meaning depends upon the matrix within which it is received. Relativism, roughly put, is the view that truth and falsity, right and wrong, standards of reasoning and procedures of justification are products of differing conventions and frameworks of assessment and that their authority is confined to the context giving rise to them, i.e. the perceived truth is in the mind of the beholder.

Although this concept has had much more exposure in the late 20th and 21st centuries, it is not really new. The history of different styles of moral and religious relativism has been reviewed by Fricker,[13] who demonstrates its history from the BCE period to the present day. In particular she quotes Montaigne (1533–1592) who foreshadows the views of Hume:

Each man calls barbarism whatever is not his own practice [because] we have no other test of truth and reason than the example and pattern of the opinions and customs of the country we live in.

Self-perceived relative truth is the complete antithesis of the traditional efforts of philosophers and theologians who concerned themselves with the search for valid argument and universal, absolute truth. One of the most controversial of modern philosophers, Richard Rorty, who combined rationalism with pragmatism, regarded the truth as a chimera. One of the most frequently quoted of his aphoristic comments is:

Truth cannot be out there – cannot exist independently of the human mind – because sentences cannot so exist, or be out there.[14]

Relativism of this nature has not escaped without criticism. After Rorty died in 2007, in an otherwise balanced obituary, Roger Scruton concluded:

However, I believe that the concept of truth is fundamental to human discourse, that it is the precondition of any genuine dialogue, and that real respect for other people requires an even greater respect for truth. . . . Rorty was paramount among those thinkers who advance their own opinion as immune to criticism, by pretending that it is not truth but consensus that counts, while defining the consensus in terms of people like themselves.[15]

When it is taken to imply that the individual is always justifiably correct, this modern form of relativism is not limited to academic exercises in philosophy and theology. It finds a virtually unlimited yet anonymous and unaccountable expression in social media that allows false respectability to emergent groups of like-minded individuals. The members can easily reinforce their own particular views and beliefs unfettered by the checks and balances inherent in everyday verbal interchange. This is particularly so in the suggestible and disaffected, whose personal and political views can easily be influenced. It is argued that social media played a significant role in the coordination of the Arab Spring,[16] which fundamentalist religious groups use for propaganda and recruitment.[17] In this way, social media not only joins people together, it can motivate them to a common purpose. Paradoxically, it can promote division, especially between those faith and lobby groups who perhaps have more interest in confirming their own beliefs and advancing their own objectives than exploring those of others.

An additional contribution to the debate on the importance of emotion in how we formulate our ideas and beliefs and make our lifestyle choices has recently come from the *Oxford Dictionary*. Their 'Word of the Year' in 2016 was 'post-truth' defined as 'relating to or denoting circumstances in which objective facts are less influential in shaping public opinion than appeals to emotion and personal belief'.[18] They made this choice because although 'the concept of post-truth has been in existence for the past decade, Oxford Dictionaries has seen a spike in frequency this year (2016) in the context of the EU referendum in the United Kingdom and the presidential election in the United States. It has also become associated with a particular noun, in the phrase post-truth politics'. This development of appeals to emotion and 'alternative facts' has not gone unnoticed in the consequences it might have,[19] and a leader in *The Economist*[20] concluded that 'the novelty of post-truth may lead back to old-fashioned oppression'. The crossover here with emotional drivers related to religious beliefs and their interplay with lifestyles and lifestyle choices (e.g., abortion, euthanasia, origin of the earth, the choice of books in education, what is studied at universities) is obvious.

It is fashionable to berate the colonial period of Britain's history forgetting about any positive features it may have had. Today, self-flagellation is seen in both written and spoken commentaries atoning for the military interventions, land-grabs, commercial exploitations and the Christian religious enthusiasms of our forefathers that accompanied British colonial expansionism. However, not all members of the Edwardian and Victorian chattering classes were untroubled by such overseas policies and there is a literature to support this. Those with insight were only too well aware of the future socio-religious dangers inherent in colonialism and they worked to anticipate and ameliorate them.

Although now largely (unfairly) relegated to the marginalia of history, Herbert Spencer (1820–1903) was the leading British philosopher and thinker as the *fin de siècle* approached. He famously coined the phrase 'survival of the fittest' with respect to Darwinism and managed to sell over one million copies of his books in his lifetime – probably still a world record for a philosopher. He was an agnostic who rejected theology and introduced a 'Synthetic Philosophy' to tackle the problems of life. In relation to religion and argument he wrote:

> In proportion as we love truth more and victory less, we shall become anxious to know what it is which leads our opponents to think as they do. We shall begin to suspect that the pertinacity of belief exhibited by them must result from a perception of something we have not perceived.

And we shall aim to supplement the portion of truth we have found with the portion found by them. . . . [we] shall not regard some men's judgements as wholly good and others as wholly bad; but shall, contrariwise, lean to the more defensible position that none are completely right and none are completely wrong.[21]

This was a very rational (but probably not widely supported) stance to take for a multi-cultural empire upon which the sun never set. Whilst Spencer was writing, others were talking. From its beginnings in 1787 as a group that rejected the doctrine of eternal hell, the South Place Institute in Finsbury, London, evolved as a centre for nonconformist and ethical debate.[22] From 1888 to 1891 it held a series of Sunday lectures designed to explain and illustrate the different religious movements of the day from across the world, delivered by people who had experience of them. These lectures were first collected together in book form in 1889 as *Religious Systems of the World* and was the surprise publication of the year, selling out within a few months. So, even at that time, people were interested in what others thought and believed. In the frontispiece of the book was an extract from the *Universal Review* of 1888. It read:

A new Catholicity has dawned upon the world. All religions are now recognized as essentially Divine. They represent the different angles at which man looks at God. . . . The old intolerance has disappeared . . . The new tolerance of faith recognizes as Divine all the creeds which have enabled men to overcome their bestial appetites with visions of things spiritual and eternal.[23]

This all looks pretty positive and forward-looking, but 130 years later religious strife continues. Where is the universal tolerance? The need to overcome beliefs which divide people and to accept and reconcile differences is now greater than ever because of the widespread international movement of people for employment, recreation and sanctuary. This need was recognized by Bertrand Russell over 50 years ago as international travel was increasing and the aftermath of two world wars was being comprehended. He said:

In this world, which is getting more and more closely interconnected, we have to learn to tolerate each other . . . put up with the fact that some people say things that we don't like . . . if we are to live together and not die together, we must learn a kind of charity and . . . tolerance.[24]

Forty years later, in a later part of the interview quoted earlier, Ninian Smart similarly advocated this theme of mutual tolerance and cross-pollination in a radio interview:

> I do believe we're moving toward a global ideology that has a place for religion and recognizes the contributions of the different traditions. Hopefully, it will have an overarching view as to how we can work together for the promotion of human values and spirituality. I would like to see an agreement that recognizes that we live on the same planet and that some interests, such as human rights, must be universal and that all religions must be respected.[25]

The contemporary moral philosopher David Wong has also tackled the issue of different groups being committed to different moral and religious standpoints across Western and Eastern cultures. He argues that:

> Moral norms need to take into account the strength of self-interest in order to accommodate that motivation and to encourage its integration with motivations that more directly lead to acting on behalf of others.[26]
>
> Given the inevitability of serious disagreement within all kinds of moral traditions that have any degree of complexity, a particular sort of ethical value becomes especially important . . . Let us call this value 'accommodation'. To have this value is to be committed to supporting non-coercive and constructive relations with others although they have ethical beliefs that conflict with one's own.[27]

Knowing the multi-cultural nature of the individuals both in society and in our caring professions, there are no situations to which the quoted comments can be more relevant than the giving and receiving of care, wherever it occurs. This is especially so when it includes the major turning points in life such as birth and death. It should be 'a given' that health and care workers are sensitive to these issues and sufficiently equipped with the relevant knowledge and insights not only to care for physical and mental illness, but also to accept and engage with the religious and cultural expectations of the patient and their family group.

Notes

1 Weber M (1991 [1922]): *The Sociology of Religion*, Beacon Press, p. 113.
2 Professor Ninian Smart was interviewed by Scott London on 'The Future of Religion' on the radio series *Insight and Outlook* in April 1999. This interview is available at: www.scottlondon.com/interviews/smart.html.

3 Herodotus (1995 [1921]): *The Histories*, 2 vols, trans Godley AD, Loeb, III.38, vol. 2, p. 51.

4 In ancient Greek geography, the western basin of the Indus River (essentially corresponding to the western territory of modern Pakistan) was on the extreme eastern fringe of the known world. They called the inhabitants Indians (those of the Indus).

5 According to *Chambers Dictionary*, 'ideology' means a body of ideas or way of thinking that forms the basis of a national or sectarian policy.

6 Hume D (1984 [1739]): *A Treatise of Human Nature*, Penguin Classics, book 1, part 4, sec. 1, p. 234.

7 *Ibid.*, book 1, part 3, sec. 9, p. 163.

8 *Ibid.*, book 1, part 4, sec. 7, p. 319.

9 *Ibid.*, book 1, part 3, sec. 9, p. 165.

10 This adage, or a paraphrase of it, is usually attributed to Francis Xavier, the co-founder of the Jesuit Order, properly known as the Society of Jesus.

11 *Whistle Down the Wind* was a 1959 novel by Mary Haley Bell which Andrew Lloyd Webber turned into a musical of the same name. 'No Matter What' is a song from the musical identifying the belief of the children which was recorded as a single by the Irish band Boyzone. The song reached number one in the UK singles chart in 1998. The lyrics are reproduced by permission of Hal Leonard Europe Ltd.

12 *The Stanford Encyclopedia of Philosophy* (2015): Relativism: Introduction and Sec. 1; available at: https://plato.stanford.edu/entries/relativism/.

13 Fricker M (2013): 'Styles of Moral Relativism: A Critical Family Tree'. In *The Oxford Handbook of the History of Ethics*, ed Crisp R, chapter 37, pp. 793–817. The quote from Montaigne is on p. 796.

14 Rorty R (1990): *Contingency, Irony and Solidarity*, Cambridge University Press, p. 5.

15 Scruton R (2007, 12 June): 'Richard Rorty's Legacy', www.opendemocracy.net/ democracy_power/people/richard_rorty_legacy.

16 Alhindi WA, Talha M, Sulong GB (2012): 'The Role of Modern Technology in the Arab Spring', *Archives Des Sciences*, Vol. 65, No. 8, August, 101–112: ISSN 1661-464X.

17 Ajbaili M (2014, 24 June): 'How ISIS Conquered Social Media', *Al Arabiya*, available at: http://english.alarabiya.net/en/media/digital/2014/06/24/How-has-ISIS-conquered-social-media-.html.

18 https://en.oxforddictionaries.com/word-of-the-year/word-of-the-year-2016.

19 Fandosjan N (2017, 22 January): 'White House Pushes "Alternative Facts". Here Are the Real Ones', *New York Times*, available at: www.nytimes.com/2017/01/22/us/politics/president-trump-inauguration-crowd-white-house.html?_r=0.

20 'Post-truth Politics: The Art of the Lie', *The Economist*, 10 September 2016, available at: www.economist.com/news/leaders/21706525-politicians-have-always-lied-does-it-matter-if-they-leave-truth-behind-entirely-art?fsrc=scn/tw/te/pe/ed/artofthelie.

21 Spencer H (1900 [1862]): *First Principles*, 6th edn, Williams and Norgate, part 1, chapter 1, sec. 3, pp. 9–10.

22 In 1929 it moved to Conway Hall in Red Lion Square, London. It is now known as the Conway Hall Ethical Society and is a centre for humanist education and research.

23 Sheowring W, Thies CW, eds (1911): *Religious Systems of the World: A Contribution to the Study of Comparative Religion*, 10th edn, George Allen & Co.

24 Interview recorded on 4 March 1959 for the BBC's programme *Face to Face* (with John Freeman).
25 London S (1998): 'Borrowing From Buddhism: An Interview with Ninian Smart', *The Witness*, Vol. 81, No. 6 (June), 8–10. Interview available online: 'The Future of Religion: An Interview with Ninian Smart', www.scottlondon.com/interviews/smart.html.
26 Wong DB (2006): *Natural Moralities: A Defense of Pluralistic Relativism*, Oxford University Press, p. 51.
27 *Ibid.*, p. 64.

Chapter 3

The characteristics of a religion or belief system

What is a religion?

Like other complex areas of life, defining what a religion is in a manner that satisfies everyone is not possible, and all the leading dictionaries vary in their emphases of different aspects. In addition, individuals and groups have their own interpretations and definitions. For instance Grayling, a humanist, emphasizes the difference between 'religions' and 'philosophies' and indicates that in his view 'what centrally constitutes the standard examples of religions . . . is faith in the existence of a supernatural, transcendent divine being',[1] whereas many people would include Buddhism, Confucianism and Taoism as qualifying to be called religions even though they do not actually depend upon a god. Some would even say that humanism itself had some of the characteristics of a religion, and there are of course other secular creeds in existence.

A concise, satisfactory definition of religion remains elusive. In 1964, Justice Potter Stewart had a similar problem in trying to define what constituted an obscene publication in the US Supreme Court. In his judgment (which is now widely quoted) he said:

> I shall not today attempt further to define the kinds of material I understand to be embraced within that description (hard-core pornography), and perhaps I could never succeed in intelligibly doing so. But I know it when I see it.[2]

And so it is with religion: impossible to define in a succinct manner, but easy to recognize when it is practised, at least in common parlance. With these caveats, and with apologies to those who will differ in their opinion, perhaps a pragmatic definition designating two acceptable broad sub-sections (within which there may be cross-over) is as follows. A religion is:

- the belief in, and worship of, one or more supernatural powers, often characterized as God or gods, the connections with one or more of which may be of a personal nature; or
- a particular system of faith, worship or belief, or a philosophy that determines a lifestyle and social construct that may or may not involve a belief in a God or gods.

The second of these could describe a religion for which a god was not essential (as mentioned above), or, at the far end of the individual spectrum, a person born as, say, a Christian or a Jew who socially practises the lifestyle but does not engage in religious worship. In some commentaries, the first of these bullet points would be referred to as 'organized religion' and the second as 'folk religion'.

The distinctive features of a religion

All religions have believers, whether in one or more supernatural gods or forces, or in a philosophy of living which governs the way they lead their lives. For a religion to be characterized as such, it has to encompass a number of recognizable traits. The following list was proposed by Alston:

- a belief in supernatural beings (gods);
- a distinction between sacred and profane objects;
- ritual acts focused around sacred objects;
- a moral code believed to be sanctioned by the gods;
- characteristically religious feelings (awe, sense of mystery, sense of guilt, adoration, etc.), which tend to be aroused in the presence of sacred objects and during the practice of ritual, and which are associated with the gods;
- prayer and other forms of communication with gods;
- a world view, i.e., a general picture of the world as a whole and the place of the individual within it, including a specification of its overall significance;
- a more or less total organization of one's life based on the world view;
- a social organization bound together by the previous characteristics.[3]

Another 'more modern looking' set of attributes which complements the above list but is more categorical is that given by Smart.[4]

The practical and ritual dimension. This implies some sort of regular events, which can be communal, as in a religious service of some sort, or personal, as in meditation, yoga or prayers. The manner of ritual is in broad terms prescribed and events are repetitive to encourage adherence.

The experiential and emotional dimension. This aspect covers phenomena such as revelations, enlightenment, a sense of being taken over by a supernatural spirit or being in a special place with mystic awe. It includes the drama of conversion and the driving out of evil spirits.

The mythic or narrative dimension. All religions have a cannon of oral or written stories which support the faith and the way of life of their followers. These can be of imagined content (e.g., creation of the world, miracles), revealed to a special individual or be historical events. Ritual and story are often bound together and in some faiths are believed to have been either inspired by, or received directly from, their god. The problems of interpretation across languages and over time are discussed in the section below on the interpretation of religion texts.

The doctrinal and philosophical dimension. These are the unquestioned core themes which provide the basic tenets upon which myths and stories are told. They represent the essences of what it is all about – the basic questions of existence and an afterlife: Why are we here? What is our destiny? What is the cosmos? And so on. Some are purely religious, for example the concept of the Trinity in Christianity and the attainment of moksha (enlightenment) in Hinduism; others are philosophical, for example the logos of the Greeks and the yin and yang of dualistic monism.

The ethical, moral and legal dimension. All religions encourage their followers to pursue a particular code of conduct throughout life. There is a large academic and religious literature covering this, much of which engages in complex argument and lexicography. In this practical text, ethical and moral principles are introduced as and when required and usually without reference to the extensive specialist literature that exists. Despite definitional complexity there are three points upon which almost everybody can agree.

- Ethical and moral codes of social conduct are often rooted in religious principles.
- At any one time, ethical and moral codes vary from place to place.
- In any one place, ethical and moral codes vary over time.

Assuming that most of our ancestors were trying just as hard as people are today to 'do the correct thing' in relation to their knowledge base and religious framework, we should perhaps not be too ready to condemn practices which we now know have no effect or, at worst, were simply barbaric. The most obvious of these is human sacrifice to please a deity, or identifying people as witches for failing to conform and causing the failure of the harvest. Others are the religious tolerance of slavery and the exclusion of women from religious offices. Analogous things happened in the history of medicine when, through ignorance, leeches were applied to the skin and holes drilled into the skull to let out evil humours.

In a number of instances, the religious code overflows from the religious realm to penetrate into domestic and international law. This can be indirect, when religious codes are absorbed into secular law (e.g., in the UK), or direct, when clerics pass judgement (e.g., sharia law in Islam). These issues will be developed further in a later section.

The social and institutional dimension. All religious movements are represented by groups of people, and these groups provide mutual support and a structure within which the religion works within society. Some groups are smaller and more regional, perhaps with unprogrammed worship, whereas others are international with well-prescribed services. All religions promote the coherence of their beliefs and activities by maintaining the integrity of their adherents.

The material dimension. Religions inevitably have a physical area set aside for devotion, whether this be in one's house or in a separate, larger building where sizeable numbers can meet. These vary enormously in their presentation from say the ornateness of a Jainist temple to the austere simplicity of the Calvinist Church. Similar variation is seen in the adoption (or not) of other material supports such as works of art and icons. There are also some geographical places that provide special powers such as the river Ganges or Uluru (Ayers Rock).

The interpretation of religious texts

The religious texts used today are the current interpretations of content handed down over generations, the number of generations differing from faith to faith.

It is well recognized that a myth or historical narrative which is passed from person to person and generation to generation by word of mouth is liable to modification and corruption, even if unintended. This is the basis of the cumulative error seen in the parlour game of 'Chinese whispers', a game in which a message is passed in a whisper from one to another in a group of people, with the result that the final version can be very different from the original. Hence non-contemporaneous transcriptions from the spoken folklore to the written word are often subject to speculation.

There are, however, problems even with the contemporaneous written word. Exegesis is the interpretation of written material, and different exegetes (translators) might interpret the same material differently, thereby allowing different inferences from the same core text. The problems can be grouped under two broad headings: the accurate meaning of the written text and the use of allegory and metaphor.

The accurate meaning of the written text

In the 1870s when Alice was talking to Humpty Dumpty and trying to get him to define the word 'glory', Humpty Dumpty replies 'When I use a word . . . it means just what I choose it to mean neither more nor less,' to which Alice replies 'The question is . . . whether you can make words to mean so many different things.'[5] Wittgenstein, regarded by many as one of the 20th century's greatest philosophers, concluded in 1953 that the meaning of words is a social-linguistic product and that the meaning of a particular word is its use in the language at the time.[6]

A good example of this is to review the word 'gay'.

- In 1755, *Dr Johnson's Dictionary* defined it as 'airy, cheerful, merry, frolick'.
- In 1933, *The Universal Dictionary of the English Language* defined it firstly as 'filled with joy and lively feeling: merry, light-hearted, cheerful', and secondly as 'immoral, dissipated [in bad taste – to lead a gay life]'.
- In 1988, *The Collins Cobuild Use of English Language Dictionary* defined it first as 'a person who is gay is homosexual', and second as 'in slightly more old-fashioned English a person who is gay is lively and enjoyable to be with'.

The progression is clear: the meanings of words can change with time.

If reading via a translation, even when the original written words are known with accuracy, there can still be problems of a different nature. Translators vary in trying to reproduce the true sense of the original. A good example is some lines in the Qur'an. One authoritative 'modern' translation (in 1930) which had wide circulation was that of Pickthall, who prefaced his translation with the cautioning words:

> The Koran cannot be translated . . . The book is here rendered almost literally and every effort has been made to choose befitting language. But the result is not the Glorious Koran . . . It can never take the place of the Koran in Arabic, nor is it meant to do so.[7]

The lines selected from the Qur'an to demonstrate the translation problem describe the attractive features of Heaven where the chosen will go after death and are from Sura 78, which Pickthall translated as follows.

31. Lo! for the duteous is achievement—

32. Gardens enclosed and vineyards,

33. And maidens for companions,

34. And a full cup.[8]

In contrast, in the Everyman Edition of the Qur'an, using the 1861 translation of Rodwell, the same lines appear as:

31. But, for the God-fearing is a blissful abode,

32. Enclosed gardens and vineyards;

33. And damsels with swelling breasts, their peers in age,

34. And a full cup.[9]

Further comment on the key differences between these two translations and their possible implications is unnecessary.

Hence it follows that the modern interpretation of words in ancient texts, which may have been written hundreds or thousands of years ago in foreign or now-dead languages, is far from straightforward.

The use of allegory and metaphor

Not only are there problems with the words themselves, whether original or translated, there is the issue of the interpretation of a phrase or passage. As written, are the words meant to say literally what they say, or is metaphor or allegory being used? Sometimes this is obvious as when Jesus says to his disciples, 'Come with me, and I will make you fishers of men.'[10] The New Testament miracles are, however, not so straightforward. As literal stories, they have been, and still are, treated with reverence by devout literalists but they have also taken a fair bashing by doubters during and since the Enlightenment.

A good example of interpretive difficulty can be found in The Gospel According to Luke.

As he approached Jericho, a blind man sat at the roadside begging . . . he shouted out, 'Jesus, Son of David, have pity on me' . . . 'Son of David, have pity on me.' Jesus stopped . . . he asked him, 'What do you want me to do for you?' 'Sir, I want my sight back,' he answered. Jesus said to him, 'Have back your sight; your faith has cured you.' He recovered his sight instantly; and he followed Jesus, praising God. And all the people gave praise to God for what they had seen.[11]

This describes one of several restorations of sight in the New Testament: the question is, was the man blind such that he was visually disabled and could not see his physical surroundings, or was he blind to the true way and the true faith?

The story is not dissimilar in structure to the interchange between Oedipus and Tiresias (the blind prophet of Apollo) in Sophocles' play *Oedipus the King*, written almost half a millennium before the birth of Jesus. In this play there is much metaphor and in particular the difference between visual and intellectual blindness. Tiresias says to Oedipus:

So, you mock my blindness? Let me tell you this.
You with your precious eyes,
You're blind to the corruption of your life,
To the house you live in, those you live with.[12]

Here the message is crystal clear. But in the miracle quoted above, was it an allegory rather than an actual medical cure? Scholars seem divided, some saying it could be both, with literalists and doubters remaining incompatible.

These problems of interpretation are returned to when necessary and as appropriate in other sections of this book.

The characteristics of a supreme being

Notwithstanding that some religions do not depend on a god, those that do have tried to characterize the nature of their divinity. Some (e.g., Greeks, Hindus, pagans) had, or still have, male and female gods and goddesses, but those with only one god (e.g., Christianity, Islam, Judaism) originally imagined her/him as male. The requirement of the godhead to be linked to the Y chromosome presumably followed the organization of society which had an almost exclusive male leadership and authorship, although there were a few notable exceptions (e.g., Boudica, Nefertiti, the Amazons). There is, however, no logical reason why god could not be a female, a married couple or, heaven forbid, a focus group. Commonly, the god or gods had the attribution of human qualities and sometimes human form – a transformation known as anthropomorphism.

The Greek and Roman system had specific gods for specific purposes (e.g., fertility, healing, love, music). Nike (of association with sporting equipment manufacture) was the Greek winged goddess of victory (both in war and in peaceful competition), with her Roman equivalent being Victoria. Religions with a single, supreme deity had to have all the qualities vested in a single source – God. The key attributes of God have been thoroughly discussed by theologians and philosophers alike. Whilst, as usual, nobody agrees on everything, the characteristics of such a single godhead could be as follows:

- almighty (omnipotent): s/he can do anything;
- all-knowing (omniscient): there is no escape;
- all-present (omnipresent): present throughout space and time;
- everlasting (eternal): s/he is everlasting and cannot choose to cease to exist;
- unchangeable (immutable): s/he is always the same, and always consistent;
- limitless (infinite): there is nothing s/he does not occupy, there are no boundaries to her domain;
- creator: s/he has created everything out of nothing (except herself);
- moral arbiter: s/he is perfectly good and morally perfect;
- transcendent and immanent: s/he has an existence outside the created world yet is present within it.[13]

Throughout time, people have searched for evidence of the existence of a god. Revelations to chosen individuals, miracles and success in war have all been cited. In the Western tradition, there are five well-rehearsed arguments.[14] Although the list below is as described in Christian texts, the principles are applicable across all religions.

- The ontological argument. This is attributed originally to St Anselm (1033–1109), who claimed that God is 'a being than which nothing greater can be conceived' and that he is 'a necessary being'. His proof depends on it being impossible to conceive of God as not existing.
- The cosmological argument. This is attributed to St Thomas Aquinas (1225–1274). His argument is that the universe cannot prove its own existence and hence a creator, God, must be inferred as a first cause. In linking with the works of Aristotle, he saw the rationality of cause and effect as the key.
- The teleological argument. This infers the existence of God from the observed evidence of order, purpose and regularity. A designer was needed for this to happen in such dependable ways.
- The moral argument. This argument, which has various forms, appeals to our higher awareness such that our conscience and sense of moral obligation would not be present if there was no God to require it.

- The religious experience argument. This recognizes that some individuals have experienced God in a personal way, and deduces that if this happens, an entity, i.e. God, must have caused it.

All of these arguments have parallels across many faiths and over the centuries have had significant supporters and significant detractors.

The basic problem of logic for non-believers is this. Is it possible for earthly beings, equipped with all their technology, who are contained within a solar system, to find evidence of a supernatural being or the way in which he or she was created, outside their own sensory limits? By analogy, it's like asking a household pet who only has its remembered life as being in a cage in the one room, to deduce that it lives in a house with several rooms that was built by Bob the Builder and the house is part of a village of similar houses, also built by Bob the Builder. An intelligent pet may speculate that the carer who supplies daily sustenance is a supreme and benevolent being who regularly crosses the limits of their perception through a door but they would have no knowledge of things beyond that perception.

Some analysts think that such simple logic is incontrovertible and renders speculation on the supernatural useless. Over recent years there have been a number of popular literature publications that try to both refute[15,16] and confirm[17,18] the existence of a wise and benevolent God or gods. So, to sum up, what is true is that there is still no irrefutable evidence to convince doubters that a supernatural being exists, and those who are devout are so principally because of belief, only some aspects of which can be supported by evidence and experience.

The problem of evil

The additional problem is that of evil, or unpleasant events. Just what is God thinking about when s/he allows awful things to occur? Perhaps s/he doesn't want evil to occur: perhaps her/his management style is rather hands off, and having given humanity free will, individuals abuse it and fail to choose the right path. Some religions, such as Zoroastrianism, have partly solved this by postulating the existence of a supernatural evil, with whom the good god is in constant conflict. If this is so, for the believers, it rather chips away at the concept of omnipotence.

God's relationship to dreadful happenings has been frequently explored in classical and popular verse. Bob Dylan was the first popular lyricist to win a Nobel Prize for Literature in 2016. In November 1978 he had a Damascene conversion in a hotel room in Tucson, Arizona when he 'sensed the presence of Jesus'.[19] Before that he was often regarded as a protest singer and in 1964 he released the album *The Times They Are A-Changin'* on which was the single 'With God on Our Side'. The lyrics address the tendency of nations, tribes or societies to believe that God will invariably side with them and oppose those with whom they disagree, thus leaving unquestioned the morality of wars fought and atrocities committed by their country. The song has nine verses, of which four are given below.

> Oh the history books tell it
> They tell it so well
> The cavalries charged
> The Indians fell
> The cavalries charged
> The Indians died
> Oh the country was young
> With God on its side.
>
> The First World War, boys
> It came and it went
> The reason for fighting
> I never did get
> But I learned to accept it
> Accept it with pride
> For you don't count the dead
> When God's on your side.
>
> In a many dark hour
> I've been thinkin' about this
> That Jesus Christ
> Was betrayed by a kiss
> But I can't think for you
> You'll have to decide
> Whether Judas Iscariot
> Had God on his side.
>
> So now as I'm leavin'
> I'm weary as Hell
> The confusion I'm feelin'
> Ain't no tongue can tell
> The words fill my head
> And fall to the floor
> If God's on our side
> He'll stop the next war.[20]

The problem of evil was considered more formally and in depth by the Enlightenment philosopher Hume whose fictional interrogator Philo excoriatingly asked: 'Is he (i.e., God) willing to prevent evil, but not able? Then he is impotent. Is he able but not willing? Then he is malevolent'.[21]

So, as with other aspects of religion, the jury is still out on the issue of evil.

Notes

1 Grayling AC (2013): *The God Argument*, Bloomsbury, pp. 16–20.
2 Potter S (1964): *Judgement in the case of Jacobellis v. Ohio.* In the archives of Cornell University Law School: Legal Information Institute. Available at www.law.cornell.edu/supremecourt/text/378/184.
3 Alston WP (1964): *Philosophy of Language*, Prentice-Hall, p. 88.
4 Smart N (1998): 'Introduction'. In *The World's Religions*, Cambridge University Press, pp. 11–22. The headings given are those of Smart, but the paragraph content and modification is the responsibility of the authors.
5 Carroll L (1871): *Through the Looking Glass*, Book Club Associates, chapter 6, p. 324. Ostensibly a children's story, there have been several 'adult' interpretations of the text.
6 Ludwig Wittgenstein's *Philosophical Investigations* was published posthumously in 1953. It is interpreted in *The Stanford Encyclopedia of Philosophy* (2014), sec. 3.3, 'Meaning as Use'. This is an open-access internet-based reference work available at https://plato.stanford.edu/entries/wittgenstein/.
7 Pickthall MW (1930): *The Meaning of the Glorious Koran*, AA Knopf. Now published by Books on Islam, p. vii.
8 *Ibid.*, p. 427.
9 Rodwell JM, Jones A (1997): *The Koran*, Everyman Edition, JM Dent, p. 406.
10 This version is taken from *The New English Bible* (1961): Oxford University Press/Cambridge University Press, The Gospel According to Matthew 4: 19, p. 7.
11 *Ibid.*, Luke, 18:35–43; pp. 128–129.
12 Fagles R (1984): *Oedipus the King*, Penguin Classics, p. 183, lines 469–472.
13 There are many sources for such a list, but the one here has been created from those in Cole P (2004): *Philosophy of Religion*, 2nd edn, Hodder and Stoughton, pp. 8–9; and Billington R (2002): *Religion without God*, Routledge, pp. 26–29. The text is the authors'.
14 Cole P (2004): *Philosophy of Religion*, 2nd edn, Hodder and Stoughton, chapters 3–7.
15 Dawkins R (2006): *The God Delusion*, Bantam Books.
16 Hitchens C (2007): *God is not Great: The Case against Religion*, Atlantic Books.
17 McGrath A, McGrath JC (2007): *The Dawkins Delusion?* SPCK Books.
18 Mayesvara dasa (2013): *God's Illusion Machine*, XLIBRIS.
19 Bell I (2014): *Time Out of Mind: The Lives of Bob Dylan*, Pegasus Books, chapter 6, p. 173.
20 Verses by Bob Dylan from the song 'With God on Our Side', from the album *The Times They Are A-Changin* (1964). Permission for reproduction from Special Rider Music.
21 Hume D (1990 [1779]): *Dialogues Concerning Natural Religion*, Penguin Classics, pp. 108–109.

Chapter 4

The range of belief paradigms

Introduction

When a god or gods, or a supernatural being, is worshipped or recognized, they can be classified by being ascribed different powers and responsibilities. Again, such classifications differ and what follows below is intended to be representative of generally agreed terminologies.[1] The order of presentation is approximately that in which belief systems evolved over time.

Polytheism

Meaning literally 'many gods', this form of belief dates from the earliest times (e.g., Egypt in 3,000 BCE, the Celts and the Norse) and continues today (e.g., Hinduism, Shintoism). The classical worlds of ancient Greece and Rome had their hierarchical pantheons of gods and goddesses each with their specific responsibilities. Paganism, common in ancient times (and by repute a growth religion today), is polytheistic and venerates nature. It is not always obvious which objects of worship are discrete beings or actually different manifestations of the one God. Gibbon summed up the situation in ancient Rome:

> The various modes of worship, which prevailed in the Roman world, were all considered by the people, as equally true; by the philosopher, as equally false; and by the magistrate, as equally useful. And thus toleration produced not only mutual indulgence, but even religious concord.[2]

Animism

This is a phenomenon which is usually a constituent of another religion and has many crossovers with pantheism (see below). Also, polytheistic religions are often linked with animism because of the worshipping of gods of nature. Animism usually expresses two main beliefs.

- All human beings possess, or actually are possessed by, souls which can exist within or independently of the body.
- Inanimate objects can, by being blessed or worshipped, come to possess special characteristics (anima), which allow them to assume a supernatural quality or essence.

In totemic animism a living being or organism (e.g., a witch doctor or magic-man), or an inanimate thing (e.g., a totem pole or religious icon), is regarded, and often venerated, as an outward symbol of an existing intimate unseen force or relation (a totem). Some religions have sacred objects or fetishes to which believers pray. The reliquaries of mediaeval cathedrals displaying the bones of saints as holy artefacts probably fit into this category. The Roman Catholic doctrine of transubstantiation, with its view that during Communion the bread and wine become the *actual* body and blood of Christ, is another example of animism. The icons of Eastern Orthodoxy are similarly regarded by some as *actual* windows into Heaven.

Animism can also link religious authority with temporal power. The story exists that, after his cremation, the left canine tooth of the Buddha was found in the remains of his funeral pyre. Following an eventful journey it became housed in the 'Temple of the Tooth' in Kandy, Sri Lanka,[3] where it has resided to the present. Kandy was the last capital of the Sri Lankan kings and the myth continues that whoever is the guardian of the tooth will rule the island.[4] Despite the fanciful nature of this belief, it did not stop the temple being attacked in 1998 by the Tamil Tigers during the Sri Lankan civil war to try to capture the symbolic tooth by using a suicide truck-bomb.

Theoretically, animism is not just a religious phenomenon and can extend to the world of superstition and lucky charms. Superstition is the belief in supernatural causality – that one event causes another without any natural process linking the two events – thus contradicting natural science. A well-known international goalkeeper would place a vial of Lourdes holy water at the back of his goal as a lucky charm,[5] and the Nobel Prize winning atomic physicist, Niels Bohr (who developed the quantum theory), had an affection for a horseshoe. The conversation with a visitor was reported as follows.

Visitor – I'm surprised to see that you have a horseshoe hanging over your door. Do you, a sober man dedicated to science, believe in that superstition?

Bohr – Of course not, but I've been told it's supposed to be lucky whether you believe in it or not.[6]

A more modern and sympathetic interpretation of animism is that man, nature and the world are all part of an interdependent complex organism each with its own 'anima' deserving mutual consideration and respect.

Monotheism

Monotheism (often referred to as just 'theism') is the belief in a single God who created the universe and continues to take an interest in its progress. It is the most common belief held in the world today (by nearly 4 billion people), because it describes the God of the Abrahamic religions (Judaism, Christianity and Islam), Sikhism and the Baha'i faith. This is a God who is both immanent (i.e., there is a divine presence within us) and transcendent (i.e., s/he is outside human knowledge and experience), who, having created the world, maintains a watching brief on the progress of his subjects who are constantly going astray and need his counsel and comfort to prevent them being overcome by sin. All three of the Abrahamic religions have holy creeds which were 'revealed' to special individuals (Moses, Jesus and Muhammed). God is all-powerful and all loving and can be terrible in his judgement of the wicked.

Pantheism

Pantheism is the belief that God is in everything or that God and the universe are one. This thesis clearly has crossover in parts with animism. Many pantheists consider God to be limited to all that lives (say from bacteria to *Homo sapiens*), whereas a more fundamental view is that he is also in the inanimate objects that make up the world. The clearest statement is made by Spinoza (1632–1677).

> Everything that is, is in God, and must be conceived through God, and so, God is the cause of all things, which are in him. . . . And then outside God there can be no substance . . . which is itself outside God.[7]

Many have challenged pantheism in that it allows for amoral and cruel acts to also be within God's purview and actions. On the other hand, the concept that a God who is within man during life yet can be expressed after death as being within nature is a comfort to the bereaved. This was the view of Shelley concerning his friend Keats, recently dead and buried.

> He is made one with Nature: there is heard
> His voice in all her music, from the moan
> Of thunder, to the song of night's sweet bird;

He is a presence to be felt and known
In darkness and in light, from herb and stone.[8]

This can be so much more consoling than taking the most basic non-believer view that after death we simply putrefy and re-enter the carbon and nitrogen cycles after being either planted or consumed by fire.

Deism

Deism is a term originating from the Enlightenment of the late 17th and early 18th centuries according to which, reason assures us, that there is a single all-powerful God who created the universe. However, thereafter, s/he does not direct how the world continues and there is no direct communication between God and her/his creatures. Prayer is useless, and the human race has to work out its own salvation.

Although often not explicitly stated it implies a rejection of prophesies, revelation and miracles.

Though only effectively designated a belief system for about 400 years, there is in fact good evidence that, as a thought process, deism existed from much earlier times by accepting a plurality of deities. Epicurus (341–270 BCE), the founder of Epicureanism, was of the opinion that humans must take responsibility for the way they live their lives. Importantly, the gods were remote and took no interest in, and did not intervene in, the world and the affairs of humans.[9]

In the Enlightenment deistic interpretation, essentially God is an absentee landlord who is used to explain the creation of the world but not what happens within it: cynically, Diderot[10] famously remarked that 'a deist is someone who has not lived long enough to be an atheist'.

Thomas Paine (1737–1809) could claim to be the first intellectual revolutionary. His writings played key roles in the French and American Revolutions and during his extraordinary life he was on speaking terms with world leaders. Having served his purpose as an idealist with his pen he was then vilified by the political class, being outlawed from Britain in 1792 and nearly guillotined in France in 1794. Following his vitriolic attacks on organized religion he was ostracized by the Americans he had helped to free and died in obscurity. He is now adopted as one of the founding sages of deism. In *The Age of Reason*, he professed his faith as follows.

> I believe in one God, and no more: and I hope for happiness beyond this life. . . . I do not believe in the creed professed by the Jewish church, by the Roman church, by the Greek church, by the Turkish church, by the Protestant church, nor by any church that I know of. My own mind is my own church.[11]

He went on in another pamphlet to say of Christianity, priestcraft was always the enemy of knowledge, because priestcraft supports itself by keeping people in delusion and ignorance.[12]

In 1859, Darwin published his *On the Origin of Species*, following which there was intense religious discussion. Some of this tried to harmonize evolution (from the 'natural selection' of successful organisms following random variation) with the rigidities of religious scholarship. It did this primarily by proposing a deistic model in which God did not interfere with a process s/he had originally conceived to meet her ultimate objectives for the human race.

Albert Einstein never denied the existence of a deity. Whilst saying 'I am not an atheist, and I don't think I can call myself a pantheist',[13] he nevertheless believed in a transcendental organizer of the universe. In response to a direct question he replied 'I believe in Spinoza's God, who reveals Himself in the lawful harmony of the world, not in a God who concerns Himself with the fate and the doings of mankind'.[14]

As such, his mixed-message comments identifying himself as a probable deist have been the subject of extensive analysis and debate. They clearly demonstrate the absence of clear definitions and the possibilities for confusion within the lexicon of the religious milieu.

Dualism

Dualism (or ditheism) proposes two gods: one who is good and one who is evil. The world as we know it is the result of the battle between these two beings. As a model it is an attempt to make sense of a world in which evil things happen and which is supposedly ruled by a benevolent god. Although evil gods are postulated in some forms of polytheism, the religion adhering strongly to dualism *per se* is Zoroastrianism with its twin gods of Ahuro Mazda (good) and Angra Mainyu (bad).

There is also an argument for regarding Christianity as being dualistic since it personifies evil in the form of Satan, who himself is eternal in his state of damnation. If Christianity claims its God to be truly omnipotent, omniscient and omnipresent, it consequently becomes necessary to assume that God is not wholly benevolent.

Another symbolic expression of dualism is the existence of 'good' and 'bad' in everyone. This is found in Hindu scriptures in the battle for the Kingdom of Bharata fought between two families, the evil Kauravas and the virtuous Pandavas as a representation of the eternal conflict of the ego with humility and higher understanding. The yin–yang philosophy of Taoism expresses dualism in a different way, postulating that 'good' and 'bad' can never exist in isolation, but only together.

Summary

There is a range of belief paradigms, each with their protagonists and their detractors. Some are mutually incompatible, others are capable of being combined to varying extents. Some religions at different times have moved from one to the other. The importance of the paradigms is that they are used to support the basic tenets of a religion and sometimes are the key to understanding the real-world demonstrations and declarations of belief.

Notes

1 This list of descriptions is extracted and paraphrased from entries in: Blackburn S (2005): *The Oxford Dictionary of Philosophy*, 2nd edn, Oxford University Press; and Billington R (2002): *Religion without God*, Routledge, chapters 2 and 3. The list is not exhaustive, but was selected as being appropriate for the book.

2 Gibbon E (2000): *The Decline and Fall of the Roman Empire*, Abridged Edition, ed Womersley D, Penguin Classics, p. 35.

3 Coomaraswamy M (1874): *The Daṭhávansa; or, The History of the Tooth-Relic of Gautama Buddha*, Trubner & Co, p. xiii and verses 44–67. Now available on Google Books in facsimile.

4 *Ibid.*, p. x.

5 www.telegraph.co.uk/men/the-filter/11208062/10-sportsmen-and-their-strange-superstitions.html.

6 Reported in the *Kingston Daily Freeman*, 28 February 1957, p. 28.

7 De Spinoza B (1994): *The Ethics*, Translation by Curley E, Penguin Classics, 1, proposition 18, p. 17.

8 Percy Bysshe Shelly (1821): 'Adonais: An Elegy on the Death of John Keats', in *Percy Bysshe Shelly: The Major Works: Oxford World's Classics*, eds Leader Z, O'Neill M, 2009. The quotation is taken from stanza 42.

9 Whitmarsh T (2016): *Battling the Gods: Atheism in the Ancient World*, Faber and Faber, chapter 12, p. 174.

10 Denis Diderot (1713–1784) was a French philosopher and a prominent figure during the Enlightenment.

11 Paine T (2009 [1794]): *The Age of Reason*, World Union of Deists, p. 2.

12 *Ibid.*, 'On the Religion of Deism Compared with the Christian Religion', p. 215.

13 Viereck GS (1936): *Glimpses of the Great*, Macaulay, p. 186.

14 In 1929, Einstein was asked by Rabbi Herbert S. Goldstein whether he believed in God and responded by telegram.

Chapter 5

What happens when we die?

Concepts surrounding death

Ideas about what happens after death, and its possible connection with how life is lived on earth, is a fundamental part of all religions. Atheists deny an afterlife, agnostics hedge their bets. Established religions differ in their acceptance of, and belief in, an afterlife. Of those that do accept it, although the details may differ, acknowledgement of an afterlife, or a different future life on earth:

- helps people to make sense of life, particularly when it seems unfair or at times of suffering (their own and others people's);
- gives support and comfort at times of loss and bereavement;
- provides a guiding framework and purpose to life.

Marcus Aurelius was the last of the 'Five Good Emperors' of Rome, a term introduced by Machiavelli in 1531 in his *Discourses on Livy*. Machiavelli has been much maligned, often by politicians, because of his brutal analysis of the elements of political ambition. He was in fact very supportive of meritocratic rather than inherited appointments and wrote:

> A Prince will also see through the reading of this history how one can organize a good kingdom: all the emperors who took the imperial throne through hereditary succession, with the exception of Titus, were bad; those who did so through adoption were all good, as were those five from Nerva to Marcus; and when the empire lapsed into hereditary succession, it came again to ruin.[1]

So much for the value of primogeniture, rules of succession and political dynasties.

Marcus Aurelius (121–180 CE), who Matthew Arnold described as 'perhaps the most beautiful figure in history',[2] was known as the philosopher-emperor who spent much of his life defending the empire. His *Meditations* is a personal diary that considers how to manage the conflicts between the pragmatic demands of the state and the philosophy of service and duty. He considers life and death frequently, and he came to terms with the transient and impermanent nature of life in the following way.

> the longest and the shortest lives are brought to the same state. The present moment is equal for all; so what is passing is equal also: the loss therefore turns out to be the merest fragment of time. No one can lose either the past or the future . . . both the longest-lived and the earliest to die suffer the same loss . . . it is only the present moment of which either stands to be deprived.[3]

George Santayana the Spanish philosopher was an atheist who contemplated the human state for many years and provided many aphorisms. His life spanned the 19th and 20th centuries. In a similar but more jocular vein, he summed up his own attitude to living as: 'There is no cure for birth and death save to enjoy the interval.'[4]

His view on the consolation of faith was that:

> Each religion, by the help of more or less myth, which it takes more or less seriously, proposes some method of fortifying the human soul and enabling it to make its peace with its destiny.[5]

All religions have, from ancient times, provided theories of cosmology that describe the creation of the earth and the universe and the humans within it and what happens to them after death. Examples include the following.

- For the ancient Egyptians, if a person had lived a just life, their ka (soul or life spirit) descended into the netherworld by boat and then ascended to a celestial plane. A pharaoh might go directly to a celestial plane and become a god.[6]
- Assyrians and Babylonians pictured a post-mortem netherworld which was a gloomy place that had a social and political structure similar to everyday life. There were no rewards for living well: the quality of post-mortem life depended upon one's status in real life and the grave goods buried with them.[7]
- The very ancient Israelites imagined the cosmos as a heaven, an earth and an underworld each occupied by gods, earthlings and the deceased

respectively. All humans shared the same fate – transfer on death to the underworld (Sheol), to live forever in a dark dusty place.[8]

- The Greeks and Romans had many models of the afterlife which changed over time. Pythagoras believed in the immortality of a soul which would try to reunite with its universal original. A spherical earth within concentric heavens allowed speculation by Ptolemy that immortality is associated with living with the stars, and Homer introduced the Elysian fields.[9]

- Believing in the creation of matter and the world by a single God, Christianity, modern Judaism and Islam envisage heaven as a sort of reward for a good life when the soul is separated from the body at death, provided that it does not end up in hell. The rewards based on earthly performance are most explicit in the Koran.[10]

- Hinduism proposes that the present universe and the lives upon it are temporary and recycled over time. It teaches that any attempt to find permanent happiness in this world is maya (an illusion). Hindus believe that a person's *atman* (spirit) is permanent and cannot change whilst the physical body is not permanent and can change. The *atman* is reborn many times: this is *samsara* (reincarnation).[11]

A penetrating insight into the mediaeval concept of the afterlife within the Western tradition is given in Dante's *Inferno*.[12] It portrays Dante, accompanied by Virgil, progressing through the levels of Hell and Purgatory to reach Heaven. The text simultaneously describes what was believed by the church together with the corruption present within the church, society and the human mind. It is also allegorical of the soul's journey towards God. Of interest is that in Canto IV, Dante placed the philosophers Socrates, Plato, Cicero, Seneca and Aristotle in a place called limbo. Limbo is the level before arriving in 'Hell Proper' and is devoted to those people who had no opportunity to choose either good or evil in terms of having faith in Christ. This circle is occupied by the virtuous pagans, those who lived before Christ was born, and by the unbaptized. For Dante, good works, virtue or morality count for nothing if a person hasn't acknowledged Christ as the redeemer.

Characteristics of individual, current religious beliefs are given in more detail in Part II of this book, but it is useful here to discuss the construct of the soul and its relationship to death as a more general concept. Perhaps we should start with what death means.

The meaning of death

In opening his short essay 'Metamorphosis' concerning the afterlife, David Eagleman speculates as follows.

There are three deaths. The first is when the body ceases to function. The second is when the body is consigned to the grave. The third is the moment, sometime in the future, when your name is spoken for the last time.[13]

This is useful thinking because it displays the variety of forms in which the word 'death' can be used and it demonstrates its lack of strict definition. Here we will consider four types of death, but in different categories and with different associations. It is appreciated that this categorization is arbitrary, but it allows the demonstration of certain characteristics and associations of the process of dying. The four categories are:

- death of the personality, or the person who existed;
- social death;
- physiological death of the human as an intact biological organism;
- the legal recording of the death of the person.

Death of the personality. This describes the time at which a person's spouse or loved one no longer recognizes the personality occupying the living soma of the person they knew. It used to be a rare event limited only to those people with a progressive intracranial neurological disorder that changed the way the person thought, behaved and interacted before they progressed to physical death. However, at least in developed nations, personality death is now a condition much more frequently seen because of the association of dementia with longevity. If fed and watered and kept warm, the physical body can live for years after the mind has ceased to be capable of an independent, self-sustaining existence. In some instances the patient is deemed 'not to have capacity' and, within the law, others can adopt responsibility for their affairs and best interests.[14]

Consequently, relatives can feel that they are keeping alive, or the nursing home is keeping alive, a physical body with whom they share no memories or love, yet they share or are linked with the same DNA. One of the authors, when a young doctor, was managing such a patient who was the father of a very well known scientist. The scientist said:

> I know that death is a process and I feel that on that continuum between life and death I said goodbye to my dad several months ago. I won't visit again – can't you just let him die peacefully?

The patient died peacefully that night (of natural causes), and the son sent a letter of thanks, believing erroneously that his father's death had been engineered. A clear case of credit given where credit's not due. The obverse of this situation (e.g., motor neurone disease), where the body is failing and weakening and the person cannot breathe in the presence of full consciousness (and presumably possession of the soul), is awful to behold. Such is life (and death) – but the situation remains that, in UK law, clinical staff cannot relieve suffering by deliberately causing physical death to occur, whether the personality is alive or clearly dead. The theoretical and theological question is: At what point does the soul leave, or does it deteriorate as well in parallel with, the body? Does only a rapid death from full mental capacity allow a soul to escape that is truly representative of the person who used to exist?

Social death is the loss of, or the change in, the social relationship with the dead person on the basis of social criteria, and is how death is made meaningful to many people. When people determine others as 'dead' when they are, or may be, still alive (e.g., in family schisms, in 'missing in action' during war,[15] in dementia, in excommunications), it is often called 'social death'. People also see others as 'alive' when they are pronounced to be brain dead (see Part III). Those who are brain dead are determined to be such by medical persons on the basis of test results that do not change the main indicators of life – pink skin colour, breathing, physical movements and facial recognition – the main and most important indicators of life for most people. This is a key reason for the reluctance to agree to organ donation.

The following is an example. Despite legislation in Japan permitting organ donation,[16] many Japanese still do not accept brain death because the source of life for them is in the heart and not the brain. This is a social belief not a medical belief. These social and cultural factors play a major role in the interpretation and meaning of death and are key perspectives in the social sciences especially sociology, anthropology and transcultural psychiatry.

Physiological death is what is conventionally meant by the death of a human. Historically, because the usual mode of death was through infection (e.g., pneumonia), organ failure (e.g., kidney disease) and fatal accidents, physiological death occurred concurrently with the death of the personality. But this is now not so straightforward. For organ transplantation to be viable, an organ that is alive has to be moved from a dead person to a live one. This involves the concept of brain death, where the brain (assumed to be the only source of consciousness of a person) is dead, yet the other organs are still viable. So, the death of the person is not the death of the whole body. For some people, 'brain death' as 'proper death' is seen essentially as a medical construction that is no more and no less than death of the brain – not death of the person – and this is why it is not always accepted by some religious groups and families.

Legal death is the time at which society records that the person is dead. It has considerable practical consequences. In the UK a person is legally dead when a person authorized to say you are dead does so. In some circumstances there may be a delay of hours or days between physiological and legal death. Particular problems continue to arise when relatives see a person pass away just before midnight, yet their legal time of death was when they were certified dead in the early hours of the following day: the relatives receive a death certificate recording the death as when it was certified, but they want to remember the day they saw them die as the date of death.

Once recorded as dead, no transactions can be carried out in the dead person's name: his or her bank accounts are frozen, his or her credit cards don't work and his or her payments to relatives cease. No further drawings may be made on his or her assets until the will has passed probate or, if there is no will, when the legal process has given authorization for the assets to be distributed to the remaining relatives. What to do with assets after death, and the issues they cause, has been a problem for centuries as seen in *King Lear* (Shakespeare), *Bleak House* (Dickens) and the victims of Agatha Christie.

Approaches to death: messages from literature

Across the world, there are approximately 150,000 recorded deaths every day. Of these, 1,500 are in the UK, meaning that 0.9% of the UK population (approximately 500,000) die annually. There are no recorded cases in history of any human managing to escape physical death. One day we are all going to die in our physical form. Hamlet, preoccupied with death, summed it up.[17]

> Thou know'st 'tis common; all that lives must die,
> Passing through nature to eternity.

Being an undertaker in the UK as the 'baby-boomer generation'[18] passes on must be one of the most secure businesses to be in. Because of the inevitability of death, there is much written, both in prose and poetry, about how individuals might prepare for the inevitable. Two poets who probably span the range of emotions are Dylan Thomas and John Keats.

Thomas's father was a confirmed atheist and Thomas himself wrote a villanelle[19] for him called 'Do Not Go Gentle into that Good Night'. It was written in 1951 to encourage his father to fight death (although there are additional interpretations). The poem is devoid of any religious imagery, perhaps in deference to his father's lack of belief. His father died in 1952. The first and last verses are:

> Do not go gentle into that good night,
> Old age should burn and rave at close of day;
> Rage, rage against the dying of the light.

And you, my father, there on the sad height,
Curse, bless, me now with your fierce tears, I pray.
Do not go gentle into that good night.
Rage, rage against the dying of the light.

In a nutshell the meaning of the words as written is a simple one – hang in there for as long as you can.

Keats on the other hand takes a much more accepting position: death is inevitable and there may be a time when we should welcome it. In his 'Ode to a Nightingale' written in 1819, in contrast to the optimism of some of his earlier work, Keats gracefully accepts the transience of life and that death is inescapable. Lines 51–56 are:

Darkling I listen; and, for many a time
I have been half in love with easeful Death,
Call'd him soft names in many a musèd rhyme,
To take into the air my quiet breath;
Now more than ever seems it rich to die,
To cease upon the midnight with no pain.[20]

This is much, much, more mellifluous than the anger of Dylan Thomas.

In contrast to these is the approach of John Donne, who little considered the approach towards death, but concentrated on what happens afterwards. Unlike Paul of Tarsus, he did not have a conversion on the road to Damascus. His early life as a bit of a 'man about town' whilst developing as one of the Metaphysical Poets was an unbelievable antithesis to his later position as the Dean of St Paul's Cathedral (1621–1631). When he was nearly 30, he secretly married his boss's niece, who was 16 at the time, and briefly found himself in prison. Although a hard and productive worker, his progress through life is perhaps worth studying as a demonstration of the value of 'who you know'. The 'Establishment'[21] was clearly alive and well in the 17th century. As a young man he wrote erotic poetry. In 'The Flea',[22] he complained to his lover that the flea could enjoy parts of her that he could not and in 'To His Mistris Going to Bed',[23] he poetically undressed her and penned the following lines:

Licence my roving hands, and let them go,
Before, behind, between, above, below.
. . .
Full nakedness! All joys are due to thee,
As souls unbodied, bodies uncloth'd must be,
To taste whole joys.
. . .

Thy self: cast all, yea, this white linen hence,
There is no penance due to innocence.
To teach thee, I am naked first; why then
What needst thou have more covering than a man.

No wonder that these poems were distributed privately and not published openly at the time. Let's hope for his sake that his subsequently adopted God accepted all-comers.

Contrast these early works with him being a proselyte, converting to Anglicanism, taking holy orders, thundering god-fearing sermons and being on speaking terms with King James I. He was a great promoter of the afterlife – that was what mattered in his view. This is well demonstrated in his Holy Sonnet 10, 'Death, Be Not Proud',[24] the beginning and last lines of which are:

Death, be not proud, though some have called thee
Mighty and dreadful, for thou art not so;
. . .
Why swellst thou then?
One short sleep past, we wake eternally,
And death shall be no more; Death, thou shalt die!

So there we have it from Donne: live well, believe and pray and you will be happy ever after.

This short section includes quotes from just five sources in a literature with hundreds that could have been chosen. It does however illustrate that people ponder death and approach it differently with different expectations. What patients and relatives read and glean from literature and the media contributes to their anticipation and interpretation of events and can sometimes have a significant impact on their behaviour and response as the pathway to death evolves.

Scepticism, exploitation and belief in an afterlife

Scepticism

In an earlier section, some primitive views on the afterlife were described, and from this we can conclude that speculation about death is an age-old, perennial problem. But first, what about those who do not believe in a god and/or an afterlife?

From reading some of today's accounts of the questioning of an afterlife it is easy to assume that 'unbelief' originated in the challenges to faith during the Enlightenment (the late 17th and 18th centuries). Whilst it is true that the growth of scepticism was very strong at this time, atheism is much older than the Enlightenment. Furthermore, atheistic beliefs were present in the earliest writings of both the Eastern and Western traditions.

In what is now India, in the sixth century BCE the materialistic Cârvâka were clear in their views.

> Be as licentious as you please; live for pleasure; there is no punishment here-after. Indulge your appetites; this is your only chance to do so. God and soul are myths; the priest is a hypocrite; the body dies and then you end.[25]

Simultaneously, in Greece some of the philosophers there were develop-ing what has come to be known as 'the symmetry argument',[26] that is, the non-experience of pre-birth is the same as death. Euripides' play *The Trojan Women* is probably the first anti-war play ever produced from the perspective of women and children. It was written in 415 BCE when Athens was slogging it out with Sparta in the Peloponnesian War. Andromarche (Hector's wife) reassures Hecuba (Queen of Troy) over the death of Polyxena (Hecuba's daughter): 'I tell you that not to be born is the same as being dead' and later, 'Polyxena is dead. It is just as if she had never looked upon the light of day. She knows nothing of her misfortunes'.[27]

The most widely cited classical arguments concerning the absence of an afterlife (that is actually experienced as such) are those of Lucretius. Lucretius (a follower of the School of Epicurus) was a Roman (probably from Naples) who wrote his famous epic poem *De rerum natura* in the first century BCE. This subsequently resulted in him being regarded as an enemy of Christianity. The cause of this, in particular, was the end of Book 3 of the poem which is an eloquent critique of the fear of death. To quote the *Stanford Encyclopedia of Philosophy*:

> The magnificent finale of book 3 (830–1094) is a diatribe against the fear of death, taking as its starting point the preceding demonstra-tion that death is simply annihilation. To fear a future state of death, Lucretius argues, is to make the conceptual blunder of supposing your-self present to regret and bewail your own non-existence. The reality is that being dead will be no worse (just as it will be no better) than it was, long ago, not yet to have been born.[28]

Fast-forwarding nearly two millennia to the Enlightenment, Boswell gives us a unique insight into the mind of the dying atheist and Scottish philoso-pher David Hume in 1777. He wrote on 3 March:

I went to see Mr David Hume who was returned from London and Bath, just adying. . . . I had a strong curiosity to be satisfied if he persisted in disbelieving a future state even when he had death before his eyes. I was persuaded from what he now said, and from his manner of saying it, that he did persist. . . . I however felt a degree of horror . . . I was like a man in sudden danger . . . And I could not but be assailed by momentary doubts while I actually had before me a man of such strong abilities and extensive inquiry dying in the persuasion of being annihilated. But I maintained my faith. I told him that I believed the Christian religion as I believed history.[29]

The belief in the absence of an afterlife and annihilation on death continues to the present. In 1927, Bertrand Russell asserted that 'I believe that when I die I shall rot, and nothing of my ego will survive'[30] and over 60 years later, in 1994, Francis Crick (who won the Nobel Prize in 1962 for discovering the DNA double helix) wrote:

You, your joys and your sorrows, your memories and ambitions, your sense of personal identity and free will, are in fact no more than the behaviour of a vast assembly of nerve cells and their attendant molecules.[31]

Not much wriggle room there for an afterlife.

In stark contrast, believers are in no doubt that they will continue in some form after death – that is one of the main purposes of their faith.

Exploitation

Other doubters have advanced arguments that people are persuaded into beliefs in an afterlife so as to give power to others. The persuasion can come firstly in the form of solace and promise, and secondly from fear.

Karl Marx addressed the former of these in a little-known 'Contribution' he wrote as an introduction to his *Critique of Hegel's Philosophy of Right*. It was published in *Deutsch–Französische Jahrbücher*, a journal produced in Paris by Karl Marx and Arnold Ruge. Only one issue, a double number, appeared in February 1844: it was discontinued partly because of the difficulties of smuggling it from France to Germany. In it, the end of the second paragraph reads as follows: 'Religion is the sigh of the oppressed creature, the sentiment of a heartless world, and the soul of soulless conditions. It is the opium of the people.'[32]

This famous quotation, born from an obscure publication, has become the watchword for those who believe that religion is a sort of suppressor that keeps the proletariat under control. The ability of religion to control the basic instincts of man was discussed in a similar vein by Freud 80 years later. Freud was in many ways an elitist and in his considerations of religions he saw them as simultaneously providing a paternal cushion with the promise of things to come whilst keeping the lower orders in check. He gave his views as follows:

> Civilization has little to fear from educated people and brain workers. In them the replacement of religious motives for civilized behaviour by other, secular motives would proceed unobtrusively; moreover, such people are to a large extent themselves vehicles of civilization. But it is another matter with the great mass of the uneducated and oppressed, who have every reason for being enemies of civilization. So long as they do not discover that people no longer believe in God, all is well.[33]

How fear incentivized the populace to behave by believing in religion was also expressed by Russell:

> Religion is based, I think, primarily and mainly upon fear. It is partly the terror of the unknown, and partly, as I have said, the wish to feel that you have a kind of elder brother who will stand by you in all your troubles and disputes. Fear is the basis of the whole thing – fear of the mysterious, fear of defeat, fear of death.[34]

Marx, Freud and Russell rejected the afterlife as a realistic possibility, but simultaneously implied that organized religion was in some way exploiting the individual by promising one.

Others have considered that religions have been manipulative, whilst nevertheless maintaining a belief in the religion itself. Two such important historical figures are Luther and the Buddha. They both recognized the exploitative potential of priests. They wanted to remove them as essential middlemen between God (or gods) and their supplicants so as to reduce the power they held over the congregation and especially over the uneducated. Neither however wanted to remove the belief in their deity or way of life: they were both devout and believing in their different ways. They wanted a direct connection between the individual and the non-earthly aspects of spiritual life uninterrupted by a go-between.

Belief in an afterlife

Human beliefs in the afterlife are probably millions of years old and most likely had major similarities with those of the hunter-gatherer societies currently in existence. These beliefs were the forerunners of those that exist today. They can be traced as an evolution of thought and opinion over the last 10,000 years or so of recorded history.

For those who do believe in a continuing existence or an everlasting peace (or torment) after the earthly life, there are many individual templates, but for the main religions, for the sake of simplicity, three basic models are defined here.

- An individual's spirit (or soul in alternative parlance) goes on a post-mortem journey undergoing a set of trials, the success of which could lead to becoming an ancestor or god, or failure of which could result in recycling or obliteration. There are normally intermediate possibilities of further cycles of life on a spectrum between these extremes.
- An earthly person dies and then their spirit achieves an ill-defined heightened state of perfect peace.
- An individual in life comprises a separate spiritual 'soul' housed in a material body that after material death continues for a time or indefinitely. The soul's eventual lifestyle and fate (e.g., to heaven, hell or limbo) may depend upon adherence to the religion's code of practice during the person's lifetime.

Some of these beliefs were briefly described for early religions in the section 'Concepts surrounding death' above and will be addressed in more detail in Part II. Here we will consider general principles by reviewing a representative sample of belief systems.

Rebirth or reincarnation as a form of the recycling of the soul from one person in the present to another in the future is characteristic of the ancient religions of India described in the Vedas in approximately 1,000 BCE. The concept is that there are a number of gods in a hierarchical structure who observe a person's life, weigh its content of goodness and badness and determine the time and quality of the next life. Each spirit will undergo many, many cycles of existence in a human body, each cycle determined by the performance in the last. Escape from the endless wheel of existence (*samsara*) into a fusion with the One Divine Being is the final, eternal objective (*moksha*),[35] which is not necessarily achieved.

Most Hindus are cremated, as it is believed that this will help their soul to escape quickly from the body. Their construct is that the present life is part of an ongoing timeless process and when the spirit has completed its passage out of the body, the mourners can continue with their lives. Death for Hindus is not the end of a person; it is the start of their rebirth.

The attainment of perfect peace is inherent in a number of religions which originated in Asia and China well before the birth of Christ. The classic example is Buddhism. In originating from Hinduism, the process of rebirth is retained, but the necessity of a Divine Being is omitted. The wheel of samsara continues to turn, but by meditation and removing desire, a state of Enlightenment can be attained and the wheel stops turning. What happens then is not defined.

In the fifth century BCE, whilst the Buddhists were reacting against Hinduism and the Jewish exiles were rethinking the nature of their God in Babylon, in China, a government official, now known universally as Confucius, was starting to have a critical look at the Chinese warlords driven by their multiple gods. Confucius taught compassion and consideration without the reward of an afterlife. There was, however, veneration of the dead. Ancestors did not cease to exist as contributors to society after death, their influence lived on, but where they were and their circumstances were obscure. As the movement of populations occurred, over the centuries, Confucianism, Taoism and Buddhism fused and intermingled and the possibility of humans who had lived a perfect existence becoming 'immortals' was surmised. Again, acceptance of the nebulous is the norm.

The independent, everlasting soul is predominantly a construct defined within the Abrahamic religions. It is least defined in Judaism, was established by Christianity and is most closely delineated in Islam. In the earlier section on 'Concepts surrounding death', other models of the afterlife in ancient religions were also described.

- Judaism conventionally believes that the primary importance of life is the way in which it is lived on earth. There are varying and conflicting views on what happens after death but the existence of a soul and the potential for its resurrection is well established. Individuals vary in their beliefs whilst still maintaining their Jewish faith. Traditional Judaism believes that when death occurs, there is an afterlife and that the righteous are treated better than the wicked: it's a sort of merit system. Souls may go to a heaven directly, after purification, or await release when the true messiah makes his or her appearance. Reform Judaism sees the faith as a continuously evolving paradigm and seeks to adapt the religion to modern knowledge and thinking. The concept of reward and punishment in the 'World to Come' is more or less abolished and the persistence of the soul has been modified to the more ambiguous 'We trust in our tradition's promise that, although God created us as finite beings, the spirit within us is eternal'.[36] Liberal Judaism, like Reform Judaism, tries to reinterpret traditional Judaism for the current times within the belief that there is a permanent direct personal relationship with God. There is no consensus on the afterlife. Most Liberal Jews reject the idea of a personal Messiah who will return to raise the righteous from the dead and also reject the idea of physical resurrection.

- Christianity regards Jesus as the Messiah predicted by Isaiah 700 years earlier.[37] Jesus promised an everlasting life – even to the wicked if they repented. This was Christianity's key 'marketing strategy'. When the body dies and is buried or cremated, Christians believe that their unique soul lives on and is raised to a new life by God in heaven. As will be described in more detail in Chapter 16, there are different views within Christianity about who exactly will be saved. Calvinism, for instance, believes the doctrine that God has ordained all that will happen (predestination), especially with regard to the salvation of some and not others.

There are many references to being saved in the New Testament, but probably the two most quoted related to Jesus are: 'I am the resurrection and the life.[38] He who believes in me will live, even though he dies' and 'God so loved the world that he gave his one and only Son, that whoever believes in him shall not perish but have eternal life'.

Matthew tells us it wasn't a good outlook if you did not believe. Jesus said 'It will be like this at the end of the age: the angels will go out and gather up the evil people from among the good and will throw them into the fiery furnace, where they will cry and grind their teeth' and later 'Then he will say to those on his left, Away from me, you that are under God's curse! Away to the eternal fire which has been prepared for the Devil and his angels!'[39]

Some Christians, including Roman Catholics, believe in Purgatory. This is an in-between state for those who were unrepentant sinners at death now queuing for heaven; it is a time of cleansing from sin and preparation for acceptance.

Interpretation of Scripture has been a cross that Christianity has had to bear since its inception and it continues today. In 2010, Pope Benedict XVI (formerly Cardinal Ratzinger) declared with *ex cathedra* authority that:

> The whole of man . . . receives eternity. . . . Christianity does not proclaim merely some salvation of the soul in a vague afterlife in which all that is precious and dear to us in this world would be eliminated, but promises eternal life, the life of the world to come.[40]

So there it is. Although different branches of the Christian Church might differ, the mainstream orthodox Roman Catholic view is unchanged over 2,000 years.

Islam, entering the scene 600 years after the birth of Christ, derives its beliefs from the Suras – the word of God spoken to Mohammed and written in the Qur'an. There are many references to heaven and hell and the criteria for admittance to both. Unlike other religions, which nowadays usually accept that there are different routes to heaven and that other religions may be accommodated, Islam, at least in its traditional form, regards its followers as privileged over others. The Qur'an expresses the beauty of Allah and emphasizes his mercy and generosity, but at times it also roars his anger at sinners and unbelievers. The earthly life when the soul and the body are together is a preparation for the hereafter. After death they may or may not separate (the soul always being eternal), and 'God created the heavens and earth for a true purpose: to reward each soul according to its deeds'.[41] After death, on the Day of Judgement, the soul will have to account for the actions of life as follows:

> And every soul will be repaid in full for what it has done. He [i.e. God] knows best what they do. Those who rejected the Truth will be led to Hell in their throngs. . . . It will be said 'Enter the gates of Hell: there you will remain. How evil is the abode of the arrogant!' [. . .][42]

> Those who were mindful of their Lord will be led in throngs to the Garden. When they arrive they will find its gates wide open, and the keepers will say to them, 'Peace be upon you. You have been good. Come in: you are here to stay'.

And, Hell, full of flames, is not a nice place.

> For those who defy their Lord We have prepared the torment of Hell: an evil destination. They will hear it drawing in its breath when they are thrown in. It blazes forth, almost bursting with rage.[43]

The price of non-compliance to the creed in Islam is high and, to be fair, this is also the belief in some Christian and other monotheistic sects.

Notes

1 Machiavelli N (2008 [1531]): *Discourse on Livy*, trans Bondanella JC and Bondanella C, Oxford World's Classics, Book 1, chapter 10, p. 49.
2 Arnold M (1865): *Essays in Criticism*, A.L. Burt Company, chapter 10, p. 260; now published by Cornell University Digital Connections; available at www.archive.org/details/cu31924013206754.
3 Marcus Aurelius (2006): *Meditations*, Penguin Classics, Book 2: 14, p. 14.
4 Santayana G (1922): 'War Shrines'. In *Soliloquies in England and Later Soliloquies*, Charles Scribner's Sons, chapter 24, p. 97.

5 Cardiff ID, ed. (1964): *The Wisdom of George Santayana: Peace with Destiny*, Philosophical Library, PUB aphorism MH-4.

6 Wright JE (2000): *The Early History of Heaven*, Oxford University Press, pp. 16–19.

7 *Ibid.*, pp. 26–41.

8 *Ibid.*, pp. 96–97.

9 *Ibid.*, pp. 100–113.

10 Abdel Haleem MAS (2016): *The Qur'an*, Oxford World's Classics, Sura 9, 72–73, p. 122, and Sura 11, 101–108, p. 143.

11 Smart N (2002): *The World's Religions*, 2nd edn, Cambridge University Press, p. 49.

12 Dante Alighieri (2012 [1320]): *The Divine Comedy: Inferno, Purgatorio, Paradiso*, trans Robin Kirkpatrick, Penguin Classics.

13 Eagleman D (2009): *Sum: Forty Tales from the Afterlife*, Cannongate, p. 23.

14 The Mental Capacity Act 2005, available at: www.legislation.gov.uk/ukpga/2005/9/contents.

15 They may have been killed, wounded or captured or had deserted.

16 Wise J (1997): 'Japan to Allow Organ Transplants', *British Medical Journal*, Vol. 314, 1298.

17 Shakespeare W: *Hamlet*; Act I, Scene 2, line 72.

18 Baby-boomers constitute the generation born when the birth rate peaked strongly in the years following the Second World War when soldiers returned home anxious to re-establish their conjugal rights. The oldest of the baby-boomers, born in 1946, are now entering their 71st year.

19 Thomas D (2014): 'Do Not Go Gently into that Good Night'. In *Dylan Thomas Omnibus: Under Milk Wood, Poems, Stories and Broadcasts*, W&N, p. 128.

20 Keats J (2007): 'Ode to a Nightingale'. In *Selected Poems: Keats*, ed Barnard J, Penguin Classics, p. 194.

21 See Jones O (2015): *The Establishment: And How They Get Away with It*, Penguin Books.

22 Donne J (1873): 'The Flea'. In *The Complete Poems of Dr John Donne*, Vol. 2, Robson & Son, p. 156, available at http://books.google.com/.

23 Donne J (1872): 'To His Mistris Going to Bed'. In *The Complete Poems of Dr John Donne*, Vol. 1, Robson & Son, pp. 223–224, available at http://books.google.com/.

24 Donne J (1873): 'Holy Sonnet 10, "Death, Be Not Proud"'. In *The Complete Poems of Dr John Donne*, Vol. 2, Robson & Son, pp. 286–287, available at http://books.google.com/.

25 Hopkins EW (1924): *Ethics of India*, Yale University Press, p. 206.

26 Warren J (2006): *Facing Death: Epicurus and His Critics*, Clarendon Press, p. 57. The pagination is from the paperback edition.

27 This translation is taken from Morwood J (2000): *Euripides: The Trojan Women and Other Plays*, Oxford World's Classics, pp. 56, 57.

28 Section 5: Ethics, available at https://plato.stanford.edu/entries/lucretius/.

29 Boswell J (1970): *Boswell in Extremes, 1776–1778*, ed Weis CM, Pottle FA, McGraw Hill, pp. 10–11.

30 Russell B (2009 [1927]): *The Basic Writings of Bertrand Russell*, ed Egner RE, Denonn LE, Routledge Classics, p. 348.

31 Crick F (1994): *The Astonishing Hypothesis: The Scientific Search for the Soul*, Touchstone, p. 3.

32 The translation is taken from Bottomore TB, Rubel M, eds (1970): *Karl Marx: Selected Writings in Sociology and Social Philosophy*, 2nd edn, Pelican Books, p. 41.

33 Freud S (1927): *The Future of an Illusion*, trans Strachey J (1961), WW Norton & Co, Sec. VII, p. 39.

34 Russell B (1986 [1927]): 'Why I Am Not a Christian'. In *Bertrand Russell on God and Religion*, ed Seckel A, Prometheus Books, chapter 3, p. 70.

35 Knott K (2016): *Hinduism: A Very Short Introduction*, Oxford University Press, 2nd edn, p. 19.

36 Reform Judaism: Modern Statement of Principles, Adopted at the 1999 Pittsburgh Convention (May 1999), available at www.jewishvirtuallibrary.org/reform-judaism-modern-statement-of-principles-1999.

37 Isaiah 7:14, 9:6.

38 John 11:25–26, 3:16.

39 Matthew 13: 49–50, 25:41.

40 Homily Of His Holiness Benedict XVI (15 August 2010), given at St Thomas of Villanova Parish, Castel Gandolfo, available at http://w2.vatican.va/content/benedict-xvi/en/homilies/2010/documents/hf_ben-xvi_hom_20100815_assunzione.html.

41 Abdel Haleem MAS (2016): *The Qur'an*, Oxford World's Classics, Sura 45: 22, p. 325.

42 *Ibid.*, Sura 39: 70–73, pp. 299–300.

43 *Ibid.*, Sura 67: 6–8, p. 382.

Chapter 6

The soul

What is it; where is it; and does it exist?

What do we mean by a soul?

The soul is a good example of a commonly used word that means different things to different people. This section discusses various problems with its interpretation and some of the efforts that have been made to prove its existence. Its use has changed over history and it is widely used in figurative language unrelated to religious significance. In the everyday use of English, it is listed as having nine separate meanings.[1] Here we will not be touching on the vexed issue of whether animals have souls, a subject of highly charged emotion and minority debate in a nation of dog-lovers.

The commonly used phrases 'in body and soul' and 'it keeps body and soul together' indicate that the two are closely linked and yet somehow separate. Most people would associate their soul as somehow representing the real kernel of their being and within their brain rather than distributed around the body as if it were in the blood. Descartes pinpointed it in the pineal gland at the base of the brain. Yet the soul is not just the self that is conscious and thinks, established as the ego of psychology: it is considerably more. This was aptly demonstrated by a T-shirt slogan given to one of the authors (PH) by a girlfriend in the 1960s decade of love and revolution when The Beatles and Rolling Stones were swapping places in the pop charts. It read:

Starve your ego
Feed your soul
And learn to live

Perhaps the message was genuine: the relationship withered soon afterwards. In addition, as evidence that they are different things, the ego dies with the person, but the soul continues on to everlasting life.

The soul is somehow descriptive of the innermost characteristics of people, either in their personality as in 'Old King Cole was a merry old soul' (i.e., his cup (or glass) was obviously always over half-full), or in the way it describes similarities and linkages at a profound level as in 'a soul-mate'. Not only individuals, but also nations are described as possessing a particular style of soul as one of their characteristics. An emerging nation in Africa would have a different type of soul to a modern industrial conurbation: you would feel the differences when you were in each place, but perhaps find it difficult to express why. The first president of Botswana, formerly the British Protectorate of Bechuanaland, made just this point.

> It should now be our intention to try to retrieve what we can of our past. We should write our own history books to prove that we did have a past, and that it was a past that was just as worth writing and learning about as any other. We must do this for the simple reason that a nation without a past is a lost nation, and a people without a past is a people without a soul.[2]

The soul recurs frequently in popular and classical poetry and drama. Judy Garland, the child star of *The Wizard of Oz*, who had an unhappy personal life and died young, left a small collection of poetry, privately published, that reveals some of her innermost feelings. In her poem about a lost love,[3] the last lines of the second verse read:

> For 'twas not into my ear you whispered but into my heart.
> ''Twas not my lips you kissed, but my soul.

Immediately the message is clear: we all understand the feeling and its nuances.

Whilst these paragraphs above describe the characteristics of the indefinable, all of which are relevant because they are facets of what constitutes the totality of what the soul means, it is necessary to return to the link with religion. For this we can employ the words of the famous bard in the history of King John.[4] Arthur, King John's nephew and claimant to the throne, either falls or jumps from the castle wall. This occasions ten lines of dramatic monologue describing his death which end with his dying words:

> As good to die and go, as die and stay.
> O me! My uncle's spirit is in these stones:
> Heaven take my soul, and England keep my bones!

And there it is – the separation of the core of the real self (the soul) from the soma at the moment of death. Perhaps Marcus Aurelius had it right when he turned the situation on its head and, agreeing with Epicurus, declared himself to be, even in life, 'A soul carrying a corpse'.[5]

The implication of the indefinable but eternal component is clear.

Arguments for and against the existence of a soul

Because of its obvious importance, there have been innumerable attempts to justify by argument or through evidence that the soul actually exists. This section will present some representative examples from the Western and Arabic traditions spanning over 2,000 years of how people have reasoned in this area. Although a soul is most closely associated with religious thought, it should be remembered that it is also a component of many other mythic belief systems.

Plato's *Republic* was written around 375 BCE, and it recounts imaginary conversations occurring in Athens at the height of the Peloponnesian War (431–411 BCE), in which Socrates (470–399 BCE) is speaking with various people. Part XI of the book deals with the immortality of the soul and the rewards of goodness. Here, Socrates is discussing things with Glaucon, Plato's older brother who was meant to represent the enthusiasm and carefree aspects of youth.[6] History teaches that Socrates, although always having the intellectual edge in an argument, was probably seriously irritating, and it was this that contributed to his eventual death sentence. The infernal questioning is well represented in this discussion that ranges back and forth about evidence, the problem of evil possibly continuing after death, and the contrary conclusions that could be reached. At the end of it there is a clear impression that despite Socrates' scepticism, Glaucon is convinced of the existence of the soul. Some of the key inferences are:

> Then if there's no evil that can destroy it [i.e. the soul], either its own or another's, it must exist for ever; that is to say, it must be immortal. [. . .]
>
> We can take that then as proved, and if so, it follows that the same souls have always existed. Their number cannot be decreased. Because no soul can die, nor can it increase; any increase in the immortal must be at the expense of mortality.

And later:

> For the truth we must look elsewhere. Where? Glaucon asked. To the soul's love of wisdom . . . Think how its kinship with the divine and immortal and eternal makes it long to associate with them and apprehend them.

These arguments were later developed by Aristotle (tutor to Alexander the Great) in his *De Anima* (written in 350 BCE).[7] To his way of thinking, the soul was in three parts, two of which ceased to exist when the body died: the third, called reason (nous), possibly continued:

> But since it is also a body . . . having life, the body cannot be soul; the body is the subject or matter, not what is attributed to it. . . . That is why the soul is the first grade of actuality of a natural body having life potentially in it. . . . That is why we can wholly dismiss as unnecessary the question whether the soul and the body are one: it is as meaningless as to ask whether the wax and the shape given to it by the stamp are one, or generally the matter of a thing and that of which it is the matter.

Despite the lack of hard evidence, the Greek scholars set most of the bases for belief for hundreds of years. At best the Greek schools can be described as providing circumstantial evidence within the scientific, astronomical and religious context of their time. To use modern parlance, their arguments were soft rather than hard in their deductive structure.

Although Socrates was unaware of it, 4,000 miles away in a distant land unknown to him (now northern India), a contemporary of his was asking similar questions and upsetting the established ideology. This was Siddhartha Gautama (485–405 BCE), better known as the Buddha. He was tackling problems such as:

> Shall I exist in the future? How shall I be in the future? . . . Where will this being go? I have a self. I have no self . . . this self of mine which speaks and feels, that experiences the consequences of good and bad actions now here and now there, this self is permanent, stable, eternal, unchanging, the same always.[8]

And: 'Is the world eternal or not? Is the world finite or not? Is the self different from the body or not?'[9] The underlying similarity of the concerns of Socrates and the Buddha identify two minds tackling the same 'Big Issues' of life and eternity at the beginnings of recorded polemic. These enigmas of the existence or not of a soul and the purpose of life are therefore not recent problems and have been addressed across continents.

Over 1,200 years later, as the 10th century turned into the 11th, the known world was in turmoil.[10] Panic spread throughout Christian countries as the first millennium portended the end of the world and pilgrimages became fashionable as a hedge against oblivion. Vladimir the Great, the Prince of Kiev, had converted from Slavic paganism to Christianity to be able to marry the sister of the Byzantine Emperor Basil II, and led the citizens of Kiev into the river Dnieper for a mass baptism to change their faith. After an effort of 12 years, the printers of Chengdu had produced a set of 130,000 wood blocks from which to print the complete works of Buddha. Lief Ericson discovered North America nearly 500 years before Columbus arrived. The Polynesians arrived in New Zealand. The Danes under King Sweyn invaded England and his son, Canute, united the two countries. The east–west split of the Catholic Church was established across the Bosphorus and in 1066 William the Conqueror of France deposed King Harold. Thirty years later, following the exhortations of Pope Urban II, the First Crusade captured Antioch, marched through what is now Syria and Lebanon to retake Jerusalem for the Christians; the Moslems had been defeated. The pre-existing claims and counter-claims for the Holy Land had become a burning dispute that survives to the 21st century.

Whilst all this tumult was going on, in what is now Uzbekistan, Avicenna (as the Europeans called him) was born in 980 CE. He grew up to be a polymath who spent much of his life in the patronage of princes and providing services as a physician. Like other great minds such as Ovid before him and Dante after him, he suffered persecution with an enforced change in location, and died at Hamadan in Iran in 1037. What interests us is that he was an assiduous student of Aristotle's *Metaphysics* and this led him to consider the soul–body problem from the perspective of a Muslim. He did this by one of the earliest uses of a 'thought experiment'.

His thought experiment[11] became known as the 'Flying Man'. The argument is in three main stages.

- If I was blindfolded and suspended, and touched nothing, I would not know I had a body
- but in my thought I would still be sure that I exist
- therefore myself, or my soul, exists as distinct from my body.

He continues to discuss that the mind can conceive of things that are not material and then draws the conclusion that the mind cannot be part of the physical body and is not destroyed when the body dies: that is the soul is immortal. This brought him into conflict with the mainstream Muslim theology of the times which presumed that, on the Day of Judgement, the whole person, body and mind, would proceed to the afterlife.

Moving forward, approximately 200 years, Maimonides,[12] the physician and rabbinic judge who was the head of the Jewish community in Cairo, questioned the wisdom of anthropomorphizing God into a being with human qualities. He saw this as a prelude to idolatry and thought it an error to take the Torah (the first five books of the Hebrew Bible) as literal truth. Maimonides concluded that God was indefinable and therefore had no recognizable attributes – clearly dangerous territory. He also believed that the body and soul were essential components of the complete human.

Then, in the 16th century, sandwiched between the end of the Renaissance and the beginning of the Enlightenment, onto the scene comes René Descartes (1596–1650). Descartes was born 60 years after Henry VIII had broken with Rome and when Elizabeth the First was on the throne and Shakespeare was writing his plays and sonnets. Elizabeth had confirmed England and Wales as Protestant, cementing the break with Catholicism for Britain as a nation and making the British sovereign the Head of the English Church.

Descartes was an intellectual who took nothing for granted. He challenged the past, and in so doing set the stage for 17th century rationalism and the Enlightenment. Despite his drive for logical integrity in all aspects of life, Descartes considered himself to be a devout Catholic and in his *Meditations on First Philosophy* (1641) he set forth proofs for God's existence. Whilst continuing to contribute in philosophy and the physical sciences (e.g., the Cartesian coordinate system, the science of optics), he persevered with an analysis of the human state and the mysteries of how we perceive and interpret the world through our senses. Descartes, like Darwin approximately 200 years later, was anxious to harmonize his religious beliefs with the new discoveries and implications of scientific progress.

Similarly to St Augustine over 1,000 years before him, Descartes tackled the issue of the inner self. He did this in both his *Discourse on Method* (1637) and in his *Meditations on First Philosophy*. In the former he wrote:

> Then, when I was examining what I was, I realized that I could pretend that I had no body, and that there was no world nor any place in which I was present, but I could not pretend in the same way that I did not exist. On the contrary, from the very fact that I was thinking of doubting the truth of other things, it followed very evidently and very certainly that I existed. . . . Thus the self – that is, the soul by which I am what I am – is completely distinct from the body . . . And even if the body did not exist the soul would still be everything that it is.[13]

This statement, which at that stage in the text was relatively unsupported by logical development, was developed further in the *Meditations* whose full title is *Meditations on First Philosophy, in which God's Existence and the Distinction between the Human Soul and the Body are Demonstrated.* In the first meditation he describes how he will test all his assertions and arguments as if they were the attacks of 'an evil mind, who is all powerful and cunning, [who] has devoted all their energies to deceiving me.[14]

Although it is in the Sixth Meditation, entitled 'The Existence of Material Things, and the Real Distinction between Mind and Body', that he argues for the permanence of the soul, it is in the Second Meditation where his famous aphorism arises when he concludes:

> To think? That's it. It is thought. This alone cannot be detached from me. I am. I exist; that is certain.[15]

Descartes' arguments are distributed throughout the text, but gathering them together as a logical thread, the sequential rationale is as follows.

- An evil demon is making me believe falsities.
- I can be certain of nothing.
- But I am able to be told falsities and think about them.
- Because I can think, I really do exist.
- The proposition: 'I am; I exist' is necessarily true.

The popular form of the conclusion of this argument is *Cogito ergo sum* – 'I think therefore I am'.

This distinction of body and soul, known as Cartesian Dualism, has a material body housing a separate incorporeal mind. It forms the basis for further speculation that there is a mortal body housing an immortal soul – a very welcome outcome for believers. In the year after the *Meditations* was first published, just to orientate within the national timelines of the 17th century, the English Civil War was getting underway with Cromwell squaring up to the Royalists. Torricelli demonstrated the existence of a vacuum and air pressure, and Tasman mapped the north and west coasts of Australia.

The evidence for the soul remained an intellectual construct until Queen Victoria was on the throne and Spiritualism arrived on the scene. It had its genesis in the 19th century and developed in the early 20th century. The great selling point of Spiritualism was that it did not just theorize about the afterlife, it actually produced the inhabitants of the afterlife to talk to living people at seances via the powers of special persons known as mediums. These sessions not only evoked images. Furniture moved and ectoplasm (later to be demonstrated on occasions to be muslin) emanated from the mouths of spirits. Photographic evidence was produced to confirm the reality of these visitors from the spirit world. Despite strong evidence (and admissions) of fraud and deception, prominent scientific thinkers such as Arthur Conan Doyle and Oliver Lodge (the inventor of the spark plug), both of whom had lost sons in the First World War, gave Spiritualism credence and support.

Proving the authenticity of the afterlife is what Conan Doyle's famous detective, Sherlock Holmes, would definitely call a 'three pipe problem', and Conan Doyle tackled it in his two-volume history and justification of Spiritualism.[16] In it he reports that:

> Evidence of the presence of the dead appeared in his [Conan Doyle's] own household and the relief afforded by posthumous messages taught him how great a solace it would be to a tortured world if it could share in the knowledge.[17]

He continues:

> Faith has been abused until it has become impossible to many earnest minds, and there is a call for proof and for knowledge. It is this that Spiritualism supplies. It founds our belief in life after death and in the existence of invisible worlds, not upon ancient tradition or upon vague intuitions, but upon proven facts, so that a science of religion may be built up, and man given a sure pathway amid the quagmire of the creeds.[18]

And:

> It is our task to do for Christianity what Jesus did for Judaism. We would take the old forms and spiritualize their meaning, and infuse into them new life. Resurrection rather than abolition is what we desire.[19]

Without wanting to besmirch his memory, this publication is a classic example of a mind continuously adjusting the interpretation of facts to fit the preconceived belief: a process completely at variance with the cutting logic of his fictional creation. As a Victorian and Edwardian opinion leader Conan Doyle had considerable impact. Such was the influence of Spiritualism that in 1931 the inter-war magnum opus of biological knowledge, *The Science of Life*,[20] allocated a chapter to 'Borderland Science and the Question of Personal Survival'. After respectfully but effectively debunking the available evidence (including that from Conan Doyle and Lodge), the authors concluded that 'upon the continuity of any individual consciousness after bodily cessation and disintegration, The Science of Life [i.e., the book] has no word of assurance, and on the other hand it assembles much that points to its improbability.[21]

Their comments presage the recent rise of neuroscience and modern concepts of consciousness with the improbability of the existence of souls. It has always been a problem to determine when a soul begins its existence (at conception, at birth, after baptism, etc.), if it is present in every human and when it leaves to begin its celestial journey. It is useful to review a few anomalies and difficulties to make the point.

In the Catechism of the Catholic Church, it states that: 'Every human life, from the moment of conception until death, is sacred because the human person has been willed for its own sake in the image and likeness of the living and holy God'.[22] This would suggest the soul begins at fertilization. On the other hand it states:

> As regards children who have died without Baptism, the Church can only entrust them to the mercy of God, as he does in the funeral rites for them. Indeed, the great mercy of God who desires that all men should be saved, and Jesus' tenderness toward children which caused him to say: 'Let the children come to me, do not hinder them,' allow us to hope that there is a way of salvation for children who have died without Baptism. All the more urgent is the Church's call not to prevent little children coming to Christ through the gift of holy Baptism.[23]

A further 'get-out clause' states: 'God has bound salvation to the sacrament of Baptism, but he himself is not bound by his sacraments'.[24]

The concept of a soul for many believers across many creeds is somehow intrinsically linked to the sentient human; but what about the non-sentient? Edward Drummond was the wrong man in the wrong place in 1843 when he was mistakenly murdered by Denis McNaughton, who believed him to be the prime minister, Robert Peel. In a celebrated case, McNaughton was found not guilty by means of insanity and the so-called McNaughton rule was established in law. So, can such a man, declared to be insane, truly possess a decent soul capable of salvation?

Although some of the details are disputed, in 1848, in a mining accident in Vermont, USA, an iron bar was driven through the left jaw and frontal brain lobes of Phineas Gage. He had previously been a solid, hard-working citizen and after the accident his personality was significantly changed, leading to the observation[25] that he was 'no longer Gage'. The concept of structural brain damage leading to functional non-responsibility was reinforced in the American Courts in 1992 when Herbert Weinstein had a charge of murder commuted to manslaughter because expert evidence said a PET[26] scan had demonstrated malfunction of brain cells around a frontal arachnoid cyst.[27] So, if the soul is, or is at least very closely related to, the mind, is it the soul before or the soul after the brain damage that counts for the afterlife?

There are further problems with brain death (see Part III), which is argued to be a process in which the legal death of the person can occur before the death of every cell. Gone is the illusion, as in Shakespeare's *King John* quoted above, that there is life and immediate death, or, as the Book of Common Prayer puts it, 'the quick and the dead'. So just when does the soul commence its journey?

These doubts, combined with progress in neuroscience, have led to more questions about the integrity of the mind as an independent unit and even whether or not we have free will at all. In the neuroscientific zealot's world there is no room for the metaphysical. In 2013, the popular science periodical *New Scientist* devoted an issue to the question of 'The Self'. There were six articles led by 'The Self: The One and Only You'.[28] A spirited defence of the sense of, and need for, conscious reality has been published to counter such neuroscientists' claims by the contemporary philosopher Mary Midgley[29] among many others. The debate rages on.

There are, however, two interesting insights to bring final twists to this discussion.

In 1950, Isaac Asimov published his iconic novel[30] *I, Robot*, which envisioned a human world in which most of the daily tasks were carried out by robots. Azimov, of course, had no knowledge then of the advances of current neuroscience. In it Susan Calvin, who is then 75 years old and retiring as a 'robopsychologist', is being interviewed by a young reporter. The text describes the growth not only of robots in number, but also in their perceptions. The crunch comes with a robot called Cutie who is different from the others in some indefinable way and demonstrates the qualities of leadership. Donovan, one of the station commanders, is in conversation with Cutie and is staggered when the robot says to him:

> I'm sorry but you don't understand. These are robots – and that means they are reasoning beings. They recognize the Master, now that I have preached the Truth to them. All the robots do. They call me the prophet.

So, the robots had developed consciousness, and with it their form of religion and belief. The parallels with the evolution of religion are obvious – perhaps within a society where people interact for mutual benefit, belief in others is a necessary construct and an inevitable end product of any form of complex neural network development.

But the penultimate word can go to Haldane, the man who gave mathematical likelihood to Darwin's theories of natural selection. Despite his lack of belief in any type of afterlife, 90 years ago he nevertheless argued logically as follows.

> It seems to me immensely unlikely that mind is a mere by-product of matter. For if my mental processes are determined wholly by the motions of atoms in my brain, I have no reason to suppose that my beliefs are true. They may be sound chemically, but that does not make them sound logically. And hence I have no reason for supposing my brain [i.e., his mind] to be composed of atoms.[31]

More recently, the neuropsychologist Broks, in a personal series of essays on what it is to be human, writes: 'Neuropsychology is the study of the relation between brain and mind. We know what the brain is. It's an organ located in the head. But what is the mind?'[32] A little later he continues:

> When we look at a picture, Palmer's Cornfield by Moonlight say, it's not the paper, the paint, the ink and the varnish we see. It's not just the depiction of a man and his dog in a wheat field under the light of the waxing crescent moon and the evening star. We are transported beyond the physical and the literal into the numinous, into a world of gods and spirits.

So, perhaps the aspirations of the fervent 21st-century neuro-boffins can also, like religious belief, never be proved by logic – perhaps they need belief as well – just that extra little bit of casuistic wizardry to push them over the edge of reason and into disbelief.

Conclusions

Because of its central importance, this chapter has reviewed a sample of arguments used to try to prove and disprove the existence and character of the soul for over 2,000 years. The soul–mind–body problem continues onwards as theologians and scientists try to analyse the subjective experience we call reality which is created by our brains from sense perception. Not to all, but to most religions and believers, a soul or some sort of eternal spirit is central to their faith. Ultimately, whatever arguments are used, both for and against its existence, none is conclusive: the essence of the soul remains as elusive as ever unless one possesses belief – one way or the other. Perhaps the very last word on the subject should again go to Haldane who, as an atheist, when answering the question as to what would happen to him after death nevertheless concluded: 'A man who is honest with himself can only answer, "I do not know".'[33]

Notes

1 *Collins Cobuild English Language Dictionary* (1988).
2 Sir Seretse Khama, first president of Botswana, in a speech at the University of Botswana, Lesotho and Swaziland, 15 May 1970, as quoted in the *Botswana Daily News*, 19 May 1970.
3 Garland J (1939): *My Love Is Lost*, available at www.jgdb.com/jgbk7.htm.
4 Shakespeare W: *King John*, Act 4, Scene 3.
5 Marcus Aurelius (2006): *Meditations*, Penguin Classics, Book 4: 41, p. 31.
6 Lee D (2007): *Plato: The Republic*, Penguin Classics, pp. 354–358.

7 The following quotation is taken from *Aristotle: On the Soul*, trans. Smith JA, Book 2, Part 1, available from the Internet Classics Archive at http://classics.mit. edu/Aristotle/soul.mb.txt.

8 Hamilton S (2001): *Indian Philosophy: A Very Short Introduction*, Oxford University Press, translation from the Majjhima Nikaya, I: 8, pp. 38–39.

9 *Ibid.*, translation from the Samyutta Nikaya, II: 223, pp. 39.

10 The examples in this paragraph are taken from: Burne J, ed. (1989): *Chronicle of the World*, Ecam Publications.

11 Goodman LE (2006): *Avicenna*, Cornell University Press, Section 3, Ideas and Immortality, pp. 155–158.

12 Seeskin K (2017): 'Maimonides'. In *The Stanford Encyclopedia of Philosophy*, ed. Edward N. Zalta, available at https://plato.stanford.edu/archives/spr2017/entries/maimonides/.

13 Descartes R (2003 [1637]): *Discourse on Method and Related Writings*, ed. Clarke DM, Penguin Classics, Part 4, p. 25.

14 Descartes R (2003 [1641]): *Meditations and other Metaphysical Writings*, ed. Clarke DM, Penguin Classics, First Meditation, p. 22.

15 *Ibid.*, Second Meditation, p. 25.

16 Conan Doyle A (2006 [1926]): *The History of Spiritualism*, Vols 1 and 2, The Echo Library.

17 *Ibid.*, Vol 2, chapter IX, p. 11.

18 *Ibid.*, Vol 2, chapter X, p. 126.

19 *Ibid.*, Vol 2, chapter X, p. 138.

20 Wells HG, Huxley J, Wells, GP (1931): *The Science of Life*, Cassell and Company, consisting of nine books.

21 *Ibid.*, Book 8, chapter 9, p. 853.

22 This is found in Article 5: The Fifth Commandment, para. 2319.

23 This is found in Article 1: The Sacrament of Baptism VI. The Necessity of Baptism, para. 1261.

24 *Ibid.*, para. 1257.

25 Harlow, JM (1868): 'Recovery from the Passage of an Iron Bar through the Head'. *Publications of the Massachusetts Medical Society*, Vol. 2, No. 3, 327–347.

26 Positron Emission Tomography.

27 Rushing SE (2014): 'The Admissibility of Brain Scans in Criminal Trials: The Case of Positron Emission Tomography'. *American Judges Association*, Vol. 50, No. 2, 62–69, available at http://neuroethics.upenn.edu/wp-content/uploads/2013/08/CR50-2Rushing.pdf.

28 Westerhoff J (2013): 'The Self: The One and Only You'. *New Scientist*, 23 February, 290–295.

29 Midgley M (2014): *Are You an Illusion?* Acumen Publishing.

30 Asimov I (1950): *I, Robot*, Voyager Classics, reprinted in 2001. The quotation is from chapter 3: Reason, pp. 54–76.

31 Haldane, JBS (2002 [1927]): *Possible Worlds: And Other Essays*, Transaction Publishers, 'When I am Dead', p. 209.

32 Broks P (2018): *The Darker the Night, the Brighter the Stars; A Neuropsychologist's Odyssey*; Allen Lane, p. 29.

33 Haldane, JBS (2002 [1927]): *Possible Worlds: And Other Essays*, Transaction Publishers, 'When I am Dead', p. 210.

Chapter 7

What does death mean to patients and their relatives?[1]

A 1986 paper[2] probably came the closest to the recognition of the crucial importance of dying as a social relationship, arguing that it is 'meaningless' to provide an answer to the question 'Is the patient dead?' outside a specific context. We need to know *who* is asking the question and *for what purpose* and *how certain* they want to be about the answer. In other parts of the literature, often not citing this more conceptual material, support exists for these ideas from more empirical and clinically oriented authors.

In 2003 a survey[3] was conducted of the determination of death by medical transport teams in the USA. With a 57% response rate from all available working teams in the USA ($N = 190$) they discovered that the key criterion for determination of death was simply unresponsiveness to advanced cardiac support. But more interesting is their finding that the key reason for not pronouncing or presuming death in their patients was 'political reasons' (71%). These political reasons included the ground crew's level of comfort, the flight crew's level of comfort, involvement in a crime scene, involvement of law enforcement officers, involvement of a child and involvement in a humanitarian mission of some sort.

Against these kinds of circumstance-led determinations, where the decision to presume death, or not to presume it, is mediated by the relationships between the patient and those others around him or her, are the prevailing social ideas about reversibility of death. In 1992 it was argued[4] that brain death is counter-intuitive because it runs against people's experience of medical rescue in the media – TV, films or newspapers. Reversibility is not only witnessed in scenes of medical resuscitation but also the rebuilding of other seemingly destroyed objects and organizations such as engines, cities or houses. The very idea of irreversibility is both ahistorical and inconsistent with everyone's contemporary social experience. It usually simply doesn't 'make sense' to people.

The experience of medical staff and families working with so-called 'brain dead' patients actually supports – not undermines – this sense of continuity. Such patients look alive – they are pink and breathing (albeit artificially);[5] they sometimes respond to surgical incision with elevated blood pressure and attempts at respiration;[6] they are capable of reproduction;[7] they develop bedsores and pneumonia (something that cadavers don't do[8]); and they move in their beds, mimicking restlessness and grasping at deliberate or accidental stimuli.[9] This is not 'confusion', 'misapprehension' or 'misconception' by the general public about those who are brain dead.[10,11,12] By most *social* criteria, the brain dead do appear alive.

Moreover, many of the brain dead resemble those asleep, a similar process that often cannot be managed without social support.[13] Little wonder there is a widespread desire by relatives and carers of the unconscious to support them, in spite of whatever medical reasons are offered for the poor responsiveness of their charges. Indeed, 'wonder' is only possible because somehow dying is viewed as a social relationship and not merely as a technical notion divorced from the everyday world of social life and its principles of interaction, reciprocity and meaning-making.

Even if death was declared and agreed by all – say, with widely observed onset of rigor mortis or even later with the onset of putrefaction – this rarely ends a social relationship. In other words, it is not only dying that is a social relationship but also death. It is not the case that death kills identity whatever legal, financial and moral changes are prompted by these bodily changes.[14] Both the social commitments and emotional attachments rarely evaporate at death. Instead, as a host of social and anthropological literature on death and dying ably demonstrates, relationships continue to evolve at the point of death.[15,16,17,18,19,20,21] This broader human context of dying and death as ongoing social relationships mean that 'determination' of death is more a determination of particular social and moral functions during bodily decline.[22]

Therefore for many patients, their families and friends, the emphasis cannot be on death purely as a cloven relationship between biology and culture, but more on the irreversibility of biologic, social and economic decline. Since 'irreversibility' can theoretically only ever be subject to mere (and fallible) technical assessment, the legal and social challenge before us is not one of consent but consensus. This brings us firmly into the world of advanced directives, participatory medical decision-making and civic law. These are debates about citizenship – legal and social discourses about rights, entitlements and obligations – not simply or solely discussions about biology or bioethics.

For most people outside the world of medicine, but briefly visiting in hospitals, death is not decided by appeals to biological argument or evidence but by a social mix of medical, legal and family consensus. As a spouse of someone with severe dementia once remarked: 'That's why I'm looking for a nursing home for her. I loved her dearly but she's just not Mary anymore. No matter how hard I try, I can't get myself to believe that she's there anymore'.[23] People stay when their loved ones appear dead; others leave when those loved ones appear fit and alive but no longer reciprocate in recognizable ways. It is the strength of bonding, opportunities for ongoing reciprocity of the relationship and the future sustainability of both that are crucial for determining whether a relationship is finished and moving into a new phase, or whether it is possible and desirable to hold onto the old one.

Medical and ethical information is necessary and important, but commonly, to the surprise and chagrin of some, not decisive. That is often because the determination of death has historically been based on the community criteria of death. Ignoring this fact about dying as a social relationship will indeed bring physicians, inevitably, predictably and unnecessarily, into conflict with families of comatose patients.[24,25]

Notes

1 This chapter is reproduced from a larger article by Kellehear A (2008): 'Dying as a Social Relationship: A Sociological Review of Debates on the Determination of Death'. *Social Science & Medicine*, Vol. 66, 1533–1544.
2 Sassower R, Grodin MA (1986): 'Epistemological Questions Concerning Death'. *Death Studies*, Vol. 10, 341–353.
3 Robinson KJ, Murphy DM, Jacobs LM (2003): 'Presumption of Death by Air Medical Transport Teams'. *Air Medical Journal*, Vol. 22, No. 3, 30–34.
4 Cole DJ (1992): 'The Reversibility of Death'. *Journal of Medical Ethics*, Vol. 18, 26–30.
5 Truog RD, Fletcher JC (1990): 'Brain Death and the Anencephalic Newborn'. *Bioethics*, Vol. 4, No. 3, 199–215.
6 Karakatsanis KG, Tsanakas JN (2002): 'A Critique on the Concept of "Brain Death"'. *Issues in Law and Medicine*, Vol. 18, No. 2, 127–141.
7 Waisel DB, Truog RD (1997): 'The End-of-life Sequence'. *Anesthesiology*, Vol. 87, No. 3, 676–686.
8 Sundin-Huard D, Fahy K (2004): 'The Problems with the Validity of the Diagnosis of Brain Death'. *Nursing in Critical Care*, Vol. 9, No. 2, 64–70.
9 Turmel A, Roux A, Bojanowski MW (1991): 'Spinal Man after Declaration of Brain Death'. *Neurosurgery*, Vol. 28, No. 2, 298–302.
10 Lizza, JP (1993): 'Persons and Death: What's Metaphysically Wrong with Our Current Statutory Definition of Death?' *Journal of Medicine and Philosophy*, Vol. 18, 351–374.
11 Siminoff LA, Bloch A (1999): 'American Attitudes and Beliefs about Brain Death: The Empirical Literature'. In *The Definition of Death: Contemporary Controversies*, eds Youngner SJ, Arnold RM, Schapiro R, The Johns Hopkins University Press, 183–193.
12 Laureys S (2005): 'Death, Unconsciousness and the Brain'. *Nature Reviews Neuroscience*, Vol. 6, 899–909.

13 Aubert V, White H (1959): 'Sleep: A Sociological Interpretation'. *Acta Sociologica*, Vol. 4, No. 2, 1–16 and 46–54.

14 Veatch RM (2005): 'The Death of Whole-Brain Death: The Plague of Disaggregators, Somaticists, and Mentalists'. *Journal of Medicine and Philosophy*, Vol. 30, 353–378.

15 Hocart AM (1953): *Encyclopedia of the Social Science*, Vol. 5, Macmillan, 'Death Customs', pp. 21–27.

16 Hartland ES (1954): *Encyclopedia of Religion and Ethics*, Vol. 4, Charles Scribner & Sons, 'Death and Disposal of the Dead', pp. 411–444.

17 Pardi MM (1977): *Death: An Anthropological Perspective*, University Press of America.

18 Riley Jr, JW (1983): 'Dying and the Meanings of Death: Sociological Inquiries'. *Annual Review of Sociology*, Vol. 9, 191–216.

19 Palgi P, Abramovitch H (1984): 'Death: A Cross-cultural Perspective'. *Annual Review of Anthropology*, Vol. 13, 385–417.

20 Howarth G (2000): 'Dismantling the Boundaries between Life and Death'. *Mortality*, Vol. 5, No. 2, 127–138.

21 Kellehear A (2007): *A Social History of Dying*, Cambridge University Press.

22 Miles S (1999): 'Death in a Technological and Pluralist Culture'. In *The Definition of Death: Contemporary Controversies*, eds Youngner SJ, Arnold RM, Schapiro R, The Johns Hopkins University Press, pp. 311–318.

23 Gubrium JF (2005): 'The Social Worlds of Old Age'. In *The Cambridge Handbook of Age and Ageing*, ed Johnson ML, Cambridge University Press, 310–315.

24 Lock M (1996): 'Death in Technological Time: Locating the End of a Meaningful Life'. *Medical Anthropology Quarterly*, Vol. 10, No. 4, 575–600.

25 Bernat JL (2005): 'The Concept and Practice of Brain Death'. *Progress in Brain Death*, Vol. 150, 369–379.

Chapter 8

Near-death experiences, deathbed visions and visions of the bereaved

Traditional religions are not the only source of beliefs in the afterlife, or God, or cosmic philosophy. In fact, there has been a long-standing set of personal experiences near death that have inspired these beliefs too. These are near-death experiences (NDEs), deathbed visions (DBVs) and visions of the bereaved (VBs).

NDEs have been recorded for thousands of years by communities around the world and figure both in early philosophical and religious texts as well as oral traditions in urban, agricultural and hunter-gatherer societies.[1,2] Over the last 50 years these have been regularly recorded in the medical and psychology literature associated mainly with resuscitation[3] or medical crisis experiences.[4] Typically, about 12–18% of patients who experience cardiac arrest and are subsequently revived tell a story about their time while ostensibly unconscious as a set of conscious experiences.[5] These stories commonly describe personal experiences of out-of-body experiences, travelling into darkness and then brightly lit spaces, feelings of peace and unconditional love, meeting a loving being of light, sometimes experiencing a life review and then meeting deceased relatives or friends. Some longer, more popular accounts have been published as best-selling books and many of these accounts detail supernatural environments that contain beautiful countryside and cities.[6] None of these contemporary examples differ substantially from those from 100 or 1,000 years ago, save that interpretations from earlier accounts were more religiously drawn and inspired.[7]

Deathbed visions have a world-wide prevalence of between 10 and 30% of dying people depending on which study one reads.[8,9] In DBVs, dying people, most commonly those dying of a terminal illness, will report seeing former (deceased) friends or relatives visit them by the bedside. Some of these will be one-off visits and others will be regular visitors to the bedside. The median time before death of these visits is estimated to be two

65

days. About half the visitors seem to be deceased parents. Conversational exchange between the visitors and the dying is common. They are nearly always viewed as comforting. Because of the stigma of 'visions' in a secular-style society with largely materialist leanings, these prevalence figures must be viewed as conservative due to expected under-reporting.

The prevalence of visions of the bereaved is extremely dependent on culture, with a variation of between 30 and over 80% depending on the country of the study.[10] VBs vary from hearing voices and smelling scents associated with the bereaved to partial and full-blown apparitions. Sometimes the apparitions do not speak or sometimes conversations can be lengthy.[11] They are not generally considered a sign of mental illness.[12]

For most people who have these kinds of experiences, the encounters are mostly evidence for the existence of an afterlife, and sometimes of a god. Although it is rare in near-death experiences for a 'Being of Light' to self-identify as a god (or an angel), it is more common for people to ascribe that type of identity to these beings. More often, however, people view these experiences as personal evidence that life continues after death.

Obviously there has been a parallel tradition of neurophysiological and psychiatric research shadowing the explosion of descriptive studies of all these exceptional experiences. Looking back upon these different studies, we can say that overwhelmingly these experiences do not seem associated with organic (e.g., brain tumour), pharmacotherapeutic (e.g., LSD) or psychiatric conditions (e.g., psychotic disorders) of the dying or bereaved person.[13] There is also no correlation between religious beliefs, education, age, medical condition or gender and these different kinds of exceptional experience.

Popular journalism and opinion as well as professional skeptics commonly argue that these are 'hallucinations'. However, aside from serious problems with the clinical criteria for deciding about hallucinations, most people are unaware that a large proportion of people see and hear things that are 'not there' (up to 25% lifetime prevalence) and less than 1 or 2% of this population meets the organic, pharmacy-related or psychiatric criteria for abnormality. NDEs, DBVs and VBs are not covered by these clinical criteria.

There have also been recurring attempts to explain these phenomena as side effects of oxygen deprivation in the dying brain – simply discredited because most of these experiences have been described by people who were not dying. Some have attempted to explain this as 'cultural reproduction' – seeing what they expect to see – but many people do not expect to see such things and are surprised and sometimes disoriented to see them. It is worth noting the famous atheist and ascetic philosopher AJ Ayer's account of his own near-death experience in May 1988. His NDE was very real to him and made him revisit the question of an afterlife. He wrote about it in the *Telegraph* and the *Spectator*, the text of both being available in full.[14]

Finally, some have questioned whether these experiences are due to drugs being taken to palliate the dying or as part of the regime of drugs given to those in surgery, or sedatives given to the bereaved. This question has also been settled by the sheer number of people reporting these experiences without any history of such drugs.

If by 'causes' we are wanting to identify a line of medical or psychiatric research that will link these to bodily processes of one sort or another, we simply do not know what causes these experiences. We are also largely at a loss to fit such experiences into conventional religious views of the afterlife. 'Heavens' and 'Hells' from the different religions are often described as eschatologies (final things or final destinations of the soul) by theologians; however, NDEs and DBVs in particular are not eschotologies but rather pareschatologies (early things that occur on the soul's journey).[15] None of these experiences give us clues to what happens next – e.g., the soul's final destination in some afterlife space or in a reincarnation. They are experiences in the borderlands of human transition from life as we know it to life as we do not know it. Because they cannot arbitrate over the different religiously constructed understandings of the afterlife, some religious theorists dismiss such experiences as without value.[16] However, for the dying and the bereaved, and for many of the families and friends who support both, these experiences are usually comforting and supportive of the empirical fact that the bonds of attachment continue between people even unto death, and sometimes beyond.

Notes

1 Kellehear A (1996): *Experiences Near-Death: Beyond Medicine and Religion*, Oxford University Press.
2 Holden J, Greyson B, James N (2009): *The Handbook of Near-Death Experiences: Thirty Years of Investigation*, ABC-CLIO.
3 Ring K (1980): *Life at Death: A Scientific Investigation of the Near-Death Experience*, Coward, McCann & Geoghegan.
4 Sabom M (1980): *Recollections of Death: A Medical Investigation*, Harper & Row.
5 Van Lommel P, van Wees R, Meyers V, Elfferich, I (2001): 'Near-Death Experiences in Survivors of Cardiac Arrest: A Prospective Study in the Netherlands'. *The Lancet*, Vol. 358, No. 9298, 2039–2045.
6 Alexander E (2012): *Proof of Heaven: A Neurosurgeon's Journey into the Afterlife*, Simon & Schuster.
7 Zaleski C (1987): *Otherworld Journeys: Accounts of Near-Death Experiences in Medieval and Modern Times*, Oxford University Press.
8 Muthumana S, Kumari M, Kellehear A, Kumar S, Moosa F (2010): 'Deathbed Visions from India: A Study of Family Observations in Northern Kerala'. *Omega: Journal of Death and Dying*, Vol. 62, No. 2, 95–107.

9 Kellehear A, Pogonet V, Mindruta-Stratan R, Gorelco V (2011): 'Deathbed Visions from the Republic of Moldova: A Content Analysis of Family Observations.' *Omega: Journal of Death and Dying*, Vol. 64, No. 4, 303–317.

10 Kellehear A (2017): 'Unusual Perceptions at the End of Life: Limitations to the Diagnosis of Hallucinations in Palliative Medicine.' *BMJ Supportive and Palliative Care*, Vol. 7, 238–246.

11 Guggenheim B, Guggenheim, J (1996): *Hello from Heaven*, Thorsons.

12 Tracy DK, Shergill SS (2013): 'Mechanisms Underlying Auditory Understanding Perception without Stimulus'. *Brain Science*, Vol. 3, 642–669.

13 Alexander E (2012): *Proof of Heaven: A Neurosurgeon's Journey into the Afterlife*, Simon & Schuster.

14 www.philosopher.eu/others-writings/a-j-ayer-what-i-saw-when-i-was-dead/.

15 Hick J (1976): *Death and Eternal Life*, Collins.

16 Kung H (1984): *Eternal Life*, Collins.

Chapter 9

The entanglement of religion, ethics and societal development

Cultural entanglements

Religions and which people practise them are often geographically determined, both internationally and locally. The spectrum spans those countries with a national faith (e.g., Iran), through to areas of cosmopolitanism, such as cities like Jerusalem, where we can speak of its Jewish, Christian, Muslim and Armenian Quarters. International military action and colonial expansionism often involves the movement of troops across the world to places with cultures and religions that many of them would otherwise never have experienced in their lives. It can also involve the translocation of civilians as workers and slaves. Such events occurred with Alexander the Great, the Romans, Napoleon and during the First and Second World Wars, and the process continues to this day. When enforced engagement happens, especially if there is subsequent military occupation, unlikely people meet and experience a range of emotions, from hatred to falling in love. This has provided the context for many operas, plays and novels. Examples are Odysseus and Calypso in 'The Odyssey' (800 BCE), Mark Antony and Cleopatra chronicled by Plutarch in 'Parallel Lives Of Noble Grecians And Romans' (100 CE), Butterfly and Pinkerton in 'Madame Butterfly' (1903), Fowler and Phuong in 'The Quiet American' (1955), and Joanna and John in 'Guess Who's Coming to Dinner?' (1967).

The properties of social groups and their dependence on custom were emphasized by the anthropologist Ruth Benedict in her groundbreaking work *Patterns of Culture*. This text emphasized the essential nature of a social group that necessarily includes culture, customs and religion: they come together as a package. She writes:

The life history of the individual is first and foremost an accommodation to the patterns and standards traditionally handed down in his community. From the moment of his birth the customs into which he is born shape his experience and his behaviour.

... today, whether it is a question of imperialism, or of race prejudice, or of a comparison between Christianity and paganism, we are still preoccupied with the uniqueness, not of the human institutions of the world at large ... But of our own institutions and achievements, our own civilization.

The distinction between any closed group and outside peoples becomes, in terms of religion, that between the true believers and the heathen. Between these two categories for thousands of years there were no common meeting points.[1]

Four years after the book's 1934 publication, the Second World War broke out; her country, the USA, entered following the attack on Pearl Harbor in 1941.

American military action across the Pacific resulted in many young American men meeting Indochinese customs and young women. Boys being boys and girls being girls, on occasions non-military action resulted. Racial, cultural and, importantly, religious differences became highlighted in the immediate postwar years.

James Michener was a lieutenant commander in the US Navy during the conflict and he wrote short stories about both military and social events in Indochina. Collected together as a book, these were published as *Tales of the South Pacific* in 1947. To the delight of the novice author, it won the Pulitzer Prize, with Rogers and Hammerstein taking up the cross-cultural problems in the musical 'South Pacific'. The latter premiered on Broadway in 1949 and was an immediate hit. During the production, significant pressure was brought to bear on the creators to tone things down, but to their credit they did not. The greatest concern focused on a song called 'You've Got To Be Carefully Taught'.[2]

An American marine, Lieutenant Cable, falls in love with a Vietnamese girl, Liat. Resentments and difficulties follow, and Cable expresses his frustrations in the following lines.

You've got to be taught
To hate and fear,
You've got to be taught
From year to year,
It's got to be drummed
In your dear little ear

You've got to be carefully taught.
You've got to be taught to be afraid
Of people whose eyes are oddly made,
And people whose skin is a diff'rent shade,
You've got to be carefully taught.
You've got to be taught before it's too late,
Before you are six or seven or eight,
To hate all the people your relatives hate,
You've got to be carefully taught!

The intended messages of this are clear and the implications for juxta-position of different religions and customs are obvious. Again, both in this song and in the work of Benedict[3] and the Jesuits (see Chapter 2, note 10), the importance of the early years is emphasized. In today's multi-cultural society there are many groups growing up cheek by jowl and then living parallel adult lives in separate sub-cultures. How many stop to think of how the others live? How many take the step of considering the other person's viewpoint?

Reinforcement and recruitment: rites and societal interventions

Many religions have practices and ceremonies to be undertaken at various points during childhood and adolescence. To the devout these are stages to be welcomed on the path to doctrinal maturity and acceptance into the family of believers. To the irreligious, they are manipulative events by which, via a corruption of influence in those they trust, the naïve are fur-ther enmeshed into a religious social structure from which escape is made more difficult. To others, they are harmless traditional observances that support the pathway into adulthood. Examples include:

- baptism and confirmation in Christianity;
- Brit Milah (circumcision) and Bar Mitzvah (aged 13 years) for Jewish boys;
- male circumcision and Shahada (for boys and girls) in Islam;
- the Amrit ceremony for Sikhs;
- Upanayana (initiation; the sacred-thread ceremony) in Hinduism.

These ceremonies allow families and communities to come together at a moment of celebration and, in doing this, the young person feels acceptance. The ceremonies also act as a reminder to the initiated that they are expected to show increased maturity, take on more responsibility than previously or start to play a more important part within their community. They also anchor the initiate's reference frame to a particular set of values and perhaps (though not necessarily and not overtly) encourage loyalty to the group first and to the wider society second. Advantages of adherence to the group are well demonstrated in other ways throughout the animal kingdom, without regard to the benefits of an afterlife.

Agnostics and atheists often do not have these ceremonies, and to this extent their children have less of a developmental socio-religious framework within which to flourish. This can be an ostensibly good thing, leading to a mature liberal outlook, but it can also leave them with less support as life's 'slings and arrows' start to hit in young adulthood. For many (including religious young people), social media now provide the first-line support matrix for their anxieties and their inner lives. The paradox of a liberal political society, designed to encourage fair play for all, is that it allows self-interest groups unfettered advancement within the limits of the law and free speech. An example of this is the Inaugural Address to the Muslim Parliament by Dr Kalim Siddiqui at Kensington Hall, London in 1992.[4]

> Under the most intense pressure ever applied by the West on Islam and Muslims, we have refused to yield on either of these flanks: we have held, extended and consolidated the moral high ground we alone occupy, and we have beaten our opponents back to re-examine the values at the core of their own existence. Liberalism has found its match; it may not survive the test we have set for it.

Although this was very probably written by someone whose views are not those of the moderate majority, it does nevertheless raise the theoretical construct that universal liberalism based on a secular humanism might be a pipe dream. The very essence of liberalism is 'live and let live', and this allows those on a mission of expansionism to influence, recruit and grow. Crusades are the same now as in medieval times. Spawned in religious fervor, they provide an unquestionable justification for interfering with other people's lives on the presupposition that the cause is just and beneficial to those who convert.

On the other hand, whatever the religion, it is difficult, even for committed non-believers, to be unmoved by religious services and ceremonies, especially those surrounding birth, marriage and death. Somehow the combination of the congregation, the music, the singing, the language, the buildings and the ceremony combine to foster a moving inner response.

Whilst such ceremony is intended to be, and usually is, a perfectly proper, caring and fulfilling experience, there are some occasions on which it is not.

In the Cold War years of the 1950s, 1960s and 1970s the struggle for international hegemony and dominance was expressed via propaganda campaigns, espionage, psychological warfare and technological initiatives such as the Space Race. In 1963, the thriller film *The Mind Benders* captured the national mood of paranoia and suspicion with the juxtaposition of spying and sensory deprivation as a prelude to brainwashing. Towards the beginning of the Cold War years in 1957, William Sargant published his classic book on mental manipulation, *Battle for the Mind*. Sargant was a psychiatrist who was a consultant for MI5. He was heavily criticized by the medical fraternity for his use of deep-sleep treatments and insulin therapy and hence is now a footnote on mainstream psychiatry's 'best-forgotten' list, but recently his work on brainwashing and conversion has had a renaissance.[5] The book was completed whilst he was convalescing from illness in Majorca and there, Robert Graves (the classicist, poet and novelist who compiled *The Greek Myths* and reportedly said 'there's no money in poetry, but then there's no poetry in money, either'), who lived on the island, helped with the editing. As a result, Graves contributed chapter 8 on 'Brain-Washing in Ancient Times', where he describes the written accounts of mystical initiations in the BCE period, thus giving a timelessness to the techniques employed.

In the foreword to his book, Sargant draws attention to a religious sermon which is worth studying in greater detail. It was delivered by George Salmon FRS, who became a theologian after a successful academic career as a mathematician sufficient to earn him an obituary in *Nature* in 1904.[6] The place was St Stephen's Church, Dublin (a Protestant church in a Catholic country), on Sunday, 3 July 1859, and the sermon[7] concerned 'The work of the holy spirit'. In it, Salmon confronts the difficult question of religious conversion. He says:

> The most violent and extensive religious excitement that history records took place in one of the darkest periods of the Church's history. I mean that which led to the Crusades; when millions of Christians thoroughly believing what they exclaimed – 'it is the will of God' – deserted their homes only to perish in heaps in a foreign land.
>
> . . . For we cannot believe that God seduced those great multitudes with false premises, and led them out to perish miserably in a distant land. *We see then that religious excitement may exist without religious knowledge* [current authors' emphasis].[8]

And later:

> And I consider it just as unlawful to produce artificially hysterical and nervous disease. Seasons of bodily depression are, no doubt, favourable to religious thoughts, yet we have no right to throw peoples' bodies into an unhealthy state in the hope of saving their souls . . . The fact is, religious excitement is good, not for itself, but for what it may lead to; and the danger of it is that it is often succeeded by a reaction which leaves the subject of it in a more unfavourable condition than before.[9]

Battle for the Mind describes the conditions needed for conversion and brain-washing and Sargant gives examples from voodoo drumming to pharmacological interventions, and cites examples from John Wesley, the Quakers and the American evangelist Billy Graham. He gives a persuasive comparison of John Wesley's conversion techniques in 1739, using charismatic public speaking to create a high emotional tension, to Grinker and Spiegel's account of battle neuroses in the North African Campaign of the Second World War in 1942.[10] Quoting from Wesley's journal, Sargant writes:

> While I [i.e., Wesley] was speaking, one before me dropped down as dead, and presently a second and a third. Five others sank down in half an hour, most of whom were in violent agonies. The 'pains' as 'of hell came about them, the snares of death over-took them'. In their trouble we called upon the Lord, and He gave us an answer of peace. One indeed continued an hour in strong pain, and one or two more for three days; but the rest were greatly comforted in that hour, and went away rejoicing and praising God.[11]

Sargant concluded as follows.

> They [men] are gifted with religious and social apprehensions . . . Therefore, the brain should not be abused by having forced upon it any religious or political mystique that stunts the reason, or any form of crude rationalization that stunts the religious sense.[12]

From the examples given in this section, it can be seen that the influence of social rites range from an innocent and constructive role through herd reinforcement to fearful conversional spectacles with potential harmful consequences. Social rites do therefore span spectra from good to evil, innocent to odious and harmless to destructive.

As a final comment, perhaps we could consider the mindset of President George W. Bush, who declared a 'War on Terror' against the 'axis of evil' as a response to the events of 11 September 2001. In 2003, God and George Bush were discussed by the *New York Times*.

> At the age of 40, Mr. Bush beat a drinking problem by surrendering to a powerful religious experience, reinforced by Bible study with friends. This kind of born-again epiphany is common in much of America – the red-state version of psychotherapy – and it creates the kind of faith that is not beset by doubt because the believer knows his life got better in the bargain.[13]

And it continues:

> Perhaps the most important effect of Mr. Bush's religion is that, for better or for worse, it imparts a profound self-confidence once he has decided on a course of action. This has been most conspicuous since Sept. 11 in the way he has talked about his mission to make the world safe for democracy. Some listeners take it as presumptuous, messianic, even blasphemous. John Green of the University of Akron, a scholar of religion in politics, sees it as a perfectly ordinary way for a religious man to understand a task history has presented him. 'For Bush to conclude that this was God's plan,' he said, 'is not a whole lot different from a plumber in Akron deciding that God wants him to serve lunch to homeless people'.

By analogy, reformed smokers are reputedly the most zealous non-smokers. Enough said.

Religion, politics and the law

Interactions between these three areas of life can occur as a choice via public opinion and the ballet box or more rigorously by integration of a religion into a governmental system. With respect to the former, it can be a facet of the emotionally driven post-truth politics described above (Chapter 2, notes 18, 19 and 20). The most forceful form of unofficial action is simple: a particular faction or lobby which could affect a politician's or a political party's fortunes desires a particular policy to be supported and makes their support contingent upon adoption of that policy. Another example would be voting for someone of the same religion irrespective of other good candidates who are standing for office. At a less significant level there are multiple routes of lobbying for the support of specific religious interests: it is done by Jews,[14] Muslims,[15] Catholics[16] and others, and, of course, the Church of England Bishops (Lords Spiritual) sit in the House of Lords in the United Kingdom. Across the world the number of lobby groups is huge and their impact is variable.

Direct interactions occur when the religion, or parts of it, are contained within the civil and/or criminal law system. It is interesting to look briefly at the history of secular codes of law. Mesopotamia was the name for the area of the Middle East contained by the Tigris and Euphrates rivers. It is often considered as a cradle of civilization in the Western world and encompasses the area of modern-day Iraq and adjoining territories. In the second millennium BCE one of its constituent parts was the Babylonian Empire. This society had belief in and worshipped multiple deities assembled into a pantheon of gods and goddesses, each representing an important aspect of earthly life. Within this polytheistic society, Hammurabi (c. 1728–1686 BCE), the sixth king of the First Babylonian Dynasty, set out his Code on the freedom of speech and civil rights.[17] His 282 edicts were later lost to history in their original until 1901, when a team of French archeologists unearthed the famous *diorite stele* (now in the Louvre, Paris), at the ancient city of Susa, Iran. Although being retributive in form ('an eye for an eye'), and penalties being dependent on social position, nevertheless no one was above the rule of law and the so-called 'Secular Tradition', often now referred to as 'separation of Church and State', was born. One's beliefs were irrelevant to the outcome of judicial and governmental decisions.

Thomas Paine, the leading Enlightenment Anglo-American philosopher, political theorist and revolutionary, wrote at length on the problems of mixing religion with politics. He was clear in his views.

> By engendering the church with the state, a sort of mule-animal, capable of only destroying, and of not breeding up, is produced, called the Church established by Law . . . Persecution is not an original feature in any religion; but it is always the strongly-marked feature of all law-religions, or religions established by law. Take away the law establishment and every religion assumes its original benignity.[18]

In 1792, a year after the publication of *The Rights of Man*, the British Government prosecuted Paine for 'libel' for his views. He was, however, not present at his own trial because he was by then in France as a honoured citizen and member of the National Assembly set up following the French Revolution.

Today, a number of countries have religion formally separated from the political system in their constitution. Examples are the USA, France, South Korea, Singapore and Italy. The USSR under Marxism introduced state atheism and discouraged all religious activities. Switzerland adopts a strange position in having separation of Church and State at federal but not at canton level. Countries such as Denmark and the United Kingdom that have significant social secularization have maintained constitutional recognition of an official state religion, but its power is minimal. In England, the original religious source of its now secular legal framework is clearly expressed in lettering at the top of one wall of the entrance hall of the Old Bailey, where it says: 'Moses gave unto the people the laws of God'.

A theocracy is a country whose rulers have both secular and spiritual authority. The only two modern countries that are true theocracies are Iran and Vatican City. In Iran, the state religion is Islam, the law is Islamic and the head of the country is the Grand Ayatollah. In Vatican City, the state religion is Roman Catholicism, and the country's leader is the Pope. Although not a theocracy, Saudia Arabia maintains Islamic courts for all aspects of law and has religious police to maintain social compliance. In some Islamic countries, such as Pakistan, Algeria, Turkey, Egypt and Sudan, it is suspected and reported by the media that fundamentalist Muslims are pushing to move to a more theocratic system of government. International theocracy is also seen as an aspiration of the terrorist organization ISIS. Major problems can potentially arise when a sector of the population responds to, or is socially controlled by, their own theocratic legal system that is operating within a democratic constitution that does not recognize it. An example of this would be sharia councils and canon law in the UK, both of which can take ecclesiastical positions at variance with the state in areas such as marriage, and in gender and sexual issues.

In the UK Human Rights Act (1998),[19] Article 9, setting out the 'Freedom of thought, conscience and religion', formalized the position of religion in British society. Section 1 says:

> Everyone has the right to freedom of thought, conscience and religion; this right includes freedom to change his religion or belief and freedom, either alone or in community with others and in public or private, to manifest his religion or belief, in worship, teaching, practice and observance.

On occasions this has been quoted by some religious groups (and individuals) to provide a reason for greater tolerance or freedom for their specific activities. Examples are problems with the wearing of Christian crosses in certain workplaces[20] and the necessity when in court to remove a face veil at the request of the judge.[21] However, what is rarely added when Article 9 is quoted is Section 2, which qualifies Section 1 as follows:

> Freedom to manifest one's religion or beliefs shall be subject only to such limitations as are prescribed by law and are necessary in a democratic society in the interests of public safety, for the protection of public order, health or morals, or for the protection of the rights and freedoms of others.

So, in conclusion, as is usual in things religious, the situation is complex and varies from place to place, over time and in individual circumstances. The ingenuity and apparent need within the psyche of some of those seeking or possessing political or theological power to require others to conform to their persuasion seems to be a timeless inbuilt attribute of the human race. There is no sign that in the modern world this is different than at any time in recorded history. Perhaps, despite its potentially divisive nature, it is a necessary constituent of the formation of effective social groups and nations; however, it also has the inevitable side effect of creating friction between those of different beliefs.

Notes

1 Benedict R (1934): *Patterns of Culture*, Mariner Books (2005). The quotations are from chapter 1, pp. 3, 5 and 8, respectively.
2 Lyrics reproduced by permission of Hal Leonard Europe Ltd.
3 Benedict R (1934): Patterns of Culture, Mariner Books (2005).
4 Available at: www.muslimparliament.org.uk/Documentation/InauguralAddress. pdf.
5 Sargant W (1957): *Battle for the Mind: A Physiology of Conversion and Brain-Washing*, Wm. Heinemann (re-issued in 2011 with an introduction by Swencionis C; Malor Books).
6 *Nature*, Vol. 69 (4 February 1904), 324–326.
7 The full published text is available at: https://archive.org/details/evidenceswork ho00salmgoog from the archives of Oxford University.
8 *Ibid.*, pp. 21–22.
9 *Ibid.*, pp. 24–25.
10 Sargant W (1957): *Battle for the Mind: A Physiology of Conversion and Brain-Washing*, Wm. Heinemann (re-issued in 2011 with an introduction by Swencionis C; Malor Books), chapter 5: 'Techniques of Religious Conversion', pp. 83–85.
11 *Ibid.*, pp. 89–90.
12 *Ibid.*, chapter 11: 'General Conclusions', p. 274.
13 Keller B (2003): 'God and George W Bush', *New York Times*, May 17.
14 Oborne P, Jones J (2009): 'The Pro-Israel Lobby in Britain', Open Democracy. available at: www.opendemocracy.net/ourkingdom/peter-oborne-james-jones/pro-israel-lobby-in-britain-full-text.
15 see MPACUK (Muslim Public Affairs Committee UK) at: www.MPACUK.org.

16 see Catholic Action UK at: http://catholicactionuk.blogspot.co.uk.
17 Ishay MR (2007): *The Human Rights Reader*, 2nd edn, Routledge, chapter 1, pp. 8–10.
18 Paine T (1791): *The Rights of Man: Common Sense and Other Political Writings*, ed. Philip M, Oxford World's Classics, 2008, pp. 138–139.
19 www.legislation.gov.uk/ukpga/1998/42/schedule/1.
20 Rudgard O (2017): 'Church of England Attacks "Troubling" European Court Ruling which says Employers Can Ban Workers from Wearing Christian Crosses", *Telegraph*, 14 March, available at: www.telegraph.co.uk/news/2017/03/14/church-england-attacks-troubling-european-court-ruling-says/.
21 Rozenberg J (2013): 'Veils in Court: This Compromise Ruling Struck the Wrong Balance', *Guardian*, 17 September, available at: www.theguardian.com/law/2013/sep/17/veil-court-ruling-wrong-balance.

Chapter 10

The uses and abuses of religions

The uses of religions

The Victorian polymath Francis Galton was Charles Darwin's half-cousin. He made major contributions in many fields of science but is usually remembered for his creation of the study of eugenics and the 'nature-versus-nurture' concept. This interest was partly inspired by Darwin's publication of *On the Origin of Species* in 1859. He is of interest to us here because he applied statistical analysis to the power of prayer.[1] Galton reasoned that if God was listening, prayer should have an effect. Since in England those most prayed for (in the past and the present) were the sovereigns and their close progeny, they should live longer than other people exposed to similar lifetime risks. The results in his paper (adapted for this essay), are shown in Table 10.1.

Although no statistical significance was calculated, it can be seen that, on average, royalty do not have the edge, and even lawyers (who probably receive very few prayers on their behalf) do rather better. Similarly, birth statistics, including stillbirths, were class-insensitive. Whilst Galton does not deny the mental support that might come from prayer, he does conclude that its efficacy cannot be proved, although it probably does no harm.

TABLE 10.1 Life expectancy and social class

Class of person	Average life expectancy in years (data from 1758 to 1843)
Members of royal households	64.04
English aristocracy	67.31
Military officers	67.6
Lawyers	68.14

Many arguments followed this publication and the debate on the effectiveness of prayer continues to the present day; in 2006 a study on 1,802 heart-bypass patients found no beneficial effect of prayer on outcomes.[2] There is, however, no doubt that for many people religion is a central plank of their existence, and that the experience of a religious component to their life is, to them, very beneficial and usually harmless to others. For some, the religious connection provides the membership of a social group of similarly minded individuals rather than necessarily allowing them to communicate directly with a deity. These factors must not be forgotten as an important component of a person's psychological health. Whether such beliefs or affiliations are required for a stable society remains debatable.

Whether driven by a self-interested belief that the commitment will favour a good afterlife, or because it is a good thing to do in itself, the work of religions for the common good has been, and continues to be, significant. Over the centuries there have been endless examples of followers from all religions who have provided alms, education and medical care to the needy and this warrants proper recognition. Although in the past there have been, and at present there still are, occasions across the world when religions have promulgated their beliefs alongside the invasion of foreign countries and colonial expansion, that does not negate the aspirations of their charity. Similarly, the abuse exposed in religiously affiliated children's care homes is an attribute of a minority of warped individuals, not of the creed. This does not of course excuse the failure of those who knew it was happening but did nothing to remedy things.

On average, since 2013, faith-based charities in England and Wales have raised £16.3 billion per annum in contributions.[3] This represents 23% of the charity sector's total income. The distribution of fundraising is shown in Table 10.2.

TABLE 10.2 Charitable income raised by faith groups

Faith group	Total income (£ millions)
Multi-faith	7.6
Buddhist	48.3
Sikh	61.4
Hindu	83.3
Quaker	104.0
Muslim	542.3
Jewish	1,012.0
Generally faith-based	3,270.0
Christian	11,208.5
Total	16,337.5

Faith-based charities make up 49% of all overseas-aid charities and 45% of human-rights charities. The faith-based sector also accounts for 39% of all anti-poverty charities. This is a huge contribution and it must be remembered that much of this aid does not only go to adherents of the donating faiths. It is clear that without faith-driven fundraising, many people would not receive the help that they do. This is a very positive feature of religious organizations.

It also cannot go without mention that religions and their ministers come into their own at a time of national crisis or following tragic occurrences. Even victims who are not religious often join with faith-based efforts to find some peace in otherwise meaningless and incomprehensible events. This compassion and the start of healing is expressed nationally, regionally and locally and increasingly across multi-faith groupings. Similarly, lapsed believers still choose religious rites to celebrate births, marriages and lives that have ended. Although these ceremonies have a mystical component related to the beliefs of the faith for the devout, they also provide a framework for non-believers to come to terms with the gift of happiness, the start of a new lifelong relationship that changes the rights of the next of kin and the knowledge that a loved one is gone forever, at least in physical form.

The abuses of religions

Unfortunately, religions also have rather a lot to answer for on the debit side of human experience; just like the charitable axis, these episodes have occurred for centuries and continue today. The damage inflicted can be personal or aimed at a group, country or on an international level. It is usually very difficult to disentangle whether the events *per se* are indeed a reflection of the scriptures, an unconscious corruption of the scriptures by the fanatically devout or a deliberate misuse of the scriptures to achieve a non-religious objective by individuals, commercial organizations or governments. As an example, a representative of the Royal United Services Institute (a British security and anti-terrorism think-tank), was recently reported as saying:

> Most Jihadists have little knowledge of Islam . . . It's the gangster excitement that fits into their sense of needing to belong.[4]

A perusal of the texts of most religions, such as the Bible and the Qur'an, will demonstrate very unpleasant sections ranging from human sacrifice via homophobia to violent expansionism. Most of these statements can be ignored, or at least re-interpreted in the light of current social norms if the religious scripts are taken to be a series of myths or stories written by people at different times. The original authors would probably have put their own interpretation and 'spin' on events and given what they thought was sound advice at the time of writing. However, in the case of Islam, there is a significant difference: the traditional belief is that the Qur'an was not the work of Mohammed, but the actual words of God transmitted through him. The Qur'an has both much kindness and much violence within it, and to an independent interpreter there are major conflicts in aspects of God's messages.

Religious wars have existed since manuscripts were written and it is always difficult to disentangle the true religious element from its corruption by power-seeking rulers. Nevertheless, religious affiliation is a lever with which to recruit forces. Examples are the conquest of Canaan by the Israelites (ca. 1400 BCE), the Muslim conquests of the 7th and 8th centuries, the Christian Crusades of the 11th to 13th centuries and the European wars of religion in the 16th and 17th centuries. Most of the Muslims in India originally gained their faith either forcefully or for the advantages adoption offered during the Mogul occupation from the 16th to the 18th centuries.

More recently, the actual role of religion in war has been questioned by Karen Armstrong, who says:

> ... so indelibly is the aggressive image of religious faith in our secular consciousness that we routinely load the violent sins of the twentieth century onto the back of 'religion' and drive it out into the political wilderness.[5]

She points out that neither of the two World Wars were fought on account of religion. To try to put some estimates on the role of religion in warfare is difficult. Analyzing the religious component of the human cost of humanity's 100 deadliest achievements results in attributing the root causes as religious to be 56.4 million in a total of 455 million deaths.[6] This of course does not account for displacements, pogroms etc. carried out in the name of religion in the absence of war or death.

Two notorious episodes in the history of Christianity and one recent one from Islam will provide examples of perverted religious fervour. The first, committed by the Roman Catholic Church, was the creation of the Spanish Inquisition. It was established in 1478 by Ferdinand II of Aragon and Isabella I of Castile and was intended to keep the rank-and-file (and especially those who had converted from Judaism and Islam to Christianity) in strict Christian adherence. The regulation of the faith of the newly converted was intensified after decrees in 1492 and 1502 that also ordered Jews and Muslims to convert or leave Spain. So concerned was the Roman Catholic Church about the later reputation of the

Inquisition that Pope John Paul II commissioned a review of its activities, which was published in 2004. This was possible because the Inquisition kept high-quality records that were still stored in the Vatican library.

The review concluded that the estimates of death and torture were significantly above the popularized figures and new estimates were published taking account of this.[7] Nevertheless, the conclusions were still seriously disturbing, and 'the Inquisition did provoke serious fear in society. Hearsay evidence and confessions after torture are well documented, as are voluntary 'confessions' to escape formal punishment. The outcome of a prosecution could take four main forms:[8] acquittal, penance, physical punishment or death by burning. Hundreds of thousands of people were charged with crimes by the Inquisition and about 3,000 were executed.[9] Even though modern interpretations tone down its reputation for extremism, it was nevertheless one of the most repressive and cruel self-governing religious bodies in history. There is no wonder Napoleon was popular in Spain when he stopped its activities in 1808.

The second black mark against Christianity (this time perpetrated by the Protestant Christians) comes in the form of the Test Acts,[10] a series of Acts of the British Parliament dating from 1661 until their repeal in 1828 which legislated that only those taking communion in the established Church of England were eligible for appointment to public office, both military and civil, or to receive a university education. This made life tough for Roman Catholics, Jews and other non-conformists. Appointees to public posts were obliged to take oaths recognizing the supremacy of the British monarch as the head of the Church of England and agreeing that there was no actual transubstantiation of the elements of the bread and wine during the sacrament of Holy Communion. Freedom and fairness for all was illusory; religious power games were a reality. Religion-based inequality was a fact of life in Christian Britain.

More recently, Islam has seriously tried to restrict the freedom of speech and, by means of this, could be seen as trying to suppress discussion on Islamic issues through terror. In 1988, Salman Rushdie published *The Satanic Verses*,[11] which subsequently won the Whitbread Award for the Novel of the Year. Within the genre of 'magical realism', the title refers to a legend of the Prophet Mohammed whereby a few verses were supposedly spoken by him as part of the Qur'an and then withdrawn.

So offended were the international Islamic community by the novel's message that there were disturbances across the world, books were burnt and booksellers, publishers and translators were threatened and harmed. On 14 February 1989, Ayatollah Khomeini, the Supreme Leader of Iran, issued a fatwa (which, after his death, can never be rescinded), calling for the death of Rushdie and his publishers. On 7 March 1989, the UK and Iran broke off diplomatic relations and what became a major international incident persisted for decades. Rushdie was forced to live under police protection for the next nine years. It is difficult to see how this was not a blatant example of intolerance being used for political purposes. In 2012, the *Guardian* published an extended article on the fatwa and its consequences in which a number of individuals active at the time defended Rushdie and lamented the religious backlash.[12]

It is also an unfortunate legacy when religions have their genesis through harm being done to others, especially when this is later celebrated. This poses a real dilemma in modern times in relation to myth versus historical fact. An example is the Feast of the Passover,[13] one of the most important events in the Jewish calendar. It celebrates Moses leading the Israelites out of Egypt to find the Promised Land. However, that is not the whole story. The voice of God told Moses to instruct his followers on a particular night to sacrifice a lamb and dab some of its blood on their doorposts and to lock their doors. That night, God went through the land of Egypt killing the first-born child of every family and the first-born of their cattle, but he knew to *pass over* the houses marked with blood, leaving them safe. Out of fear of God's power, Pharaoh then allowed the Jews to leave Egypt. This is not a story of universal love and compassion, but a story identifying a chosen group – an exclusivity which in the minds of some persists to this day.

This illustrates well the incompatibility of myth and historical fact. The arguments are as follows.

- If the story was a myth and the annual Passover celebrations were symbolic of the early growth of a religious group, this is easily accepted by everybody, both Jews and gentiles alike.
- If this was a myth, then probably much more of the Old Testament is mythical, and is historically inaccurate.
- If that is the case, then interpretation of the Torah should be in the spirit of what was written, and not taken as if all of it is literal truth.
- If the stories are accepted as allegories, then members of the group will understand that they are perhaps not 'chosen' above others in God's eyes and can regard all other humans as being of equal value, with equal claims.

A counter-argument is as follows.

- If the story is regarded as historically accurate, the group is superior to others in the eyes of God because he gave them preference and, together with other covenants, promised them a tract of land.

- If this is the case, they deserve special advantages.
- Since God is eternal, their preferential status continues indefinitely.
- Therefore, some people are more equal than others – forever.
- This is a view that is unacceptable to most and incompatible with the United Nations Declaration of Human Rights.

The obvious conflict between these two patterns of reasoning, both of which are internally consistent, demonstrates how those who wish to can generate animosity and demand a twisted loyalty to their cause. It should, however, be made clear that there are elements of the New Testament and the Qur'an that could have been selected to generate the same incompatibilities with human rights. There are, in every religion, literalists and modernists who battle it out over their scriptures. Unfortunately, 'pick 'n' mix' does not improve the logic of a faith; it simply increases the cynicism of non-believers.

So, in summary, throughout history, religions have been put to good and bad uses. There seem to be no indications that this will change in the future. The whole confused landscape will continue to meander along with various groups having hegemony over others at various times – and those without belief looking on at the convoluted machinations. Military activity fought in the name of religious sects is often a sublimation of different earthly objectives. Somehow, in the final analysis of their motivations, no matter how well they started out, temporal leaders tend towards power and immortality rather than altruism and obscurity. On occasions, with weapons and terrorism involved, innocents meet their deaths in an untimely fashion. The support and finance for these activities unfortunately frequently originates from foreign powers with anything but religious conviction. The young left behind are at best turned against the aggressor's nominal faith and at worst respond by returning violence with violence. Before immediately criticizing the latter, one has to ask, if this is their only chance of survival, who can blame them?

Notes

1 Galton F (1872): 'Statistical Inquiries into the Efficacy of Prayer'. *Fortnightly Review*, Vol. 12, 125–135. Reprinted in *International Journal of Epidemiology*, Vol. 41, No. 4 (2012), 923–928. Available at: https://academic.oup.com/ije/article/41/4/923/689380/Statistical-inquiries-into-the-efficacy-of-prayer.

2 Benson H et al. (2006): A Study of the Therapeutic Effects of Intercessionary Prayer (STEP) in Cardiac Bypass Patients: A Multicenter Randomized Trial of Uncertainty and Certainty of Receiving Intercessionary Prayer', *American Heart Journal*, Vol. 151, 934–942.

3 Bull D, de Las Casas L, Wharton R (June 2016): *Faith Matters: Understanding the Size, Income and Focus of Faith-Based Charities*, New Philanthropy Capital Ltd. Available at: www.thinknpc.org/publications/faith-matters/.

4 The Economist (2017): 'In the Eye of the Storm', *The Economist*, 1 April 2017, pp. 28–29.
5 Armstrong K (2015): *Fields of Blood: Religion and the History of Violence*, Vintage, p. 1.
6 White M (2012): *Atrocitology*, Cannongate. The figures given are calculated by the authors from various sections of the text.
7 Kamen H (2014): *The Spanish Inquisition: A Historical Revision*, 4th edn, Yale University Press.
8 *Ibid.*, p. 248.
9 *Ibid.*, p. 253.
10 Charles II (1672): 'An Act for Preventing Dangers which may Happen from Popish Recusants'. In *Statutes of the Realm: Volume 5, 1628 – 80*; pp 782–785. Available at: www.british-history.ac.uk/statutes-realm/vol5/pp782-785.
11 Rushdie S (1988): *The Satanic Verses*, new edn 1998, Vintage.
12 *Guardian* (2012): 'Looking Back at Salman Rushdie's *The Satanic Verses*', *Guardian*, 14 September. Available at: www.theguardian.com/books/2012/sep/14/looking-at-salman-rushdies-satanic-verses.
13 Exodus 12:1–14.

Part II

Managing death in different faiths and doctrines

Apart from Chapters 11 and 12, which are sectioned individually, all these chapters have standard sub-divisions of: 'Description of the religion', 'Care of the dying', 'Management of death', 'Autopsy and organ transplantation' and 'Further reading'.

Chapter 11

An introduction to religions and belief systems

Basic concepts

Religions, belief systems and other spiritualties are notoriously difficult to describe and classify. In order to aid interpretation, this section attempts to set out some significant current groupings.

Records of religion and secular persuasions, intended to determine how to live and to explain the purpose of life and any afterlife, are as old as written history; however, in fact, evidence of thought about life and any afterlife extends further into pre-history.

Archeological evidence from Africa, Australia, Canada, the USA, South America, Japan, Malaysia, Laos and Indonesia dating back over the whole length of human history (1–1.5 million years) indicates that hunter-gatherer religions such as animism, pantheism, shamanism etc. have always existed (see Appendix 11.1). These have formed the foundational nuclei of all subsequent religions and are still demonstrated today in places where the so-called 'indigenous', 'aboriginal', 'hill' or 'desert' peoples are to be found. They evolved into 'modern' theistic beliefs when nomads settled in communities and became gardeners and farmers after the last ice age.[1]

It is unlikely that NHS staff will have to deal with such very early traditions; however, it is important to recognize this long legacy and cultural ancestry for the modern smorgasbord of ideologies. Since written history, the development of beliefs has reflected the life and times of the period. For example, multiple Anglo-Saxon, Greek, Roman and Norse gods have been worshipped, some for fertility, some for rain, some for beauty etc. Also, traditions of medieval European ideas about anti-Christianity and witchcraft may still be expressed in movements such as paganism and New Age ideologies.

What we experience today in a varying pattern across the world is a complex inheritance of ideology, modification, rejection and re-discovery. This brief introduction tries to make sense of how these factors are expressed in the 21st century, and also tries to put perspective on connections across time and geography.

The religions and life systems surviving to the present and seen in the UK have principally evolved from antiquity in China and Japan, the Indian subcontinent and the Middle East. Originally these developed along separate lines until travel (both commercial and military) linked them together. Over time they have migrated across the world, been modified and split into denominations. During the 20th century it is necessary to add 'non-belief' ethical ways of living and what is termed 'New Age spirituality' or 'cosmic humanism'. The latter, whilst not embracing traditional religious thinking, nevertheless recognise a link to the wholeness of things and the natural world.

It is within this categorization that this introduction will continue. The details of each of the religions will be expanded and placed within a paradigm of healthcare and death in the subsequent chapters of Part II of the book.

Chinese and Japanese beliefs

There are three philosophical systems of importance in China and Japan: Shintoism, Taoism and Confucianism. All have been in existence for over 2,500 years and have been major influences in the development of China, Japan and other countries of the Far East. They are best thought of as wise systems of life that have directed societies and linked variously with other religious faiths. They do not necessarily depend upon a single paternal supernatural being who has to be prayed to and who will determine the nature of the afterlife, if any. Their characteristics are summarized in Figure 11.1.

Religions of the Indian subcontinent

These religions are often termed 'Dharmic religions' in textbooks. Dharma has no exact translation in English (and its exact meaning varies in Indian scholarship), but it implies the eternal law of the cosmos, inherent in the very nature of things, together with ideal behaviour including duties, rights, laws, conduct and virtues. Hinduism, the oldest of these religions, is often thought of as the 'parent faith' because of its antiquity and because the other religions probably separated off to rid themselves of what they saw as defects and limitations whilst making other improvements.

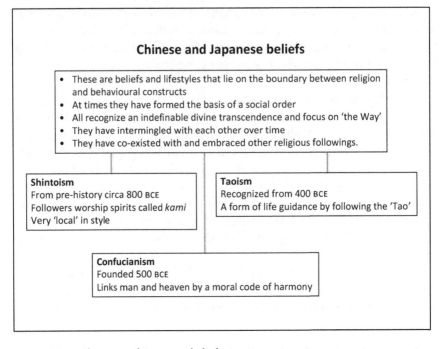

Figure 11.1 Chinese and Japanese beliefs

The characteristic of these faiths is belief in the continuing cycle of life with the present conditions determined by the life that went before. One can move up and down the social ladder with each generation; this provides some logic for position in the caste system as a consequence of prior effort. As such, one's future depends on today's adherence to the rules and performance in life. Their characteristics are summarized in Figure 11.2.

Religions of the Middle East

These can be categorized as Zoroastrianism and the Abrahamic faiths.

Zoroastrianism was historically a very important faith in the area of what is now modern-day Iran that combined belief with lifestyle. It is probably the world's oldest monotheistic religion (opposed by a destructive spirit) and was the official religion of Persia (Iran) from 600 BCE to 650 CE. An outline of the faith is given in Figure 11.3.

The Abrahamic faiths, Judaism, Christianity, Islam and the Baha'i faith all originated in the area that is now Palestine and Israel. All have come into existence as revelations to one or more prophet-like persons. They are set out in Figure 11.4. Judaism, Christianity and Islam are faiths that have tried to convert non-believers, both by peaceful persuasion and (less commonly)

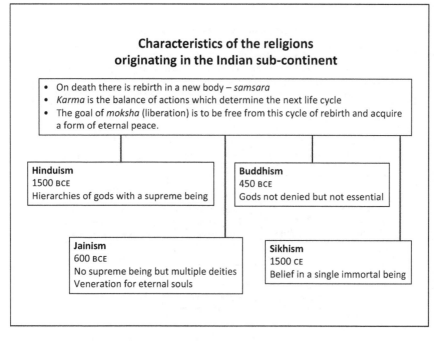

Characteristics of the religions originating in the Indian sub-continent

- On death there is rebirth in a new body – *samsara*
- *Karma* is the balance of actions which determine the next life cycle
- The goal of *moksha* (liberation) is to be free from this cycle of rebirth and acquire a form of eternal peace.

Hinduism
1500 BCE
Hierarchies of gods with a supreme being

Buddhism
450 BCE
Gods not denied but not essential

Jainism
600 BCE
No supreme being but multiple deities
Veneration for eternal souls

Sikhism
1500 CE
Belief in a single immortal being

FIGURE 11.2 Religions originating in the Indian subcontinent

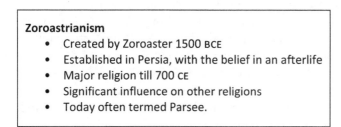

Zoroastrianism
- Created by Zoroaster 1500 BCE
- Established in Persia, with the belief in an afterlife
- Major religion till 700 CE
- Significant influence on other religions
- Today often termed Parsee.

FIGURE 11.3 An outline of Zoroastrianism

by enforcement. When enforcement has occurred, there have been those who have converted (proselytes), and those who have paid lip service to the aggressors but have kept their own beliefs alive. These are usually termed crypto-Christians, crypto-pagans etc.

Secular ethics and new faiths

Atheism and agnosticism have been around for over two millennia, but the numbers of their adherents are increasing in the 21st century. Within

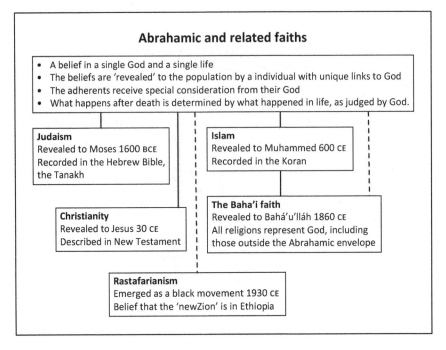

FIGURE 11.4 Abrahamic and related faiths

them are a number of defined life systems based around ethical values and a respect for one's fellow man, e.g., humanism. Both atheists and agnostics may be part of an additional spiritual movement. Many of these interface easily with secular Buddhism. A summary is set out in Figure 11.5.

New Age beliefs seek a unity with mankind and nature and possibly a transcendental life force. To some extent they are a return to a pantheism that tries to make sense of how we interpret the human state and the world around us. A summary is given in Figure 11.5.

Summary

This short section has set out the major faiths and life systems of the present world in a slightly artificial fashion so as to try to systematize and clarify the origins and links between them. Many of those included above will be described individually in the rest of Part II, but it may be useful from time to time to refer to Figures 11.1–11.5 above to see how a particular faith 'fits in' and relates to others. It is important to remember that many religions and belief systems are in a constant state of change and evolution; a good example of this are the Quakers, who grew out of Christianity 400 years ago but whom today also find meaning and value in other faiths and traditions.

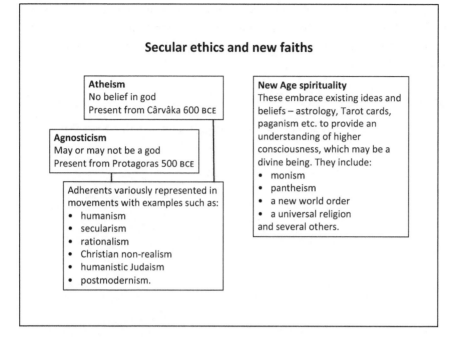

Figure 11.5 Secular ethics and new faiths

Appendix 11.1 Approximate timeline of religions described in this text

Timeline	China and Japan	Indian subcontinent	Middle East	Secular philosophies and other belief systems
Pre-history	Archaeological evidence from Africa, Australia, Canada, the USA, South America, Japan, Malaysia, Laos and Indonesia dating back over the whole length of human history (1–1.5 million years) indicates that hunter-gatherer religions such as animism, pantheism, shamanism etc. have always existed.			
2000–1000 BCE		1500: Hinduism	1750: Judaism 1500: Zoroastrianism	Uncertain origin: Paganism
1000 BCE – 0 CE	800: Shinto 500: Confucianism 550: Taoism	600: Jainism 450: Buddhism		600: Atheism 500: Agnosticism
0–1000 CE			30: Christianity 600: Islam	
1000–2000 CE		1500: Sikhism	1860: Baha'i faith 1920: Rastafarianism	1896: Union of Ethical Societies formed (humanism) 1960: New Age movements

This time chart shows the relative birth periods of the religions covered in Part II of the book. By the nature of the records available, many of the dates given are approximate, but give a relativity to the development of different beliefs.

Note

1 Kellehear A (2007): *A Social History of Dying*, Cambridge University Press.

Chapter 12

The landscape of religions worldwide and in the UK

The distribution of religions across the world

A comprehensive demographic study by the Pew Research Centre's Forum on Religion and Public Life, published in 2012,[1] showed that as in 2010 worldwide, more than eight in ten people identified themselves with a religion. Of the total population of 6.9 billion, 5.8 billion (84%) reported affiliation to one of the religions. Consequently, the study also revealed that a significant proportion (16%) of the world population, approximating 1.1 billion in total numbers, did not identify themselves with any religion.

Based on the numbers alone, five major world religious groups, as estimated in the year 2010, were:

- Christians (2.2 billion; 32% of world population)
- Muslims (1.6 billion; 23%)
- Hindus (1 billion; 15%)
- Buddhists (500 million; 7%)
- Jews (14 million; 0.2%).

In addition, 6% of the total world population (400 million) practised various folk or traditional religions, which included:

- African traditional religions
- Chinese folk religions
- Native American religions
- Australian aboriginal religions.

Less than 1% of the world population (58 million) affiliated themselves with the other religions such as the Baha'i faith, Jainism, Sikhism, Shintoism,

Taoism, Tenrikyo, Wicca, Zoroastrianism and many others. It ought also to be noted that the proportion of world population that remained unaffiliated to any religion formed the third-largest group, following Christians and Muslims. In general, people from religious groups tend to live in the countries where their religious group makes the majority. Only 27% of total world population live as religious minorities.

Various religious groups have different patterns of geographic distribution globally (see Table 12.1). The Christians tend to be more evenly dispersed around the world. The Muslims are concentrated in the Asia-Pacific, Middle East-North Africa and sub-Saharan Africa regions. Many religious groups, including Hindus, Buddhists, the folk religions and other religions, as well as the unaffiliated, are concentrated in the Asia-Pacific region. Jews are concentrated in the Middle East-North Africa region and in North America.

Points of note are as follows,

- Amongst Christians, nearly 50% are Catholics, 37% Protestants, 12% Orthodox and 1% are those who view themselves as other types of Christians, including Christian Scientists, Mormons and Jehovah's Witnesses. Table 12.1 shows that Christianity has spread far from its historical origins (in the Middle East). With the exception of the Asia-Pacific region and the Middle East, Christians now live in various major regions of the world as majority religious groupings. Of the 232 countries and territories studied in 2010, Christians lived as a majority in 157 countries.
- Worldwide, 87% of Muslims are Sunnis and 13% are Shi'as. Muslims live as majority religious groupings in 49 countries, mainly in the Middle East, Asia-Pacific and sub-Saharan Africa regions.
- Less than 1% of Hindus live outside the Asia-Pacific region. They are in the majority in India and Nepal, where they constitute 80% of the population.
- Buddhists, like Hindus, are mainly concentrated in the Asia-Pacific region, the area of their origin and development. Nearly half of the world's Buddhists live in China. The countries where Buddhists live in a majority are Cambodia, Thailand, Burma, Bhutan, Sri-Lanka, Laos and Mongolia.
- Jews are geographically concentrated in North America and the Middle East. They live as a majority religious group in Israel.
- Folk religions include African traditional religions, Chinese folk religions, Native American religions and Australian aboriginal religions. They are concentrated in the Asia-Pacific region, and are less institutionalized than

TABLE **12.1** The percentage distribution of a faith's adherents in the six major regions of the world

	Regions of the world					
	North America	Latin America and Caribbean	Europe	Sub-Saharan Africa	Asia-Pacific	Middle East and North Africa
Global Population	5%	8.6%	10.8%	11.9%	58.8%	4.9%
Religious groups						
Christians	12.3%	24.4%	25.7%	23.8%	13.2%	0.6%
Muslims	0.2%	0.1%	2.7%	15.5%	61.7%	19.8%
Hindus	0.2%	0.1%	0.1%	0.2%	99.3%	0.2%
Buddhists	0.8%	0.1%	0.3%	<0.1%	98.7%	0.1%
Jews	43.6%	3.4%	10.2%	0.7%	1.5%	40.6%
Folk religions	0.3%	2.5%	0.3%	6.6%	90.1%	0.3%
Other religions	3.8%	1.7%	1.6%	3.3%	89.2%	0.4%
Unaffiliated	5.2%	4.0%	12.0%	2.4%	76.2%	0.2%

the other religions. In Taiwan and Vietnam, they are present in a significant proportion (approximately 40% of the population). However, they do not represent a majority group in any of the countries of the world.

- The groups of other religions are also concentrated in the Asia-Pacific region. They do not represent a majority religious group in any of the countries in the world. These are all minority religions such as the Baha'i faith, Jainism, Sikhism, Shintoism, Taoism, Tenrikyo, Wicca, Zoroastrianism and many others.

- The large group of religiously unaffiliated people includes atheists, agnostics and others who do not identify with any religion; some may believe spiritually in the existence of God or a higher power. The vast majority of this group are concentrated in the Asia-Pacific region, followed by Europe. They make a majority group among the population of the Czech Republic, North Korea, China, Estonia, Japan and Hong Kong.

More recent general estimates and future projections

In the year 2015, the population of the world was estimated to be 7.3 billion (compared with 6.9 billion in the year 2010). The relative proportion of different religious groups across the world was as follows.[2]

- Christians: 31.2%
- Muslims: 24.1%
- Hindus: 15.1%
- Buddhists: 6.9%
- Jews: 0.2%
- Folk religions: 5.7%
- Other religions: 0.8%
- Unaffiliated: 16%.

By the year 2060, the world population is expected to increase by 32% to 9.6 billion. In the projections made by the Pew Research Centre, in the coming years, Muslims will see the fastest growth, being the religious group with the relatively youngest population and highest fertility. Their population is projected to increase by 70%. Over the same time period, the number of Christians will grow by 34%. This relative difference in growth rates of the two religions will result in Christians and Muslims being in the same proportion (approximately 30% each) of the world population by the year 2060.

All other religious groups and the unaffiliated have been projected to have a growth rate lower than the world average, with Buddhists having a negative growth. This will result in decreases in their relative proportions of the world population.

TABLE **12.2** The projected percentage growth among different religious groups by 2060

Percent growth by 2060	
Global	+32%
Christians	+34%
Muslims	+70%
Hindus	+27%
Buddhists	−7%
Jews	+15%
Folk religions	+5%
Other religions	0
Unaffiliated	+3%

Demographics of religion in the UK

The distribution of faiths recorded in the 2011 census in England and Wales[3] is set out in Table 12.3.

Scotland reported an even higher proportion of people unaffiliated to any religion (36.7%) and a lower proportion of Muslims (1.4%).

Compared with the previous census conducted in the year 2001, the most notable trend in 2011 for England and Wales was a significant increase in the proportion of population declaring no religion from 14.8% in 2001 to 25.1% in 2011. The proportion of Christians decreased from 71.7% in the year 2001 to 59.3% in 2011. There was an overall modest increase in the proportion of minority religions, the most notable being that of Muslims increasing from 3.0% in 2001 to 4.8% in 2011. Various recent surveys and reports[4] (not census) suggest that the current trend is towards a relative decrease in the proportion of Christians and an increase in the proportion of unaffiliated

TABLE **12.3** Distribution of faiths in England and Wales in 2011

Belief system	Proportion of the population in England and Wales (%)
Christian	59.3
No belief	25
No religion stated	7
Muslim	4.8
Hindu	1.5
Sikh	0.8
Jewish	0.5
Buddhist	0.3
Other	0.3

groups. According to one recent survey in the year 2017,[5] more than half of the population of Britain affiliates to no religion.

Demographics of religion among the health service workforce in the UK

The available statistics on the religious profile of the NHS hospital and community health service workforce in the UK date back to the year 2013.[6] The data are also limited to England. According to the data, among the workforce, 19% were Christians, 6% Muslims, 6% Hindus and 4% other religions. Approximately 7% were atheists and 57% reported no religion or did not choose to disclose any religion.

These data have significant mismatches with those of the general population in Table 12.3, especially in the categories of no or undisclosed religious belief (57% compared with 32%). This reinforces the need for an understanding by health care workers of the belief systems and religions of those whom they look after.

Notes

1 Pew Research Center (2012): *The Global Religious Landscape: A Report on the Size and Distribution of the World's Major Religious Groups as of 2010*, December, www.pewforum.org/2012/12/18/global-religious-landscape-exec/.
2 Pew Research Centre (2017): *The Changing Global Religious Landscape*, April, www.pewforum.org/2017/04/05/the-changing-global-religious-landscape/.
3 Office for National Statistics (2011): *Religion in England and Wales 2011*, www.ons.gov.uk/peoplepopulationandcommunity/culturalidentity/religion/articles/religioninenglandandwales2011/2012-12-11.
4 National Centre for Social Research (2015): *British Social Attitudes: Church of England Decline has Accelerated in Past Decade*, May, www.natcen.ac.uk/news-media/press-releases/2015/may/british-social-attitudes-church-of-england-decline-has-accelerated-in-past-decade/.
5 National Centre for Social Research (2017): *British Social Attitudes: Religious Affiliations 2017*, http://natcen.ac.uk/our-research/research/british-social-attitudes/.
6 Health and Social Care Information Centre (2013): *NHS Hospital and Community Health Service Workforce in Each HEE Region – Provisional Statistics*, October, https://digital.nhs.uk/data-and-information/publications/statistical/nhs-workforce-statistics/nhs-workforce-statistics-july-2017-provisional-statistics.

Chapter 13

The Baha'i faith

Description of the religion

Numbers practising the religion

Baha'i is the youngest of the Abrahamic faiths, with 6 million followers worldwide and 6,000 in the UK. Although subject to discrimination, it remains the largest minority group in Iran.[1]

Origin and beliefs

The Baha'i community emerged from Shi'a Islam in what is now Iran in the 1860s as a faction within Babism (founder: the Bab, 1819–1850).[2] The Baha'is believe there to be one genderless omnipotent God whose power can never be appreciated on a human level. The universe and all creation belong to him. He gives to all human beings a soul that lives forever.[3] Its originator was the Persian Mirza Husayn Ali Nuri (1817 – 1892) who, after a revelation whilst imprisoned, subsequently became known as Baha'ullah (which translates as 'the Glory of God')[4]. Baha'is believe that Bahá'lláh is the most recent prophet of a supreme God[5]. The Baha'i faith is not a branch of Islam (that regards it as apostasy[6]), and has had a missionary component from the end of the 19th century[7].

Baha'is accept the divine nature of the missions of Abraham, Moses, Zoroaster, the Buddha, Jesus and Muhammad. They believe each one was a further stage in the revelation of God.[8] Because of this and its birth in an Islamic culture the Baha'i faith is usually regarded as one of the Abrahamic faiths (see Chapter 11, Figure 11.4). The Baha'i religion is unique in accepting all other faiths as true and valid.[9] Bahá'u'lláh taught that God intervenes throughout human history at different times to reveal more of himself through his messengers and the idea of progressive revelation is of fundamental significance for the Baha'i faith.[10] The Baha'i faith construct is that of a process defined by Divine Will marked by the appearance of prophets: in time more will appear.[11]

Bahá'u'lláh thought that different religions had different ideas of God because they were built out of their own experiences and cultures, i.e., there is a relativity about religion.[12] A central tenet is that of unity across the countries and acceptance of ethnic groups of the world.[13] Individually, Baha'is should live a good and honest life similar to that of the 'virtuous life' of the ancient Greeks and Roman stoics. Baha'is believe that different peoples should work together for the common benefit of humanity with the final objective of creating a peaceful global community. All human beings are different, but equal; there should be no inequality between races or sexes.[14]

Worship and lifestyle

The Baha'i faith has obligatory prayers[15] but virtually no rituals because rituals can overwhelm the importance of prayer and contemplation. The faith has no clergy, sacraments or individuals in a religious hierarchy[16] or leadership positions, and is administered by elected bodies at local, national and international levels. The international headquarters is in Haifa, Israel.[17] The lack of ritual means that major personal events, such as weddings and funerals, can be arranged by Baha'is as they wish. They may incorporate elements of local tradition. This is permissible as long as these traditions do not imply adherence to another religion.

Baha'i services are simple with readings from the scriptures, and prayers recited by an individual on behalf of all who are present. There are only three recognized rituals:[18]

- Obligatory daily prayers. These can be offered personally if unable to attend the temple or house of worship. Prayer is essentially a private duty.
- Reciting the Prayer for the Dead at a funeral.
- The simple marriage rite.

Every year there is a fast of 19 days (from which the sick, elderly and pregnant are exempted) preceding the Baha'i New Year[19] which is celebrated on approximately 21 March.

According to Baha'i teachings the purpose of life in the physical world is to live with spiritual qualities such as love, patience, compassion, justice, wisdom and purity. In the physical world, humans prepare themselves for the next world. After death, the spiritual entity continues to progress and the ultimate aim is to unite with God. Heaven or Hell, according to Baha'is, represents how near or far an entity is from God.

Care of the dying

Standard clinical care is appropriate. Normally Baha'is will accept the usual routines and treatment whilst recognizing the role of the spirit, prayer and communion with God. Palliative care is accepted. They will wish to continue their normal daily religious activities, which include reading from the Baha'i scriptures and daily prayers; for this they will need a quiet room.

Baha'is have freedom with their diet but alcohol and mind-altering drugs are prohibited. Most, in practice, are vegetarian. If a patient is fasting, arrangements need to be made for the provision of food before dawn and after dusk.

When dying there is no requirement for priests, but they like to have their family around them. The approach to death is personal rather than specified by scripture.

Suicide is prohibited, but if it occurs, the person is treated compassionately.

Management of death

Because of the belief in a soul, care of the body requires great respect. Baha'is are usually happy to accept last offices from healthcare staff, but in some countries in the Middle East (or by personal choice), there may be family washing and wrapping of the body in one or more white sheets. Often a burial ring, inscribed, 'I came forth from God, and return unto Him, detached from all save Him, holding fast to His Name, the Merciful, the Compassionate', is placed on the forefinger if aged 15 years or over. The wrapped body is then placed in a coffin.

Simple funerals are held, usually in consultation with the local Baha'i community. The only obligatory part is to recite the Baha'i Prayer for the Dead. Burial is very strongly preferred and cremation and embalming are traditionally forbidden. The body must be buried as soon as is practicable (24 hours preferred) within one hour's journey from the place of death (by any transport, from foot to airplane). The deceased's feet should point to the tomb of Baha'u'llah near Acre (the Quiblih).

Autopsy and organ transplantation

There are no objections to modern medicine, so voluntary autopsy and organ transplantation are personal issues.

Further reading

- Rutty J: 'Baha'i', in *E-Learning for Health*, Royal College of Pathologists, 'Faith Considerations Part 1: Abrahamic Faiths', published on the web by Health Education England NHS (undated), available at; www.e-lfh. org.uk/programmes/medical-examiner/.
- Maceoin D (2010): 'Baha'ism', in *The Penguin Handbook of the World's Living Religions*, ed. Hinnells JR, chapter 16, pp. 621–645.
- BBC (2009): 'Introduction to Baha'I Beliefs and God'. www.bbc.co.uk/ religion/religions/bahai/beliefs/god.shtml
- DK (2013): *The Religions Book*, UK edn, Doling Kindersley, 'We Shall Know Him through His Messengers', pp. 308–309.

Notes

1 Maceoin D (2010): 'Baha'ism', in *The Penguin Handbook of the World's Living Religions*, ed. Hinnells JR, chapter 16, p. 621.
2 *Ibid.*, p. 620.
3 'Introduction to Baha'i Beliefs and God'. www.bbc.co.uk/religion/religions/ bahai/beliefs/god.shtml.
4 Smart N (1998): *The World's Religions*, 2nd edn, chapter 20, 'Islam Passes through the Shadows', p. 497.
5 DK (2013): *The Religions Book*, UK edn, Dorling Kindersley, 'We Shall Know Him through His Messengers', p. 309.
6 Smart N (1999): *Modern Islam in World Philosophies*, Routledge, chapter 12, p. 303.
7 Maceoin D (2010): 'Baha'ism', in *The Penguin Handbook of the World's Living Religions*, ed. Hinnells JR, chapter 160, p. 620.
8 DK (2013): *The Religions Book*, UK edn, Dorling Kindersley, 'We Shall Know Him through His Messengers', p. 309.
9 *Ibid.*
10 Maceoin D (2010): 'Baha'ism', in *The Penguin Handbook of the World's Living Religions*, ed. Hinnells JR, chapter 160, pp. 624–625.
11 Smart N (1998): *The World's Religions*, 2nd edn, chapter 20, 'Islam Passes through the Shadows', p. 498.
12 Smart N (1999): *Modern Islam in World Philosophies*, Routledge, chapter 12, p. 303.
13 DK (2013): *The Religions Book*, UK edn, Dorling Kindersley, 'We Shall Know Him through His Messengers', p. 309.
14 Smart N (1999): *Modern Islam in World Philosophies*, Routledge, chapter 12, p. 303.
15 'Baha'i Prayer'. www.bbc.co.uk/religion/religions/bahai/customs/prayer_1.shtml.
16 Holloway R (2016): *A Little History of Religion*, chapter 37, 'Opening Doors', pp. 219–220.
17 Leith B (2003): *The Baha'i Faith in World Religions*, 2nd edn, ed. Gill D, p. 21.
18 'Baha'i Rituals'. www.bbc.co.uk/religion/religions/bahai/customs/worship.shtml.
19 'Baha'is and Fasting'. www.bbc.co.uk/religion/religions/bahai/customs/fasting. shtml.

Chapter 14

Buddhism

Description of the religion

Numbers practising the religion

Buddhism today has around 500 million followers (8–10% of the world's population), the majority being in East and Southeast Asia. It is also the most popular Eastern philosophy in Western countries, with 150–250,000 Buddhists in the UK,[1] where the number is growing.

Origins and beliefs

Buddha is a title for the one who is 'enlightened' or awakened. Buddhism is based on the teachings of the Buddha (see below). It focuses on personal spiritual development and honest self-analysis and strives for a deep insight into the true nature of life and its purpose,[2] with the ultimate objective of removing suffering in the world.[3] Morality, wisdom and meditation are fundamental,[4] as is *Ahimsa*, the principle of inviolability of life.[5] Buddhism is not a revealed religion with an all-powerful God but is based wholly on empirical human experience; indeed, some consider it not to be a religion in the normal sense.[6] In its purest form there is an acceptance of constant change in all things, with no worship of gods or deities.[7] The objective is to be at inner peace, having removed all desires (which are the basic cause of suffering) from the mind[8] and to follow 'the middle way' between excess and nihilism.[9] The Buddhist universe is distinguished by cyclical change: by the endless process of craving and gratification, the repeated sequence of life and death, and the creation and destruction of matter.[10]

The early centuries of Buddhism were characterized by verbal transmission and there was no attempt made to chronologically describe the

Buddha's life until the *Pali Canon* was written about 500 years after his death.[11] Although this makes accuracy difficult, the message he promulgated is so invariant that the spirit of his core teachings is clear. What follows in this section is a brief account intended to be representative of the sources available.

Tradition has it that Siddhartha Gautama, a Hindu prince, was born in India at a place known as Kapilavastu (just inside the borders of modern Nepal), in 563 BCE, and died in Kusinagara (now in Uttar Pradesh, India) in 483 BCE, lying on his right side between two sal trees, which miraculously bloomed out of season. As a prince, Gautama witnessed pain and suffering in his subjects and at the age of 29 left his home, his wife and his baby son with a view to discovering the ultimate truth that would alleviate man's pain and torment. After travelling around seeking answers, he embraced 'the middle way' between denial and indulgence. Age 35, he meditated alone at Bodh Gaya under the Bodhi Tree. After remembering his former lives he achieved 'enlightenment' and mental peace and put an end to his pain of rebirth. As 'the Enlightened One' or 'the Buddha', he then preached his first sermon and Buddhism as a religion (and philosophy) was born. For the rest of his life he was a nomadic teacher spreading the *Dhamma* (the teaching) and acquiring an ever-increasing following. To help with this spiritual task a *Sangha* or monastic order (including nuns as well as monks), was formed.[12] Buddhism then began to be decentralized and was spread internationally by Buddhist monks, nuns and laypersons.

Buddha's teachings centre on seeing things the way they are, thus overcoming frustrations, imperfections and unpleasantness. During his life he emphasized that each person should think for him/herself on how best to live. As he was dying, Buddha's last words were 'Decay is inherent in all things: be sure to strive with clarity of mind (for nirvana)'. He then passed through several stages of meditation and entered into the final *Nirvana* as he died.[13] His wishes were that there should be no central source of doctrine and authority, but that behaviour should be a personal matter.[14] However, following his death, various councils were held to develop the faith,[15] and at present, in practical terms, different schools have their own authorities. At an international level, to promote cohesion, organizations such as the World Fellowship Of Buddhists[16] (founded in 1950) and the International Buddhist Confederation[17] (founded 2012) have been established.

The Buddha did not deny the existence of gods but for him the goal and reward of enlightenment and final *Nirvana* was not in any way to attain an eternal supernatural state. *Nirvana* is the attainment of a tranquil and perfect mind with the fusion of virtue and wisdom. After death you do not then have the pain of being reborn. *Nirvana*, as originally envisaged, was not a form of Buddhist heaven; it is the complete ending of greed, hatred and ignorance by living a good life.[18] This led the Christian Bishop Bigandet, who was a leading Victorian Buddhist scholar, to declare 'by an inexplicable and a deplorable eccentricity this system [Buddhism] merely promises men as a reward for their moral efforts the bottomless gulf of annihilation'.[19] It is perhaps this lack of dependence on a benevolent supernatural deity and eternal life that has enabled the moral lifestyle of Buddhism to be developed within secular Western philosophies.

Worship and lifestyle

Buddhism was spawned from a primitive Brahmin culture (early Hinduism) and preserves many of its beliefs. It rejected the hierarchical authority of the Brahmin priests[20] and the concept of sacrifice to the gods,[21] disallowed the caste system[22] and was persuaded to elevate the position of women (a radical step in its time).[23] The retained beliefs are as follows.

- We are all subject to reincarnation and pass through many human and non-human lives[24] in preparation and development towards achieving release from the pain of life, the state that Buddhism calls *Nirvana* (see above).
- The process of repeated rebirth (as in Hinduism) is called *samsara*. There can be movement up into more favourable states, or down into lower states. Conventionally there are various 'realms' of rebirth and most descriptions have a wheel with three good rebirths (humans, gods and titans), and three unpleasant rebirths (animals, ghosts and hell).[25] The Buddha saw *samsara* as an eternal grind of deaths and rebirths until the cycle was broken.[26]
- The doctrine of *karma* holds that the circumstances of future births are determined by the goodness of the present life that is ending. Humans have free will and *karma* is determined by moral actions and choices and the events consequent upon them. It can accumulate or diminish throughout life.[27]
- *Dharma* has a variety of meanings, but is essentially a 'natural law' that covers the order and behaviour of natural phenomena (cause and effect) including the idea of a universal moral law. *Dharma* is 'visible' to enlightened beings such as a Buddha. Practically, *Dharma* is active in the law of *karma* when one's deeds are weighed over a lifetime.[28]

The core doctrinal teachings address the issue of suffering. They are described by the Four Noble Truths.[29]

1   Life is suffering.
2   Suffering is caused by ignorance – not realising the way the things really are (i.e., impermanence) and thus craving to either hold on to them or 'fix' them.
3   Suffering can be ended when one is 'enlightened' to the reality of impermanence and craving ceases.
4   There is a path (the Noble Eightfold Path) which leads to the end of suffering.

The Noble Eightfold Path (known as 'the middle way') is as follows:[30]

1   the right belief
2   the right resolve
3   the right speech
4   the right action
5   the right livelihood
6   the right effort
7   the right mindfulness
8   the right meditation.

It is believed that ultimately, following the Noble Eightfold Path will lead to emancipation from rebirth.

The Buddha insisted that he was not a god and asked people not to worship him but to practise his teaching.[31] However, after his death, with the spread of Buddhism and the evolution of thought, an enormous number of Buddhist scriptures have led to many controversies of authority and interpretation. A major split (the Great Schism) occurred in the third century BCE over the rules of monasticism, which eventually created the two major schools of Mahāyāna Buddhism (the great vehicle), and Hīnayāna (the lesser vehicle).[32] Developments since his death have produced significant changes to his original principles, leading to a new 'Buddhology' with an eternal heavenly state.[33] Many Buddhist followings now have venerated images and statues of Buddha to which they pray,[34] and concepts of a pantheon of celestial deities emerged in the Mahāyāna school.[35] The best-known Celestial Buddha is *Amitabha*, who is said to have established a paradise ('the pure land') for anyone who remembers his name at the moment of death.[36] There are clear analogies here with the icons and prophets of other religions, but they are not features of the original Buddha's teachings.

The spread of Buddhism

Buddhism spread steadily from its inception in northern India (see Figures 14.1 and 14.2) through adjoining countries and reached all parts of Asia and the Far East. There it co-existed easily with endogenous philosophies/religions. In the land of its birth it enjoyed mixed fortunes and in the 10th century came under attack from the Muslim Turks in campaigns justified by the ideals of *jihad*. From these it never recovered, despite the reintroduction of religious tolerance by the Moguls in the 16th century.[37] This led to the paradoxical situation, which still pertains, that Buddhism was spread across distant countries whilst it had all but disappeared from the land of its birth.

The growth and spread of Buddhism has produced a confusing variation in the detail of beliefs. Whilst respecting the central tenets of the Buddha's *Dhamma*, the characteristics of present-day Buddhism vary hugely across the world. It is easy to misrepresent and mis-label the diversity that occurs. What follows below is meant to be a balanced description[38] and reference should be made to Figures 14.1 and 14.2.

Mahāyāna (East Asian) Buddhism is characterized by the Bodhisattva ideal,[39] the aim of each person to become a Buddha with the recognition of the original Buddha as a super-human transcendental anima set within an accompanying philosophy. Lay people are very important and the doctrine emphasizes a common search for universal salvation with the possibility of eternal salvation. Mahāyāna Buddhism has subsets such as Zen, Pure Land and Tibetan Buddhism and is dominant in Tibet, China, Taiwan, Japan, Korea, Vietnam and eastern Mongolia.

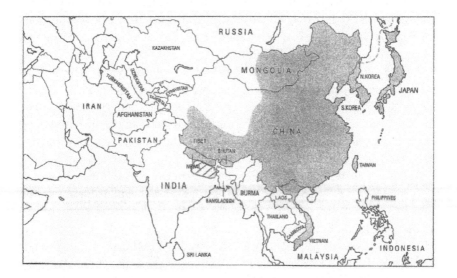

FIGURE 14.1 Mahāyāna Buddhism in Asia. Reproduced under license from Keown D (2013): *Buddhism: A Very Short Introduction*, Oxford University Press, p. XVI. The hatched area shows where the Buddha taught and lived.

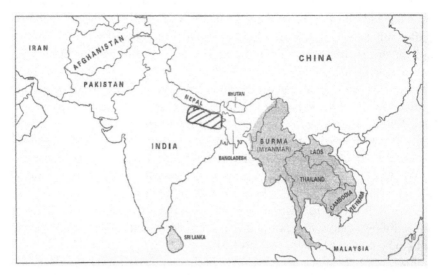

FIGURE 14.2 Theravāda Buddhism in Asia. Reproduced under license from Keown D (2013): *Buddhism: A Very Short Introduction*, Oxford University Press, p. XV. The hatched area shows where the Buddha taught and lived.

Theravāda (Southern) Buddhism follows the Buddha's original teachings, observing the *Pali* Canon. It is a conservative movement promoting meditation that adheres closely to the ethos of the original Buddha and does not offer supernatural solutions. Each person has to make the path to enlightenment by their own efforts to arrive at the non-theistic ideal of self purification in *Nirvana*. It is the dominant religion of Sri Lanka, Myanmar (Burma), Thailand, Laos and Cambodia.

Tibetan (Northern) Buddhism, a sub-set of Mahāyāna is practiced in Tibet, Mongolia, Bhutan, and neighbouring areas and has many complex rituals, symbols and procedures. It represents a small minority of the total number of Buddhists. This form of Buddhism is for many people the western face of Buddhism because of its leader the Dalai Lama who has lived in exile since the Chinese invasion in 1959.

Buddhism in Western Countries. Buddhism came to the west through the academic work of 18th- and 19th-century scholars and from immigration. It had a considerable lift from the work of Christmas Humphreys (1901–1983), an English judge who founded the Buddhist Society in 1924. Buddhism as a philosophy meshes well with ethical liberalism and is not in conflict with developments in science. Against the potential nihilism of quarks, quanta and the ever-increasing entropy of the universe it provides a set of guidelines and allows personal reflection to find a rational matrix within chaos. In the west there are now many schools of Buddhism and the main adherents are middle class white converts. In the 2011 UK census there were nearly a quarter of a million people who declared themselves Buddhists.[40]

Care of the dying

Patients will usually accept normal clinical care with adaptations as below. Buddhism approaches health from a holistic perspective as a harmonious balance of the body, mind, emotion and spirituality. The majority are vegetarian and may be helped by peace and quiet for meditation. Some may embrace alternative therapies which they wish to be continued alongside conventional medical pathways.

It is useful to be aware of the type of Buddhism followed by the patient and their relatives and friends. According to Buddhist tradition, at death the body ceases but the ever-flowing consciousness and its mental accompaniments continue into another body. Thus, death has a special significance to the Buddhist because of the idea of rebirth. Buddhists regard the state of mind in the approach to death as very important because it influences the future rebirth. They may have concerns that disease will increase 'bad Karma' which needs to be countered by right understanding and mindfulness. Because of this they may want details about likely timescales etc., to enable them to prepare and some may refuse sedatives or analgesics. It is thus very important for the dying patient and family to be in a quiet place during this time to enable wholesome thoughts and for past good deeds to be reflected upon. Visits from other Buddhists or a priest or a small shrine placed in the patient's vision may be requested and chanting from texts dealing with the impermanence of life may occur.

There remain divisions of opinion on such subjects as brain death and euthanasia possibly because of *Ahimsa*, the principle of inviolability of life. Attitudes to suicide vary depending on the individual and their school of belief.

Management of death

Last offices by healthcare staff are appropriate. There are no formal Buddhist funeral rites but sometimes the body is left to rest for a few hours before moving it. It is customary for cremation within three to seven days. Any form of service can be used provided it is not Abrahamic or accepting of a single deity. Family and friends usually arrange a form of personal memorial service and the giving of 'alms'. Pregnant women may stay away from a funeral as it may bring bad luck to the baby.

Autopsy and organ transplantation

There is no scriptural objection to autopsy or organ donation, so these are personal matters, but serving others is a component of Buddhism. The exceptions are if a small child dies or if there is a sudden death, because then, the mind would not have been prepared for rebirth.

Further reading

- Rutty J: 'Buddhism', in *E-Learning for Health*, Royal College of Pathologists, 'Faith Considerations Part 2: Dharmic Faiths', published on the web by Health Education England NHS (undated), available at; www.e-lfh.org.uk/programmes/medical-examiner/.
- Keown D (2013): *Buddhism: A Very Short Introduction*, Oxford University Press.
- Eckel MD (2005): *Buddhism: In Eastern Religions*, ed. Coogan MD, Oxford University Press, pp. 110–211
- DK (2013): *The Religions Book*, UK edn, Dorling Kindersley, 'Finding the Middle Way', pp. 132–163.

Notes

1 BBC (2009): 'Buddhism at a Glance'. See: www.bbc.co.uk/religion/religions/buddhism/ataglance/glance.shtml.
2 BBC (2009): 'Buddhism at a Glance'. See: www.bbc.co.uk/religion/religions/buddhism/ataglance/glance.shtml.
3 DK (2013): *The Religions Book*, UK edn, Dorling Kindersley, 'Escape from the Eternal Cycle', pp. 142–143.
4 Keown D (2013): *Buddhism: A Very Short Introduction*, Oxford University Press, chapter 7, pp. 96–111.
5 *Ibid.*, pp. 113–114.
6 *Ibid.*, pp. 3–5.
7 DK (2013): *The Religions Book*, UK edn, Dorling Kindersley, 'The Enlightenment of Buddha', pp. 134–135.
8 *Ibid.*, 'Escape from the Eternal Cycle', pp. 139.
9 DK (2013): *The Religions Book*, UK edn, Dorling Kindersley, 'The Enlightenment of Buddha', pp. 133.
10 Keown D (2013): *Buddhism: A Very Short Introduction*, Oxford University Press, p. 56; and BBC (2009): 'The Buddhist Universe'. See: www.bbc.co.uk/religion/religions/buddhism/beliefs/universe_1.shtml.
11 Keown D (2013): *Buddhism: A Very Short Introduction*, Oxford University Press, pp. 18–19.

12 The above paragraph is based on Keown D (2013): *Buddhism: A Very Short Introduction*, Oxford University Press, 'The Buddha', pp. 17–31; and Goonewardene AD (1996): 'Buddhism: The Life of Gotama Buddha', in *Six World Faiths*, ed. Cole WO, Cassell, pp. 111–122.

13 Keown D (2013): *Buddhism: A Very Short Introduction*, Oxford, pp. 30–31.

14 *Ibid.*, p. 30.

15 Goonewardene AD (1996): 'Buddhism: History and Development', in *Six World Faiths*, ed. Cole WO, Cassell.

16 See: http://wfbhq.org.

17 www.ibcworld.org.

18 Cousins LS (2010): 'Buddhism', in *The Penguin Handbook of the World's Living Religions*, ed. Hinnells JR, Penguin, chapter 8, pp. 402–403; and Keown D (2013): *Buddhism: A Very Short Introduction*, Oxford, pp. 48–50 and 56–57.

19 Macdonald F (1911): 'Buddha and Buddhism' in *Religious Systems of the World*, eds Sheowring W and Conrad WT, Allen and Unwin, pp. 156.

20 Smart N (1998): 'South Asia' in *The World's Religions*, 2nd end, Cambridge University Press, chapter 2, pp. 57–68.

21 Keown D (2013): *Buddhism: A Very Short Introduction*, Oxford University Press, pp. 113–114.

22 Batchelor S (1997): *Buddhism in World Religions*, ed. Gill D, Collins, p. 25.

23 Goonewardene AD (1996): 'Buddhism: The Life of Gotama Buddha', in *Six World Faiths*, ed. Cole WO, Cassell; and Murcott S (1991): *The First Buddhist Women: Translations and Commentary on the Therigatha*, Parallax Press, p. 4.

24 Keown D (2013): *Buddhism: A Very Short Introduction*, Oxford University Press, p. 32.

25 *Ibid.*, pp. 34–35.

26 Eckel MD (2005): *Buddhism in Eastern Religions*, ed. Coogan MD, Duncan Baird Publishers, pp. 194–195.

27 Keown D (2013): *Buddhism: A Very Short Introduction*, Oxford University Press, chapter 3, 'Karma and Rebirth', pp. 32–47; and Cousins LS (2010): 'Buddhism', in *The Penguin Handbook of the World's Living Religions*, ed. Hinnells JR, Penguin, chapter 8, p. 398.

28 Keown D (2013): *Buddhism: A Very Short Introduction*, Oxford University Press, pp. 112–113; and Cousins LS (2010): 'Buddhism', in *The Penguin Handbook of the World's Living Religions*, ed. Hinnells JR, Penguin, chapter 8, p. 379.

29 Keown D (2013): *Buddhism: A Very Short Introduction*, Oxford University Press, chapter 4, 'The Four Noble Truths', pp. 48–60.

30 DK (2013): *The Religions Book*, UK edn, Dorling Kindersley, 'Escape from the Eternal Cycle', pp. 140–141; and Keown D (2013): *Buddhism: A Very Short Introduction*, Oxford University Press, pp. 58–60.

31 Goonewardene AD (1996): 'Buddhism: The Life of Gotama Buddha', in *Six World Faiths*, ed. Cole WO, Cassell, p. 120.

32 Keown D (2013): *Buddhism: A Very Short Introduction*, Oxford University Press, p. 61; and Eckel MD (2005): *Buddhism in Eastern Religions*, ed. Coogan MD, Duncan Baird Publishers, pp. 122.

33 Keown D (2013): *Buddhism: A Very Short Introduction*, Oxford University Press, pp. 62–64.

34 DK (2013): *The Religions Book*, UK edn, Dorling Kindersley, 'Buddhas and Bodhisattvas', p. 154; and BBC (2006): 'Buddhist Worship'. See: www.bbc.co.uk/religion/religions/buddhism/customs/worship_1.shtml.

35 Eckel MD (2005): *Buddhism in Eastern Religions*, ed. Coogan MD, Duncan Baird Publishers, p. 135.

36 *Ibid.*, p. 137.
37 Keown D (2013): *Buddhism: A Very Short Introduction*, Oxford University Press, pp. 77–78.
38 This is a very abbreviated meld of information in Keown D (2013): *Buddhism: A Very Short Introduction*, Oxford University Press, chapter 6; Batchelor S (1997): *The Spread of Buddhism in World Religions*, ed. Gill D, Collins, pp. 31–36; and Cousins LS (2010): 'Buddhism', in *The Penguin Handbook of the World's Living Religions*, ed. Hinnells JR, Penguin, chapter 8, pp. 391–440 – but the responsibility of what is written falls to the present authors.
39 A Bodhisattva is someone who takes a vow to work tirelessly over many lifetimes to lead others to *Nirvana*. They have six perfections: generosity, morality, patience, courage, meditation and wisdom.
40 Hard data on UK Buddhism are hard to find, but those interested may wish to consult: www.thebuddhistsociety.org. See also Chapter 12 of this book.

Chapter 15

Chinese religions

Description of the religions/philosophies

Introduction and numbers practising

Religions and life philosophies have played an important role in Chinese society for thousands of years and their influence has spread to neighbouring countries such as Korea, Vietnam and Japan. The system is difficult to classify from a Western perspective because it does not express the same clear demarcations between different faiths and is an integral part of community life. The term for religion in China is *tsung-chiao*, which literally means a lineage of teachings. Many of the Chinese embrace three intertwined philosophies:

- Confucianism for the ethics of public life
- Taoism for rituals and attitudes towards nature
- Buddhism for salvation and the afterlife.[1]

All have had enormous influences on the Chinese throughout history.

Taoism, Confucianism and Buddhism have peacefully co-existed for centuries with each borrowing and incorporating ideas from the others.[2] As an example, the term Neo-Confucianism[3,4] describes a mixture of thought from both Buddhist and Taoist elements assimilated into Confucianism that was established around 1000 CE.

In the modern context, Chinese religion is festive, defined by the stages of life, i.e., birth, maturation, marriage and death and the annual cycle of festivals.[5] The establishment of the Republic of China (1912) and the Cultural Revolution (1966) greatly diminished the importance of Confucianism[6] but it is now having a renaissance.[7] At present, as a Communist country, China has no official religion but the government does formally recognize five religions. These are Buddhism, Taoism,[8] Islam, Catholicism and Protestantism. In addition to these there is an increase in secular (often called lay) movements.

Because of the inseparable and variable nature of these religions/ philosophies and the lack of any census data, it is impossible to give accurate numbers of adherents but they will number in the hundreds of millions, if not billions. There is also increasing interest among Western countries in the Chinese approach to life and its problems.[9]

In this chapter we will consider Taoism and Confucianism together since they are so intimately linked. Buddhism (which is also frequently imported into a mixed belief paradigm), Christianity, Islam, and secular movements are described in Chapters 14, 16, 18 and 22, respectively.

Confucianism

In ancient China, polytheism was common and there were ceremonies to pray to the gods for good fortune. In parallel were a plurality of evil demons who needed to be scared off with fireworks. Religion was really about getting things achieved and maintaining a balance in nature. On earth there were frequent rivalries between competing warlords.[10] Into this confusion, in 551 BCE was born a man named Kong Fuzi, whose Latinized name is Confucius. He was well educated, occupied several civil administrative posts and around the age of 30 years became a full-time teacher and thinker, later becoming a nomadic sage.

He saw Heaven as the source of moral order and that instead of violence, war and chaos, people should seek to work constructively with others and develop sincerity, diligence, kindness and seriousness within a spirit of humaneness called 'Ren'.[11] He wanted politicians and leaders to focus on the well-being of their peoples, not on individual ambition.[12] All persons should practice patience, compassion, courtesy and seek an understanding of the complexities of the human condition. Although he wrote little, his philosophy of life was set down after his death by his followers in five major texts, later expanded to seven with the addition of the two well-known texts the *Analects* and the *Classic of Filial Piety*. Confucius emphasized the importance of ancestor respect and the five constant relationships: sovereign-subject; father-son; husband-wife; brother-brother; and friend-friend.[13]

When he died in 479 BCE, it appears that little had changed in the government but his legacy of teachings on how the individual should live continued. Following Confucius, Mencius (300 BCE) and Xun Zi (250 BCE) developed the philosophy.[14] Later, under the Emperor Han Wudi, who ruled from 141 to 87 BCE, Confucianism was institutionalized. Wudi established the Imperial Academy to promote Confucian philosophy and it remained the dominant philosophy of China for nearly 2,000 years until the imperial system was overthrown in 1912 CE.[15]

Confucius' views on familial bonds did not stop at death. The dead are mourned intensely, sometimes for years, and there are family rites to commemorate them. The dead do not cease to exist; they retain a continuing presence in our lives. Ancestor tablets, kept in shrines in the family home, maintain the veneration over generations. Ideas about the exact nature of any soul in the ancestor tablets are vague and there is supposed fluidity between the living and the dead. Beliefs about death vary depending upon the school of Confucian thought followed.[16]

Taoism

The foundation of Taoism is attributed to LaoTse (born circa 600 BCE, died 524 BCE), who produced *The Book of the Way*. It is a philosophy that recognizes the unity and interdependency of everything from the concept of the universe down to the detailed phenomena of nature. Overseeing this whole cosmology is the Tao, an incomprehensible metaphysical essence. Individuals attain peace when they align their lifestyle to be in harmony with the natural world. The ultimate objective is to acquire serenity and subsequently immortality.[17] Over time, depending on geography, Taoism has absorbed many folk beliefs, along with aspects of Shintoism, Buddhism and Confucianism.[18] In regard to spirits, fortune-telling and geomancy, a form that has become popular in the Western world is feng shui.[19]

LaoTse introduced the concept of *yin and yang* (which was also recognized in some schools of Confucianism), with its well-known *taijitu* graphic (Figure 15.1). The symbol shows a balance between two opposites with a portion of the opposite element in each section. Yin and yang can be thought of as complementary (rather than opposing) forces that interact and mutually contain elements of each other to form a dynamic system in which the whole is greater than the assembled parts.[20] For instance, there is no shadow without light; all men have a female component; the friend in the enemy etc. Hence insight and tolerance are virtues.[21]

LaoTse differed significantly in his analysis of social systems. Whereas Confucius taught compliance to a set of rules, LaoTse thought that humans lose balance when they feel compelled to control others. The reality does not meet their psychological need and they are in a constant state of irritation. He advised that they should relax and follow nature: just go with the flow. LaoTse's approach was described by *wu-wei*: doing by not-doing: letting things be, letting things happen. Individuals should have as much freedom as possible to live the best life without constraint.[22] Taoism applied these values to women as well as men, with women priests and scholars.[23]

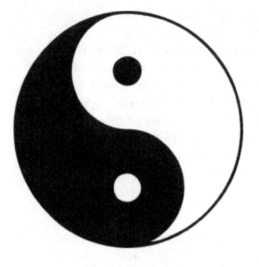

FIGURE **15.1** The *taijitu* symbol of yin and yang: yin is associated with darkness, water and the female, yang with light, activity, air and the male.

On death, the vital force of life, called *Qi*, is lost. Taoists have a firm belief in the afterlife and an assembly of male and female gods led by the Tao and the Celestial Worthies who were created when the universe came into existence. Humans themselves could become 'Immortals' through meditation and alignment with 'The Way'. Priests help to transform the dead into benevolent ancestors: immortals enjoy deathlessness and release from the constraints of human existence. Although there are a variety of interpretations of death, the commonest is that there are two souls, the *hun* and the *po*. The *hun* soul is made of *yang qi*, which will reside in ancestral tablets, and the *po soul* made of *yin qi* will settle peacefully into the grave. If the souls are not satisfactorily settled they can descend into the underworld, or hell, that has a structure similar to a Chinese bureaucracy.[24]

Care of the dying

There is a wide range of approaches to illness and death in the Chinese depending on social background, education, family values etc. This can range from a typical Western approach through to very traditional beliefs. Where a patient and their relatives are on this spectrum needs to be established. The Chinese can also be subject to superstitions such as 'good' and 'bad' bed numbers and other non-medical influences. Jade is often worn as a good-luck charm. Flowers of all colours are used for funerals and if brought as a present may be interpreted as a bad omen.

Traditionally, in terms of belief, to maintain health, humans have to conform to the natural rhythms of the universe. Life is venerated and respected. Harmony between yin and yang, the free flow of chi (breath of life) and balance among the five elements (metal, wood, water, fire and earth) are important in understanding the traditional Chinese concepts of health and illness. Disharmony between these components (deficiency or excess of chi, emotional excesses, mismatches of yin, yang and the five elements) disturbs the nourishing cycle from being in phase with nature and results in disease. Death can be interpreted as a complete separation of the yin and the yang. Both Taoism and Confucianism understand death and dying as a flow of life back to its origin, from being to non-being. Humans can make a choice to die well rather than make a non-virtuous effort to preserve life. The withdrawal of life support is a difficult and controversial issue so needs sensitive management. Chinese patients often prefer to die at home, where they have a sense of safety and belonging.

Common aspects of traditional Chinese medicine include acupuncture, herbal practice, nutrition therapy, cupping, meditation and exercise. There may be daily devotion to mind-body exercises, even in old age and with physical disability. These need to be accommodated within a hospital setting.

For both religions routine clinical care allowing access to family, priests and holy men is appropriate. The presence of the family at the bedside is an understood duty and the dying or dead person will be venerated by the younger members of the family.

Suicide is a tragedy but not in itself sinful.

Management of death

Confucianism

Funeral and mourning customs differ from family to family, so it is important to enquire in each individual case. Traditionally the family cry out at death to inform others and may begin mourning by wearing clothes of rough material.

The body is washed by healthcare staff or the funeral directors and traditionally put in a coffin usually with food and personal objects of the deceased, e.g., lucky charms. Doing this is important to the families and incense and gifts may be brought by the mourners. A Buddhist, Taoist or even Christian priest may perform the burial service. Friends and family follow the coffin to the burial site with a willow branch symbolizing the soul of the dead person. The willow branch is taken back to the family altar where it is used to install the soul of the deceased. Liturgies are performed on the seventh, ninth and forty-ninth days following the burial and on the first and third annual anniversaries of death.

Some of the deceased are buried, others cremated.

Taoism

After death, the relatives will clean the body using incense, so often there is not much role for healthcare staff. Some are embalmed. To represent purification and protection from influences after death, paper money or other talismans may be put on the body. A deceased child would be dressed in new clothes.

Ritualistic funeral rites and a priest provide support for the family determining the right time and place for burial, although nowadays many relatives prefer cremation. A traditional belief is that the deceased only realizes that death has occurred on the seventh day. The funeral is led by a Taoist priest and special hell notes, paper houses and other goods may be burnt to allow the soul to pray for escape from hell. Traditionally, after ten years the bones are exhumed, cleaned and buried in a place chosen by a feng shui expert.

Autopsy and organ transplantation

Confucianism

There is no prohibition, although traditionalists may be suspicious or unhappy with desecration of the body.

Taoism

Traditionalists are superstitious about autopsy. They believe it is critical to appease the evil spirits and ghosts who are everywhere. Because the heart is central to all aspects of life, examination of this may be refused. Other organs are less important. Although it is an individual decision, many adherents will permit organ donation, usually excluding the heart.

Further reading

- Rutty J: 'Confucianism and Taoism in Far Eastern Faiths', in *E-Learning for Health*, Royal College of Pathologists, 'Faith Considerations Part 3: Far Eastern Faiths', published on the web by Health Education England NHS (undated), available at: www.e-lfh.org.uk/programmes/medical-examiner/.
- Saso M (2010): 'Chinese Religions', in *The Penguin Handbook of the World's Living Religions*, ed. Hinnells JR, chapter 9, pp. 447–480.

- DK (2013): *The Religions Book*, UK edn, Dorling Kindersley, 'Accept the Way of the Universe', pp 66–67.
- DK (2013): *The Religions Book*, UK edn, Dorling Kindersley, 'Virtue is Not Sent from Heaven', pp. 74–77.

Notes

1 Saso M (2010): 'Chinese Religions', in *The Penguin Handbook of the World's Living Religions*, ed. Hinnells JR, chapter 9, p. 447.
2 Smart N (1998): *The World's Religions*, 2nd edn, Cambridge University Press, chapter 3, 'China', pp. 106–107.
3 *Ibid.*, pp. 106–107.
4 Oldstone-Moore J (2005): 'Confucianism', in *Eastern Religions*, ed. Coogan MD, Duncan Baird Publishers, p. 238.
5 Saso M (2010): 'Chinese Religions', in *The Penguin Handbook of the World's Living Religions*, ed. Hinnells JR, chapter 9, p. 447.
6 Smart N (1998): *The World's Religions*, 2nd edn, Cambridge University Press, chapter 3, 'China', pp. 106–107.
7 DK (2013): *The Religions Book*, UK edn, Dorling Kindersley, 'Virtue is Not Sent from Heaven', p. 77.
8 Taoism is used interchangeably with Daoism.
9 Bell DA, Chaibong H (eds) (2003): *Confucianism for the Modern World*, Cambridge University Press.
10 Smart N (1998): *The World's Religions*, 2nd edn, Cambridge University Press, chapter 3, 'China', pp. 112–113.
11 DK (2013): *The Religions Book*, UK edn, Dorling Kindersley, 'Virtue is Not Sent from Heaven', p. 74.
12 *Ibid.*, p. 75.
13 *Ibid.*, p. 76.
14 Oldstone-Moore J (2005): 'Confucianism', in *Eastern Religions*, ed. Coogan MD, Duncan Baird Publishers, p. 324.
15 Smart N (1999): *Chinese Philosophies in World Philosophies*, Routledge, p. 74.
16 Oldstone-Moore J (2005): 'Death and the Afterlife in Confucianism', in *Eastern Religions*, ed. Coogan MD, Duncan Baird Publishers, pp. 396–405.
17 DK (2013): *The Religions Book*, UK edn, Dorling Kindersley, 'Accept the Way of the Universe', p. 66–67. 7
18 Saso M (2010): 'Chinese Religions', in *The Penguin Handbook of the World's Living Religions*, ed. Hinnells JR, chapter 9, pp. 449–450.
19 Oldstone-Moore J (2005): 'Sacred Space in Taoism', in *Eastern Religions*, ed. Coogan MD, Duncan Baird Publishers, p. 275..
20 Saso M (2010): 'Chinese Religions', in *The Penguin Handbook of the World's Living Religions*, ed. Hinnells JR, chapter 9, pp. 452, 455; and Smart N (1999): *Chinese Philosophies in World Philosophies*, Routledge, p. 69.
21 Holloway R (2016): 'The Way to Go', *A Little History of Religion*, Yale University Press, chapter 15, pp. 84–85.
22 *Ibid.*, p. 85.
23 *Ibid.*, p. 86.
24 Oldstone-Moore J (2005): 'Death and the Afterlife in Taoism', in *Eastern Religions*, ed. Coogan MD, Duncan Baird Publishers, pp 294–303.

Chapter 16

Christianity

Description of the religion

Numbers practising the religion

Christianity represents the world's largest religious grouping at over 2 billion followers (approximately 30% of the world's population). From inception its importance in society has ebbed and flowed. On several occasions Christianity's success has been helped by alliances with earthly political powers, with mutual benefits to each.[1] In the 21st century, with the march of Western secularism and the revival and growth of Christianity in Latin America, Africa and parts of Asia, Christianity has shifted its majority numbers and its centre of growth southwards,[2] away from Europe and North America.

Origin and beliefs

The faith is based on a belief in the teaching of Jesus, the Messiah, who lived in the Holy Land 2,000 years ago. Jesus was born as a Jew to Jewish parents. Traditional teaching says that his mother Mary became pregnant by the direct intervention of God without any contribution from his earthly father Joseph.[3] At 30 years old he was baptised as a Jew by John the Baptist and on emergence from the river Jordan heard God calling him his 'beloved son':[4] his mission had started. John also proclaimed him as the long-awaited Messiah of the Jews, who would lead them from persecution and oppression.[5] 'Christos' is the Greek word for Messiah, or 'the anointed one' – hence the common translation as 'Christ'. Jesus differs from all other prophets, soothsayers and oracles in that he claimed he was Jesus the God-man,[6] i.e., that he was actually the progeny of God, the exact nature of his essence being a source of much theological division.

Yet Jesus escapes definite descriptions. He spoke in riddles, metaphors and parables, laid down few clear rules, created no institution, had no contemporaneous scribes,[7] and there are no contemporary accounts of his life.[8] We are left with compound exegeses and the expositions of hermeneutics around the central themes of love, an all-embracing God and promises of an everlasting life. His life and ministry comprise the New Testament.

Jesus became a preacher and healer who offered eternal salvation and the pardoning of sin to all who repented, whilst criticizing existing religious practices. His powerful message was perceived as a threat to both the Roman and religious (Jewish) authorities. He was arrested and tried, and Pontius Pilate, the Roman Governor, sentenced him to death by crucifixion. Some interpreters see his death as part of God's master plan; others don't.

It was after the death of Jesus that the unique beliefs of Christianity were established. After being taken down from the cross his body was placed in a tomb and a heavy stone rolled into position to block the entrance. The next day, just after sunrise, three women (Mary Magdalene, Joanna and Mary the mother of James) came to anoint Jesus' body. They found the stone rolled away and the tomb empty apart from the grave-clothes. Then (depending on the Gospel version), in the tomb, either one[9] or two angels,[10] or one[11] or two[12] young men, said that Jesus had risen from the dead. Afterwards, for a period of 40 days, he made various appearances to the apostles,[13,14] including making plans to see them at a specified time in Galilee – an appointment that he kept. Hence, he had cheated death – there really was life everlasting. In Christianity, Good Friday remembers Jesus' crucifixion, and Easter Sunday his resurrection from the dead.

Jesus' message to his apostles after resurrection was that they should stay together until his final return when, effectively, he would lead a new world order as prescribed by God. The apostles waited for his return, but he never came, and still hasn't. Had it been left to the apostles, Christianity may simply have withered as another minor Jewish sect. However, because Jesus had appeared to a Roman called Saul (who was not one of the original apostles) in a vision on the road to Damascus, the whole situation changed. Saul, who was now Paul, castigated the existing apostles and commenced on what was to prove a very successful missionary programme. His zeal and enthusiasm caused the others to follow his lead and Christianity, with its message of universal forgiveness and eternal life, spread across the Roman world.[15]

Christianity then progressed, sometimes covertly and unwanted by the Romans, as a sub-set of Judaism. Christianity's first big break came with Emperor Constantine, who legitimized Christianity in 313 CE and in 380 CE Emperor Theodosius made Christianity the official religion of the Roman Empire. For the first but not the last time, Christianity was linked with a secular government.[16] Under the leadership of Prelates (like bishops), the religious Sees of Rome, Constantinople, Alexandria, Antioch and Jerusalem were established, of which the first two were the most important. Christianity's evolution to its present state over 2,000 years is summarized in Figure 16.1.

In an effort to unify and clarify the diverging faith groups the Romans pressed for a fundamental statement of dogma to be drawn up, called the Nicene Creed, but their well-intentioned efforts ultimately backfired. Over the next 600 years the religion developed and spread with geographical and doctrinal differences developing. The biggest rift was between the Sees of Rome and Constantinople. Rome saw itself as the senior See; Constantinople saw Rome's position as only honorary, without doctrinal authority.

It should be noted that Figure 16.1 is only a summary diagram. Other churches, such as the Armenian, broke from mainline doctrine after the Council of Chalcedon in 451 CE.[17]

The Christian doctrine of the Trinity teaches the significance of the Father, Son and Holy Spirit as three facets of one God. Problems came to a head when the so-called 'filoque clause' (meaning 'the son') was introduced into

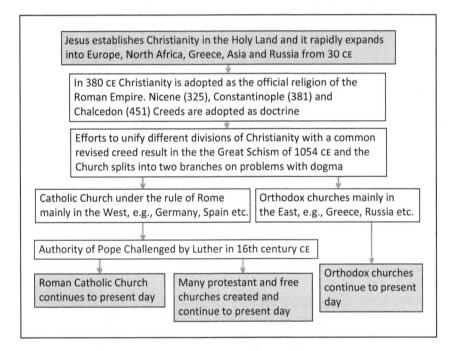

FIGURE **16.1** An outline of the history of the Christian faith

the Nicene Creed and adopted by the See of Rome in 1014 CE.[18] Originally, as crafted in 381 CE, the Creed states:

> We believe in the Holy Spirit, the Lord and Giver of Life, *who proceeds from the Father*, who with the Father and Son together is worshipped and glorified. . .

The *filoque clause* is a small but (apparently) fundamental addition made in 1014 CE to make it read:

> We believe in the Holy Spirit, the Lord and Giver of Life, *who proceeds from the Father and the Son*, who with the Father and Son together is worshipped and glorified. . .

There were other differences with things such as the types of bread for communion and the forms of service, but the *filoque clause* was the deal-breaker. In 1054, the Bishops of Rome and Constantinople mutually excommunicated each other[19] and the Church split along doctrinal, theological, linguistic, political and geographic lines. The addition of three words had become the reason, or excuse, to fracture the Christian world dogmatically and geographically.

As shown in Figure 16.1, the orthodox faiths continue today, but the Roman Catholic Church suffered another major split in the 16th century. In 1521, Martin Luther challenged papal authority, the purchasing of forgiveness through indulgencies, the lack of vernacular texts and the interposing of a priest between man and God. In summary, the victory was Luther's, academically, doctrinally and practically. His activities spawned the Protestant and Non-Conformist faiths. Because there was no clear single alternative being offered to Roman Catholicism, the new churches had no common doctrine and many different denominations emerged. Academically these are now described in three divisions.[20]

- Church Christianity – worship centred around a church subject to its interpretation of the scriptures with buildings and rituals.
- Biblical Christianity – the scriptures, direct to God, form the basis of prayer and faith rather than going through a priestly mediator.
- Monastic or mystical Christianity – this locates Christianity in the spiritual experience of the individual.

In observance, there are many overlaps in these divisions of understanding, interpretation and practice.

Over the intervening years the fortunes of different sections of Christianity have waxed and waned and today's still-moving canvas is the legacy of all these events. The picture varies across the globe. The major sub-divisions are described below in a proportionate manner relevant to medical care in the UK. It is not possible to cover all the individual variations.[21]

Christian denominations today: worship and lifestyle

The Roman Catholic Church

The Roman Catholic Church with over 1 billion members is the largest Christian community. It has the Pope as the head of a hierarchy of bishops and priests and is administered from Vatican City (an independent state), in Rome.

Literally for some, symbolically for others, the Pope is the true apostolic successor to Saint Peter, who was the first Bishop of Rome. The Church has seven defined sacraments to formalize the characteristics of its faith: Baptism, Eucharist, Confirmation, Reconciliation, Anointing of the Sick, Marriage and Holy Orders. The confession of sins, accompanied by genuine regret, sometimes punished with a penance, is a fundamental part of the faith.

Catholics believe that life on earth is the first chapter of eternal existence. From the moment of conception, through birth until death, a person prepares for eternal life. After death God invites followers into His life in Heaven. Purgatory is an intermediate state after physical death in which some of those ultimately destined for Heaven must further prepare themselves to achieve the necessary qualities. To die with mortal sin without repentance and rejecting God can lead to eternal Hell.

Protestant (Anglican) Churches

There are many protestant faiths, but in the UK 'Protestant' is generally used to mean 'Anglican'. This is a worldwide association of churches and the third-largest Christian communion in the world, having 85 million members related to the Church of England, with the Archbishop of Canterbury as its head. Although he is symbolically recognized across the world, unlike the Pope he has no formal authority or jurisdiction throughout the Communion.

Anglicans share many Catholic doctrines, but they reject the power of the Pope. Their practices and liturgy evolved into the Church of England following the Protestant Reformation of the 16th century and the fusion of Church and State by Elizabeth I in 1559. There are many churches within the Anglican Communion, such as the Church of Ireland, the Scottish Episcopal Church, the American Episcopal Church, with others in Africa, Australasia and the Asia-Pacific region, each with their own variations on doctrine and liturgy. Some of this geographical spread reflects past British colonialism.

Anglicans believe that everyone baptised will share in Christ's resurrection and eternal life after death through a soul that transcends to the afterlife.

Orthodox Churches

Eastern Orthodoxy, or officially the Orthodox Catholic Church, is the second-largest association of Christian Churches, with over 250 million members worldwide. The Church has no formal central doctrinal or governance authority, but the Patriarch of Constantinople is recognized as the senior bishop and the Church of Constantinople (since the Great Schism of 1054) has an accepted precedence. The Orthodox Churches share with the other Christian churches the belief that God revealed himself in Jesus Christ and in his resurrection, but differ substantially in the way of life and worship, and in certain aspects of theology.

They practice the original Christian Faith as set out in the original Nicene Creed. They believe that their faith is passed down through a sacred tradition from one generation to the next and that its bishops are analogous to Christ's apostles. Fasting as a preparation for prayer can be important. The majority of Orthodox Christians live in Eastern Europe, Greece, the Caucasus and Russia. All are areas in which the Church also has an important social role.

There are Orthodox churches of varying denominations across the UK, but compared with Roman Catholics and Anglicans, the numbers of Orthodox Christians in the UK is small.

Modern Christian movements (Pentecostal, Liberal, Evangelical and Charismatic Christianity)

These are worldwide Protestant movements that believe in eternal salvation through faith in Jesus and his atonement. Most believe in conversion or the 'born-again' experience.

The USA has the largest concentration of evangelicals in the world, who represent 25% of the nation's population, based principally in the 'Bible Belt' states. In the UK, modern Christian movements are represented mainly by the evangelical Anglicans, and in the Methodist and Baptist communities. Developing countries have especially embraced this style, where modern Christian movements are the fastest-growing aspect of Christianity.

Non-conformist or Free churches

A 'Free' or 'non-conformist' Christian church or faith does not conform to, or see itself as part of, the bigger established faiths with their centralized dogmas and traditions. Neither are they linked to state control. The Church of Scotland, which is Protestant and Presbyterian, has an unusual position in that it remains the national church, but it has complete independence in spiritual questions and appointments. It does not recognize the authority of the Archbishop of Canterbury.

The majority of members regard themselves as Protestants. Examples of Free churches include:

- Methodist
- Baptist
- The Salvation Army
- Quaker (Religious Society of Friends)
- Seventh-Day Adventist
- Pentecostal
- Plymouth Brethren
- The United Reform Church
- The 'Afro-Caribbean Community', in the main involving Anglican, Methodist and Pentecostal churches
- The Free Church of Scotland (the 'Wee Frees').

They each have their Christian principles and practices that often place less emphasis on the administration of sacraments. Such is their variability that attitudes towards death need to be explored individually with the patient and relatives to prevent confusion.

The Church of Jesus Christ of Latter-Day Saints (Mormon Church)

The Mormon Church was founded in 1830 by the self-declared prophet Joseph Smith. The Book of Mormon is understood as a holy scripture comparable to the Bible. There are over 11 million members worldwide today. Mormons embrace the idea that they have reinstated the Church as created by Christ where other Christian churches have deviated.

Mormons believe that there are three stages to life:

- pre-existence as a spirit child (prenatal)
- probation on earth
- eternal life with the Heavenly Father.

Death is thought to be a blessing and an entry to eternal existence. At some time after death, the spirit and the body will reunite and be resurrected to the spirit world, which has both a Paradise and a Spirit Prison where unrighteous spirits live in darkness.

Jehovah's Witnesses

These are a Christian religious group of approximately 10 million adherents founded in 1872 by the American clergyman Charles Taze Russell in Pennsylvania. Followers are baptised when of an age of understanding. If a child dies, it is protected by the baptismal state of the parents.[22] There is belief in Armageddon and the re-appearance of Jesus Christ's personal reign on earth. The religion rejects secular law where it conflicts with divine law and only recognizes the faith and one's duty to Jesus Christ. Witnesses do not normally celebrate birthdays or religious festivals. Jehovah's Witnesses refuse blood because of several scriptural references, the most important being from Acts 15:29:

> that you abstain from things offered to idols, from blood, from things strangled, and from sexual immorality. If you keep yourselves from these, you will do well.

Failure to observe this has sometimes resulted in expulsion from the group. There is now a considerable guidance literature available discussing blood and blood products, and sometimes active participation in hospital lay committees by adherents.

Christian Scientists

Mary Baker Eddy, who had a revelation that allowed her to recover from spinal injuries, founded the Church of Christ Scientist in Boston (USA) in 1879. There are now branches in over 80 countries. Their belief is that illness is an illusion that can be cured by belief in Jesus as the Healer. This differs from other branches of Christianity in that the faith's followers rely on God for healing rather than on medicine.

Care of the dying

Christianity has always had problems with evil, justice, divine omnipotence, sin, human sexuality and abortion and the meaning of pain and suffering. Each is interpreted and managed differently by the individual sub-sections of Christianity so it is important to record the individual's specific denomination in their notes and to follow their specific wishes. Palliative care and euthanasia are other difficult areas but the majority have a measured approach to death based on the alleviation of suffering when death is inevitable. Most would hold that it is religiously wrong to deliberately accelerate death, but that it is not ethically wrong to use sufficient medicines to minimize suffering. There is no longer any religious shame associated with suicide in most denominations, with the body being treated as any other deceased Christian, including burial in consecrated ground. Jehovah's Witnesses and members of the Church of Latter-Day Saints believe the outcome of suicide is in the hands of God. Afro-Caribbean adherents usually still regard suicide as a stigma.

Baptism, recognizing the individual's entry into a Christian faith is a fundamental rite of all denominations and can be done at any age. The Sacrament of Baptism is often called 'The door of the Church'. Baptism is usually done by a priest of the appropriate persuasion, but in an emergency or in the absence of a minister, anyone already baptized may perform a baptism. The sign of a cross is made on the person's forehead, a little water poured onto it (or another accessible part of the body), with the words '[Name], I baptize you in the name of the Father and of the Son and of the Holy Spirit. Amen'. Should a child die without being baptized, some parents may feel that their child will be prevented from entering the family of God and children can be baptized even at or after death if necessary.

Many regular churchgoing Christians of all denominations welcome a visit from a minister, and the 'Sacrament of the Sick' may be appropriate. Some Anglicans might welcome 'anointing' in the time before death. Death rites are especially important for Roman Catholics. There are a number of Catholic sacraments related to the dying or deceased person:

- Reconciliation (Confession or Penance)
- Holy Communion (Eucharist)
- Anointing of the Sick (Last Rites).

A Catholic priest should always be called in good time to enable these sacraments to be given, although they are sometimes administered up to several hours after death. The last rites are meant to prepare the dying person's soul for death, by providing absolution of sins, sacramental grace, prayers for the relief of suffering through anointing and the final administration of the Eucharist (also called Holy Communion, Mas, or the Lord's Supper). At death a prayer of commendation of the soul may be offered.

Followers of Christian Science are often cared for in Christian Science nursing homes, although they may be admitted to hospital for accidents, childbirth or treatment. The decision of whether or not to accept medical intervention lies with the individual, including organ transplantation. Some accept supportive care in hospitals but reject drugs or surgery. Alcohol and tobacco are not allowed and blood transfusions are traditionally rejected.

Management of death

After death, for the vast majority of Christians routine last offices by hospital staff are appropriate. Both burial and cremation are acceptable. Aspects relevant to particular denominations are given below. As usual, sympathetic questioning of the patient and relatives as to what they would prefer prevents many difficulties.

Roman Catholics

The mourning period will vary depending on which culture the family and deceased are from. For example, the Irish Catholic community has a tradition, now dying out, called the 'wake'. This is where the deceased is kept in the home overnight before the funeral so that relatives and friends can spend time remembering the person's life. Rather than a sad time, it is considered a joyful time to remember and celebrate the person's life, and to give the deceased a 'good send off'.

The Afro-Caribbean community

Last offices are ideally performed by a healthcare worker from the same background. The Afro-Caribbean community believes that the body should be intact for the afterlife and so disfigurement is distressing as the body may be viewed before and during the funeral service, particularly by the Pentecostal community. Embalming may be preferred if the funeral is delayed.

Burial is preferred over cremation and some of the deceased are returned to the island of their birth for burial. The funeral is important for the family and friends and may be postponed until they can arrive. The funeral procession usually starts at the home of the deceased.

Latter-Day Saints

Routine last offices are appropriate but if the deceased has a sacred garment it must be replaced on the body. The body may be viewed before the funeral at the church meeting house. Burial is preferable but cremation is not ruled out.

Christian Scientists

Routine last rites are appropriate but a female body should be handled by female staff. Cremation is usually preferred.

Autopsy and organ transplantation

With the majority of Christians, there are no problems with either. Some of the commoner exceptions are set out below.

The Afro-Caribbean community

Organ donation is not welcomed by the older traditionalists, but is likely to be more acceptable to younger people. The older generation believes that the body should be left intact for resurrection, so only coroner's autopsies are permitted. Organs retained until after the funeral can cause distress and may require a second burial.

Latter-Day Saints

Mormons will pray before making a decision about donation, but it is not objected to in principle. Permission for autopsy is similar.

Jehovah's Witnesses

Organ donation is a matter for individuals, but if it is practised, all blood must be drained from the organ first. Blood cannot be stored or re-used in any way.

Autopsy is an issue for individuals, but blood tests are usually not permitted.

Christian Scientists

They object to autopsies. Organ and tissue donation is an issue that is left to the individual church member.

Further reading

- Rutty J: 'Christianity', in *E-Learning for Health*, Royal College of Pathologists, 'Faith Considerations Part 1: Abrahamic Faiths', published on the web by Health Education England NHS (undated), available at; www.e-lfh.org.uk/programmes/medical-examiner/
- Woodhead L (2014): *Christianity: A Very Short Introduction*, Oxford University Press.
- Young J (2010): *Christianity: An Introduction*, McGraw-Hill C Inc.
- MacCulloch D (2010): *A History of Christianity*, Penguin Books.

Notes

1 Woodhead L (2014): *Christianity: a Very Short Introduction*, Oxford University Press, p. 42.
2 *Ibid.*, p. 89.
3 Matthew 1:18–25 and Luke 1:26–38.
4 Matthew 3:13–17; Mark 1:9–11; Luke 3:21–23.
5 John 1:29–34.
6 Woodhead L (2014): *Christianity: a Very Short Introduction*, Oxford University Press, chapter 1, pp. 3–20.
7 *Ibid.*, p. 3.
8 The first written evidence is a letter from Paul to the Corinthians in about 55 CE (25 years after Jesus' death) and the other gospels of Mark, Matthew, Luke and John have been timed from 60–120 CE. These texts are both complementary and at times conflicting.
9 Matthew 28:1–3.
10 John 20:11–12.
11 Mark 16:1–8.
12 Luke 24:1–12.
13 John 20:19–31.
14 Acts 1:1–5.
15 Holloway R (2016): *A Little History of Religion*, Yale University Press, chapter 20, pp. 116–118.
16 The first state religion was in Armenia in 301 CE, followed by Ethiopia in 330 CE.
17 MacCulloch D (2010): *A History of Christianity*, Penguin Books, part II, p. 187.
18 Young J (2010): *Christianity: An Introduction*, McGraw-Hill C Inc., chapter 16; pp. 306–307.
19 This was not revoked for 900 years. See MacCulloch D (2010): *A History of Christianity*, Penguin Books, part IV, p. 174.
20 Woodhead L (2014): *Christianity: A Very Short Introduction*, Oxford University Press, chapters 4 and 5, pp. 57–88.
21 What follows is a meld from Woodhead L (2014): *Christianity: A Very Short Introduction*, Oxford University Press; Young J (2010): *Christianity: An Introduction*, McGraw-Hill C Inc.; and MacCulloch D (2010): *A History of Christianity*, Penguin Books. The responsibility for the content rests with the authors.
22 1 Corinthians 7:14.

Chapter 17

Hinduism

Description of the religion

Numbers practising the religion

Hinduism has over 900 million adherents worldwide and is practised on all continents. It is the religion of approximately 80% of the people in India and Nepal, and there are just under 1 million Hindus in the UK.[1]

Origin and beliefs

Hinduism is so called because it originated in the Indus valley (Persian name *Sindhu*) in northern India.[2] Hinduism can trace its roots back to at least 2000 BC, making it the oldest existing religion in the world. Over time, because of dissatisfactions with it, it spawned Buddhism (5th century BCE), Jainism (6th century BCE) and Sikhism (16th century CE). At the time of the formation of Buddhism and Jainism, although the heredity Brahmin priesthood was formed, Hinduism as we know it today with its complicated caste system and temple complexes had probably not developed.[3]

Because of its beginnings in pre-history there is no recognized original source for the faith and controversy over whether 'Hindu' represents a religion or an Indian way of life continues. Half-a-century ago, in trying to resolve this issue, to the chagrin of religious groups, the India Supreme Court in 1966 said:

> When we think of the Hindu religion, we find it difficult, if not impossible, to define the Hindu religion or even adequately describe it. Unlike other religions in the world, the Hindu religion does not claim any one prophet, it does not worship any one god, it does not subscribe to any one dogma, it does not believe in any one philosophic concept, it does

not follow any one set of religious rites or performances, in fact, it does not appear to satisfy the narrow traditional features of any religion or creed. It may broadly be described as a way of life and nothing more.[4]

This legal view has been re-confirmed by further judgements in 1995[5] and 2016.[6] However, these decisions, which encompass definitional complexities, were taken in the context of political uses of the term and on a day-to-day basis at personal and community level, the practice of Hinduism as the indigenous religion continues as it always has. As practised, Hinduism is hugely variable. The historical evolution both in Asia and in its diaspora has produced both minor and major groupings set out on a spectrum of which one end is virtually unrecognizable from the other.[7] What follows is an attempt to steer a middle course amongst this variability.

The basis of the doctrine is *Sanatana Dharma*.[8] *Sanatana* means eternal but there is no exact English equivalent for *Dharma*. It is perhaps best thought of as a concept relating to the nature and moral order of man that implies right conduct, religion, duty, quality of life, law, justice and welfare with the absence of negative feelings and self-abasement.[9] Hindus may be polytheistic, monotheistic or monistic. Characteristically, there is a belief in a single supreme being Brahman[10] (please note the difference from Brahmin, which represent upper caste), who pervades the whole of nature as the absolute reality[11] and is represented in humans as *atman*, a sort of personal essence[12] often thought of as an eternal soul.[13] God can be manifest in many forms. These forms can be human or non-human and Brahman can be taken to oversee a pantheon of over 1 million different gods. Since Victorian times this has led scholars to interpret the core of Hinduism as a form of pantheism expressed by individuals as a polytheism through devotion to their chosen and physically represented deities.[14] Important figures below Brahman and close to the top of this pyramid are called the 'Hindu Trinity' or *Trimurti*.[15] These comprise Brahma, Vishnu and Shiva representing the categorical concepts of creation, preservation and destruction, together with personal gods and goddesses such as Krishna, Rama or and Ganesh. As one descends the pyramid, a myriad of others are found. The religion allows wide freedom in the details of personal belief: individuals can worship their preferred gods in various forms of prayer and custom.[16] Over centuries, many features of religious practice have changed. Animal sacrifice is now obsolete, the power of the Brahmins is substantially reduced and there are many social challenges.[17] It is a religion that over centuries has survived by continual adaptation to place and time, almost in a Darwinian way. Miraculously, throughout it all, the cow has remained as the dynamic symbol of the Indian nation: a mother producing products of goodness and purity.[18]

The Hindu scriptures are divided into two parts, the *shrutis* (truths divinely revealed to the early sages by gods), and the *smritis* (human compositions that are 'remembered' or narrate past events). The most important *shrutis* are the *Vedas* (of which there are four) and the *Upanishads* (of which there are six principle ones), and their scriptures originate from between 1500 BCE and 300 BCE. Collectively they contain hymns and mantras, moral stories, aphorisms and mythological tales.[19] The early Brahmins used to accurately remember the content of these writings and pass them down the generations. The British administrators of the 18th century were amazed to find that Brahmin students learnt the scriptures from oral transmission from their elders rather than from reading texts.[20]

Worship and lifestyle

Although there are temples for community services, the home is perhaps the most important place of worship (*puja*[21]). Most dwellings will have a room, corner or alcove set aside with pictures, statuettes or other images of their chosen god appropriately decorated and cared for.[22] Worship is traditionally a daily routine, morning and evening, preceded by ritual cleansing. Hinduism is a way of life steeped in culture but what actually counts is conduct rather than the minutiae of belief.[23] Associated with the Hindu religion are many festivals and holy days, the most well known of which is Diwali, the Festival of Lights.[24]

Hindu society developed within class and caste systems. Traditionally there were four social classes (*varna*) and four stages of life (*ashrama*).[25] The classes are as follows.

- Brahmin: priests, teachers, performance of religious ceremonies, interpretation of texts.
- Kshatriya: warriors, rulers, maintenance of law and order.
- Vaishya: traders, farmers, breeders.
- Shudra: servants, labouring classes; these support the other three.

However, even in Victorian times it was recognized that apart from the Brahmins, the others are not in practical use as castes but remain as classes. In practice there are a great many number of castes (*jati*), sects and tribes,[26] which rise and fall on the social scale.[27] Sitting below them all were India's *Dalits* or 'untouchables', who have suffered routine violence and discrimination for centuries as a 'polluting' presence.[28]

The attribution of 'pure' or 'impure' to a particular caste depends upon those making the judgement.[29] The touch of a lower-caste person on a Brahmin necessitated ritual purification and menstruating women were also polluting. A woman should keep focused on the home and family and bearing sons was her virtue.[30] The norm was that you would live, socialize, marry and eat within your caste.[31] Marriages were arranged with the interests of both parental families in mind and after marriage it was the custom for the wife to move into the home of the husband's family.[32] However, in all these areas one must be careful of generalizations because with industrialization, human rights and feminism, things are changing rapidly,[33] particularly in urban areas.

Untouchability was officially abolished in 1950 with the setting out of the Indian Constitution,[34] which requires that the state:

> shall not discriminate against any citizen on grounds only of religion, race, caste, sex, place of birth or any of them.

There has been subsequent strengthening legislation. Dowry was prohibited in 1961, but the practice continues, and the gender:birth ratio in 2011 of 1.09 males to 1.00 females points to continued selective abortion. Although there has been great progress (female and Dalit pressure groups have scored successes, and there have been two Dalit presidents of India), old habits die hard. Many people in the modern Dalit and women's movements have turned to secular lifestyles to obtain equality and this raises the issue of whether modern Hinduism may have to reject the teaching of the *shrutis* and the *smriti* because of the nature of the duty of women and Untouchables and the concepts of purity and pollution. The situation of many of India's Untouchables continues as a social ill in need of repair.[35]

Hinduism as a religion traditionally regards an earthly human as having an eternal soul living in a temporary body that is continuously recycled indefinitely. Hindus believe that existence is a cycle of birth, death and rebirth (*Samsara*) governed by *Karma*. The ultimate aim of these rebirths is to attain *moksha*, or fusion with God. Life is believed to have different goals according to a person's stage of life and their position in the social structure. *Karma*'s literal meaning is 'action'. Good or virtuous actions in harmony with Dharma will have good reactions: bad actions against Dharma will have the opposite effect. A person, to be a proper Hindu, does have to act – idle meditation is not 'good Karma' but 'good Dharma' is. What you do is the key. At the end of one's life the good and bad Karma are weighed and the result determines one's position in the next life, or whether one attains *moksha*. This process of cyclical reincarnation may continue through many, perhaps thousands, of earthly lives. The soul is reborn over and over again according to the law of Karma and the physical host can be an insect, an animal or a human. The goal of liberation (*moksha*) is to make us free from this cycle of action and reaction, and from rebirth.[36] Death, like sleep, can be interpreted as simply an interval between periods of consciousness.[37]

Care of the dying

In Britain, during medical treatment only very rarely are there problems with caste differences between the patient and healthcare staff (and *vice versa*). The Hindu understanding of illness varies from traditional to sophisticated depending on the patient and family. The traditional approach is called *Ayurveda* and promotes optimal wellbeing and longevity through a lifestyle that addresses mind, body, behaviour and environment.[38] There is no 'official' religious view on suicide but suicide and euthanasia can be difficult subjects because they might be thought to interfere with the balance of Karma. Fasting may affect medical and nursing plans. Determining the position of the patient with respect to traditional beliefs and including the family in therapeutic decisions is clearly important. Avoid medical interventions during times of prayer or meditation. Putting Hindu scriptures on the floor is regarded as insulting.

Most Hindus will not eat beef and hold the cow (the provider of milk) in reverence. Some will not eat chicken or eggs and many are vegetarians. The exact dietary requirements of the patient and family need to be clearly established. Handwashing before and after eating is mandatory. Tobacco and alcohol are not usually accepted, but there are an increasing number of 'secular Hindus'.

Hindus prefer to wash in free-flowing water, e.g., a shower, as baths are considered unhygienic by many. If there is no shower, ask the patient if they would like a jug to use in a bath. Modesty is important to Hindu women and they may prefer female nurses. Jewellery usually has a religious significance, e.g., a woman's bangles are only removed on her husband's death, and some Hindu boys wear a silk thread across their torso. These religious symbols need to be respected and only removed if necessary.

Dying in hospital can be deeply distressing to the family. To the majority of Hindus there is great religious significance in being able to die at home, and they may wish to be moved to the floor to be next to Mother Earth. Some will even prefer to return to India to die at the sacred city of Varanasi on the north bank of the River Ganges. The patient's family may wish to have a Hindu priest to read from the Hindu holy books or to perform holy rites.[39] The latter may include tying a thread around the wrist or neck. As the person nears death, large numbers of family members will probably be present. Before death (before the soul leaves the body), there may be chanting and a few drops of Ganges water, the leaves of the sacred tulsi plant and a piece of gold may be placed in the dying person's mouth while prayers are recited.

Management of death

Antyesti is the funeral oblation. Last offices by healthcare staff are not usually necessary because it is customary for the relatives to bathe, dress and wrap the body in a new cloth. Sometimes the body will be taken home to do this. If there is no family immediately available, gender-specific healthcare staff should wear gloves and touch the body as little as possible to ensure minimal contact. The eyes should be closed, the limbs straightened and the body wrapped in a plain sheet with no emblems or artefacts. Jewellery, religious threads and other religious objects should be left in place. The body will be washed later by relatives or morticians. If the body has to be left overnight in a room, a candle or low light should be left burning.

Disposal of the body is by cremation, as soon as possible after death. Only the soul is needed for reincarnation. There may need to be provision made for the rapid issuing of a Medical Certificate of Cause of Death to allow registration to proceed quickly. If there are delays to this, e.g., reporting to the coroner, a sensitive explanation is required. Traditionally the eldest son lights the funeral pyre, with the modern equivalent being attending the coffin as it enters the cremation furnace. The ashes are scattered on the third day, preferably in the Ganges, but there are designated river-bank sites in the UK. Sometimes the ashes are split so that a proportion can return to India. *Shradda* is the last rite to be performed, which is meant to support the spirits of the dead in their pilgrimage to their new life. The rite is performed between the tenth and thiry-first days after cremation, when the eldest son makes offerings of rice balls and milk. The first annual death anniversary is observed by a *shraddha* ceremony that enables the deceased (*preta*) to be admitted into the assembly of forefathers.

Autopsy and organ transplantation

There is no specific contradiction to either, as set out in the religion, but with the exception of blood donation and transfusion, autopsy and organ donation remains unpopular. If an autopsy or organ donation does occur, ritual preparation of the body will commence immediately afterwards.

Further reading

- Rutty J: 'Hinduism', in *E-Learning for Health*, Royal College of Pathologists, 'Faith Considerations Part 2: Dharmic Faiths', published on the web by Health Education England NHS (undated), available at; www.e-lfh.org.uk/programmes/medical-examiner/

- Knott K (2016): *Hinduism: A Very Short Introduction*, Oxford University Press.
- Weightman S (2010): 'Hinduism', in *The Penguin Handbook of the World's Living Religions*, ed. Hinnells JR, Penguin, chapter 5, pp. 263–311.
- DK (2013): *The Religions Book*, UK edn, Dorling Kindersley, 'Hinduism', pp. 90–125.

Notes

1 Knott K (2016): *Hinduism: A Very Short Introduction*, Oxford University Press, p. 94, box 4.
2 Pancholi N (1996): 'Hinduism', in *Six World Faiths*, ed. Cole WO, Cassell, p. 13.
3 Smart N (1999): *South Asian Philosophies in World Philosophies*, Routledge, p. 14.
4 Supreme Court of India judgment. SASTRI YAGNAPURUSHADJI & ORS V. MULDAS BRUDARDAS VAISHYA & ANR [1966] INSC 12; AIR 1966 SC 1119; 1966 (3) SCR 242 (14 January 1966).
5 Supreme Court of India 11/12/1995 Civil Appeal 2835 of 1989, p. 27 of 34. Available at: https://sci.gov.in/jonew/judis/10197.pdf.
6 Anon (2016): 'Will Not Re-Visit 1995 Judgement on "Hindutva": Supreme Court'. *The Economic Times* (India Times Ltd), 26 October. https://economictimes. indiatimes.com/news/politics-and-nation/will-not-re-visit-1995-judgement-on-hindutva-supreme-court/articleshow/55063539.cms'
7 Weightman S (2010): 'Hinduism', in *The Penguin Handbook of the World's Living Religions*, ed. Hinnells JR, Penguin, chapter 5, pp. 263–264.
8 DK (2013): *The Religions Book*; UK edn, Dorling Kindersley, 'A Rational World', p. 94.
9 Weightman S (2010): 'Hinduism', in *The Penguin Handbook of the World's Living Religions*, ed. Hinnells JR, Penguin, chapter 5, pp. 281–282.
10 Brahman (the ultimate reality), should not be confused with Brahma (a four-headed male god) or brahmin (a priest of the highest caste). Although the context usually makes it clear, there is further confusion because brāhman is sometimes used interchangeably with brahmin.
11 DK (2013): *The Religions Book*; UK edn, Dorling Kindersley, 'Brahman is My Self within the Heart', pp. 103–104.
12 Knott K (2016): *Hinduism: A Very Short Introduction*, Oxford University Press, p. 25.
13 BBC (2009): 'Hinduism'. See: www.bbc.co.uk/religion/religions/hinduism/concepts/concepts_1.shtml.
14 Lyall A (1911): *Hinduism in Religious Systems of the World*, eds Sheowring W and Conrad WT, George Allen and Unwin, p. 113; and Knott K (2016): *Hinduism: A Very Short Introduction*, Oxford, p. 55.
15 DK (2013): *The Religions Book*; UK edn, Dorling Kindersley, 'A Rational World', p. 97.
16 Knott K (2016): *Hinduism: A Very Short Introduction*, Oxford University Press, p. 55.
17 Knott K (2016): *Hinduism: A Very Short Introduction*, Oxford University Press, chapter 7, 'Challenges to Hinduism: Women and Dalits', pp. 74–87.
18 Knott K (2016): *Hinduism: A Very Short Introduction*, Oxford University Press, p. 107.

19 Knott K (2016): *Hinduism: A Very Short Introduction*, Oxford University Press, pp. 12–15, and see table 1, p. 13.
20 Knott K (2016): *Hinduism: A Very Short Introduction*, Oxford University Press, p. 16.
21 DK (2013): *The Religions Book*, UK edn, Dorling Kindersley, 'We Speak to the Gods through Daily Rituals', pp. 114–115.
22 Pancholi N (1996): 'Hinduism', in *Six World Faiths*, ed. Cole WO, Cassell, p. 21.
23 DK (2013): *The Religions Book*; UK edn, Dorling Kindersley, 'The Four Stages of Life', p. 108.
24 Knott K (2016): *Hinduism: A Very Short Introduction*, Oxford University Press, p. 58, box 2.
25 Knott K (2016): *Hinduism: A Very Short Introduction*, Oxford University Press, p. 18, table 2.
26 Lyall A (1911): *Hinduism in Religious Systems of the World*, eds Sheowring W and Conrad WT, George Allen and Unwin, p. 114.
27 Pancholi N (1996): 'Hinduism', in *Six World Faiths*, ed. Cole WO, Cassell, p. 43.
28 Knott K (2016): *Hinduism: A Very Short Introduction*, Oxford University Press, pp. 82–83.
29 Weightman S (2010): 'Hinduism', in *The Penguin Handbook of the World's Living Religions*, ed. Hinnells JR, Penguin, chapter 5, p. 282.
30 Knott K (2016): *Hinduism: A Very Short Introduction*, Oxford University Press, p. 75.
31 Pancholi N (1996): 'Hinduism', in *Six World Faiths*, ed. Cole WO, Cassell, pp. 43–44.
32 Pancholi N (1996): 'Hinduism', in *Six World Faiths*, ed. Cole WO, Cassell, pp. 17–20.
33 Knott K (2016): *Hinduism: A Very Short Introduction*, Oxford University Press, chapter 7, 'Challenges to Hinduism: Women and Dalits', pp. 74–87.
34 The Constitution of India (1950): Part III; Fundamental Rights; Art. 15(1). Available at: www.india.gov.in/sites/upload_files/npi/files/coi_part_full.pdf.
35 Knott K (2016): *Hinduism: A Very Short Introduction*, Oxford University Press, 'Daughters, Dowry and Sex Determination', pp. 79–81, and 'Untouchability and the Rise of Dalit Identity', pp. 82–83, 18–19.
36 Weightman S (2010): 'Hinduism', in *The Penguin Handbook of the World's Living Religions*, ed. Hinnells JR, Penguin, chapter 5, p. 284; Knott K (2016): *Hinduism: A Very Short Introduction*, Oxford University Press, 'Karma, Yoga and the Self', pp. 32–37; and DK (2013): *The Religions Book*; UK edn, Dorling Kindersley, 'Brahman is My Self within the Heart', pp. 104–105.
37 Lyall A (1911): *Hinduism in Religious Systems of the World*, eds Sheowring W and Conrad WT, George Allen and Unwin, p. 121.
38 Sharma et al. (2007): 'Utilisation of Ayurveda in Health Care: An Approach for Prevention, Health Promotion and Treatment of Disease; Part 1 – Ayurveda, the Science of Life'. *Journal of Alternative and Complementary Medicine*, Vol. 13, No. 9, 1012.
39 Traditionally brahmins are not involved in the actual disposal of the body because it is regarded as a polluting task. See Knott K (2016): *Hinduism: A Very Short Introduction*, Oxford University Press, p. 17.

Chapter 18

Islam

Description of the religion

Numbers practising the religion

The current distribution of Muslims across the world is set out in Table 18.1.[1] The different sections of Islam are described later.

Whilst Muslims are found on all five inhabited continents, more than 60% of the global Muslim population is in Asia and about 20% is in the Middle East and North Africa. However, the Middle East and North Africa regions have the highest percentage of Muslim-majority countries. Countries with Shi'a majorities usually have a substantial Sunni minority and vice versa.

More than 300 million Muslims, or one-fifth of the world's Muslim population, live in countries where Islam is not the majority religion. These minority-Muslim populations are often quite large. India, for example, has the third-largest population of Muslims worldwide. China has more Muslims than Syria, while Russia is home to more Muslims than Jordan and Libya combined.

TABLE 18.1 The current distribution of Muslims across the world

Division of Islam	Sunni	Wahhabi	Shi'a
Worldwide numbers (estimates)	1.5 billion	5 million	300 million
Main geographical locations	Saudi Arabia, Pakistan, India, Indonesia, Egypt, Bangladesh, Syria, Turkey, Nigeria, Libya, Tunisia and Sudan	Saudi Arabia, the United Arab Emirates and Qatar	Iran, Azerbaijan, Bahrain and Iraq

Origins and beliefs

It is conventional to time the birth of Islam from 610 CE, when the Word of God began to make itself known to the prophet Muhammad by the Angel Gabriel. An alternative view is that Islam was always the intended religion for man, it's just that the earlier efforts to enact it through prophets such as Abraham, Moses and Jesus distorted the message and never completed God's purpose.[2] In either case, for Muslims, Muhammad was the final prophet who established the religion of Islam as the true way of life and belief in the eyes of a one true God. 'Islam' in Arabic means 'to submit', specifically to God,[3] and a Muslim is 'one who submits'. Muslims worship God, not Muhammad; he is not the equivalent to Jesus in Christianity. This is made clear in the central article of faith, 'There is no god but God, Muhammad is the Messenger of God'.[4]

The scriptures and the law

Muhammad was born in Mecca in 570 CE, and as an adult he used to go to caves near the city on Mount Hira to meditate. During one night in 610 CE, the Angel Gabriel commanded him to remember and recite what he said. The first divine revelation had occurred, and they would continue over the next 22 years (until his death in 632 CE).[5] Muhammed remembered them word-perfectly and passed them on orally to his followers, who in turn memorized them. These statements are regarded as co-extensive with God's actual words and many are in the first person.[6]

When collected together as the 114 suras (literally rows), or chapters, they form the Qur'an.[7] For the vast majority of Muslims they are believed to be the actual speech of God, not human interpretations of God as in the Bible and other holy books.[8] Current scholarship agrees that most of his utterances were recorded in Muhammad's lifetime but it was only after his death during the Third Caliphate of Uthman (approximately 650 CE) that a formal codex was set down to ensure a uniform message and interpretation. This 'Uthmanic Codex' has remained as the only canonical text of the Qur'an that exists, recognized by both Sunnis and Shi'as throughout the Muslim world.[9] In terms of volume, beliefs occupy the largest part, followed sequentially by morals, rituals and laws.[10] The core belief of Islam is that there is one God (Allah) who is the creator and ruler of the universe, being all-powerful with no equal.

In addition to God's direct words, Muhammad was a preacher and sage and his own wise sayings, actions and anecdotes interpreting the Qur'an in practical terms were also recorded, first orally and then in written form.[11] It is these sources to which a curious person should go to answer the question 'What does Islam say about . . .'[12] Several written versions of such advice exist. From these emerged the Sunna and the Hadiths, two terms which are often used synonymously but which do have differences. Sunna literally means a path, way or example, i.e., the actions, sayings and tacit approvals of Muhammad[13] that are the second most important source of Islamic law and life. It can be said that if the Sunna controls the interpretation of the Qur'an, then consensus controls the interpretation of the Sunna.[14] The Hadiths are a wider collection of statements concerning the actions of Muhammad and his followers which often contain Sunna but also encompass broader issues. There are several versions of each collected over the early centuries of the religion.[15] Many of the supposed quoted requirements of the Qur'an are in fact man-made interpretations quoted from the Sunna and the Hadiths. Debate over the authenticity and authority of the Hadiths continues unabated.[16,17]

Ruthven, in trying to put into perspective the controversy of truth versus interpretation, says 'Muhammad . . . is a bridge between myth and history, the realms respectively of divine and human action. He inhabits a world where historical activity is surrounded by supernatural forces, where the numinous constantly interpenetrates the dull sublunary world of common sense. To grasp this world in its fullness must lie beyond our capacities as moderns'.[18]

Hadith scribes and scholars were aware from the outset that spurious stories were invented to support rival positions in disputes within Islamic law and eventually 'two sound versions' were set down in 870 CE and 875 CE. In the 19th century modernist scholars questioned their authenticity and Chirag (1898) took the view that the 'vast flood of traditions soon formed a chaotic sea. Truth and error, fact and fable mingled together in an indistinguishable confusion'.[19] Accurate or otherwise, the Sunna and Hadiths (in addition to the Qur'an), became the model from which to lead a Muslim life.

Islam has its own legal system called the Shari'a which both upholds the good of society and helps humans to attain salvation. It is thought of as the unchanging and everlasting will of God. Shari'a has four sources of guidance.

- *The Qur'an*, as the direct and unmodified will of God is the primary source – it represents His word.
- *The Sunna* contains a much larger quantity of legal material recorded in the Hadith literature based on the Prophet's recorded words and his own legal judgments.

- *The Ijma* can be thought of as a form of common law of precedent based on past interpretations by Muslim scholars and achieved through consensus.
- *The Qiyas* is a form of logical reasoning when situations arise that are not explicitly covered in the above guidance.

With this system, five schools of jurisprudence emerged.

Jihad[20] is a word that has entered modern parlance through an unfortunate association with terrorism. Its traditional intention is to mean 'exertion' or 'struggle'. In the Hadiths the Prophet distinguished between the lesser jihad of war and the greater jihad against evil. The greater jihad is the struggle that devout Muslims are engaged in throughout life to do good and live by Islamic law. However, the concept of the lesser jihad was enhanced during the centuries of conquest (see below), and it is this aspect that often remains at the forefront of modern minds, reinforced by terrorism and suicide bombers.

The divisions within Islam

After Muhammad's death there were three caliphs who carried the faith forwards, but problems struck with the fourth, who was assassinated (see Figure 18.1), and a schism occurred. The dispute was over leadership and interpretation of the religion and resulted in internecine conflict which continues to the present. In the tradition that became Sunni Islam, the community as a whole, represented by the *ulema* (the Muslim scholarly class), was heir to Muhammad. Their collective interpretation of Islam, expressed through consensus (*ijma*), was as definitive as the Qur'an or the Prophet's edicts.[21] The tradition that would become Shi'ite Islam believed that the family of the Prophet had inherited Muhammad's authority, which was held by select members of the family known as Imams.[22] These early disputes were largely concerned with power rather than differences in doctrine.[23] The Shi'ite Hadith tradition differs greatly from its Sunni counterpart.[24] In Islam there is still no central religious authority similar to the Vatican or Church of England, so national, regional and local interpretations of the faith are the norm.

The Shi'a community was originally led by selected members of Muhammad's descendants, called Imams. This inheritance passed successfully till the eleventh generation, who died without an apparent heir in 874 CE. However, there was belief in a hidden son with whom contact was established by special clerics called 'ambassadors'. They themselves died out in 941 CE.[25] Since then, the Shi'a community, as it is today, has been led by living scholars called mujtahids who act as the representatives of the Hidden Imam on earth. The most senior of these progress to become an Ayatollah and above them Grand Ayatollahs act as 'models to be imitated'.[26]

The nomenclature of Sunni Islam is also complex and varied.

- An Imam is today commonly used to refer to the official that leads the prayers at a mosque (not to be confused with the inherited Shiite Imams).[27]
- A Grand Mufti refers to the highest official of religious law in a Sunni Muslim country.

Across the world there are several variations in nomenclature. Both Sunni and Shi'a divisions have sects within them and their details are complex. Identified in Figure 18.1 (and in Table 18.1) are the Wahhabi, who were founded in the 18th century. They follow an austere form of Islam that insists on a literal interpretation of the Quran and have been closely associated with the royal family and politics of Saudia Arabia.

Sufism emphasizes the mysticism of the holy books and seeks to experience the reality of God's power and grace through direct experience.[28] Its adherents can come from both Sunni and Shi'a divisions.[29]

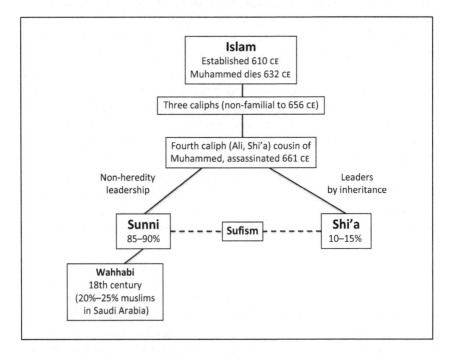

FIGURE 18.1 The main divisions of Islam

The geo-political expansion of Islam

From its early beginnings, Islam, like its predecessor Christianity, aspired to universality so it had a missionary and political component. The rapid expansion of Islam in the two centuries after the Prophet's death are illustrated in Figure 18.2.[30]

This was first achieved under a single caliphate but soon rival factions drained the caliphate of legitimacy and no single authority had universal acceptance. A mosque, The Dome of the Rock, was built on the site of the ruined Temple of Solomon in Jerusalem (see Chapters 16 and 20). From 1095 to 1291, Islam came under attack from a series of Christian crusades blessed by the Roman Catholic Church to regain control of the Holy Land. In 1099, Jerusalem was re-captured by the Christians. The mosque was given to the Augustinians and converted back to a church, only to be recaptured by the Muslim Ottomans in 1187.

Over time different regional leaders and caliphs (both Shi'a and Sunni) came and went but in 1517, as the *de facto* leaders of Islam, the Ottomans claimed the caliphate with their headquarters in Constantinople. Throughout, Islam was associated with major advances in science, medicine and philosophy. Religious leadership as a political force was finally disestablished by Atatürk, when he made Turkey a secular state in 1924, although it has since been re-established in other countries such as Iran.

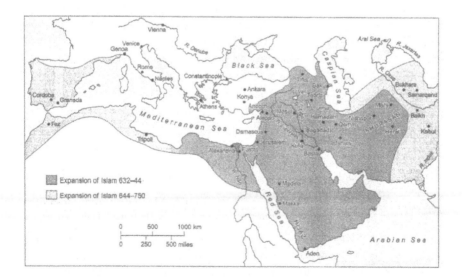

FIGURE **18.2** The rise and spread of Islam. Reproduced under licence from Ruthven M (1997): *Islam: A Very Short Introduction*, Oxford University Press, p. XIII

Worship and lifestyle

Adherents to the Islamic faith demonstrate their beliefs by living their lives according to the traditional duties of the five pillars of Islam. These are as follows.

- *Shahadah*: sincerely reciting the Muslim profession of faith.
- *Salat*: performing prayers in the proper way five times each day. *Wudhu* is the ritual washing performed by Muslims before prayer.
- *Zakat*: paying an alms (or charity) tax to benefit the poor and the needy.
- *Sawm*: fasting during the month of Ramadan.
- *Hajj*: pilgrimage to Mecca.

Carrying out these obligations provides the framework of a Muslim's life, and weaves their everyday activities and their beliefs into a single framework. The holy day for visiting the mosque is Friday. Islam regards it as pointless to live life without putting faith into action and practice. How well a life is lived will influence the afterlife. Generally, Muslims hold that death is part of God's overall plan. The Qur'an states 'We belong to God and to Him we shall return'.[31] Life on earth is a preparation for the afterlife. It is believed that everyone is judged after death and will then go either to Paradise or the Fire, based on their good and bad actions during their lifetime. Life after earthly death will be determined by the judgement of God.[32]

Islam originated in medieval times and translating the norms of those times onto modern society is difficult, as it is in Hinduism (see Chapter 17). Some verses of the Qur'an, such as: 'Men are the managers of the affairs of women. . .'[33] fly in the face of gender equality and no subject is more fraught than the position (and duties) of women.[34] The current situation is that both between and within countries there is huge variation in the expression of Islam in the modern world: this ranges from strict fundamentalism to relaxed tolerance and multi-faith liaison.

Care of the dying

The variability of individual lifestyles within a Moslem context requires healthcare staff to determine just what a patient and their relatives believe and expect. It is also useful to establish at the outset if any Muslim festivals will occur during the likely period of terminal illness.

All meat eaten should be halal and pork is forbidden. Fish and eggs are allowed and alcohol is prohibited. Clinical staff need to discuss these requirements with the patient and family since there is diversity in practice. Some pharmaceutical products contain non-halal components and the patient may ask about this. In cases of necessity prohibited things may become permissible (*halal*) for the duration of the emergency or need, as Islam puts a priority on life over death.[35]

During Ramadan, when there is fasting before sunrise till after sunset, the sick are exempted. If they wish to observe the fast, then food needs to be available at the appropriate times. Essential drugs and other medicines can be administered in the normal way.

During terminal illness, the norms of Muslim life should be observed. The patient should be assisted in ritual washing before prayer (*Wudhu*, see above) with washing water in the same location as the WC. The hands, mouth, nose, face, arms and feet are cleaned in order. Patients prefer to wash in free-flowing water, e.g., a shower, and baths are considered unhygienic. If withdrawal of life support becomes a possibility, this needs to be approached with care since it can be interpreted as assisted suicide, and the latter is prohibited in Islamic law.

Muslim women (and their male family members) may prefer their care to be delivered by female staff and although not always possible this should be aim. Women or men may wear or have with them a locket, charm or a copy of the Qur'an for support and these should not be removed unless absolutely necessary.

The dying Muslim may wish to sit or lie with his/her face towards Mecca. The bed might need to be moved to achieve this orientation. The family, with or without a local imam, may recite prayers around the bed. When Muslims are dying, they (or someone on their behalf) recite the Islamic declaration of faith, the Shahada: 'There is no God but Allah and Muhammad is the Messenger of Allah'. They may try to say the last words of Muhammad: 'Allah, help me through the hardship and agony of death'. If possible, before a Muslim dies, the call to prayer should be whispered into the person's ear, so it is the last thing a Muslim hears before death.

Management of death

Muslims believe that at the Day of Judgement there will be a physical resurrection. Death should not be feared as it is assumed that an observant Muslim will achieve salvation, and so extreme grief is often suppressed. Traditionally, cremation is forbidden because there is belief in total-body resurrection and there is huge respect for dead bodies. Muslims try to bury the dead person as quickly as possible, within 24 hours and facing Mecca. There is therefore a need to complete the death certification process as soon as is practicably possible.

Normally the body is ceremonially washed three or more times by relatives or qualified Muslims and then wrapped with three pieces of white cloth (*kafan*).

Healthcare staff only need involvement if the family or funeral directors are not available. If it becomes necessary to do last offices they should be limited to:

- gender-specific attendants
- disposable gloves
- body not washed nor nails or hair cut
- jaw supported so mouth closed
- body straightened
- head turned to right shoulder (so that it can face Mecca after burial)
- body wrapped in a white sheet.

Delay to the funeral causes distress, so if it becomes a coroner's case, time should be taken to explain the reasons for its necessity.

Although there is some variation in cultural interpretation of customs and rituals before, at and after death, there are traditionally three official days of mourning during which time family and friends offer their condolences. After this period, condolences should not be offered because this will reawaken the pain of the death within the family. Instead, life should return to normality; life must go on.

A widowed wife is expected to mourn for 130 days and to dress simply, with no jewellery. She is also traditionally confined to the home during this time, leaving only when it is absolutely necessary. Following this period she will resume her place in society and is encouraged to remarry.

Autopsy and organ transplantation

Autopsies are prohibited within the traditional Islamic faith. The family may wish to have a scanning autopsy (see Chapter 20, Judaism) if this will reveal the cause of death. The rituals of after-death care begin when examination of the body is complete.

There are no religious objections to blood transfusions. For solid organ donation there is much variation in belief and practice across the world. The body is thought to belong to God, so some Muslims are against donation. If donation is approved, the organs should be transplanted as soon as possible and not stored for long periods.

Further reading

- Rutty J: 'Islam', in *E-Learning for Health*, Royal College of Pathologists, 'Faith Considerations Part 1: Abrahamic Faiths', published on the web by Health Education England NHS (undated), available at; www.e-lfh. org.uk/programmes/medical-examiner/.

- Ruthven M (1997): *Islam: A Very Short Introduction*, Oxford.
- DK (2013): *The Religions Book*, UK edn, Dorling Kindersley, 'Islam', pp. 250–291.

Notes

1 These data are taken from the Pew Research Centre, available at: www.pew forum.org/2009/10/07/mapping-the-global-muslim-population/.
2 Holloway R (2016): *A Little History of Religion*, Yale University Press, chapter 23, p. 133.
3 ibid: pg. 131
4 Ruthven M (1997): *Islam: A Very Short Introduction*, Oxford University Press, p. 20.
5 *Ibid.*, pp. 21–22.
6 Haleem MA (2011): *Understanding the Quran*, I.B.Tauris, p. 3.
7 For a modern interpretation of the Quran, see *ibid.*
8 Ruthven M (1997): *Islam: A Very Short Introduction*, Oxford University Press, p. 21.
9 Haleem MA (2011): *Understanding the Quran*, I.B.Tauris, pp. 4–5.
10 *Ibid.*, p. 6.
11 Ruthven M (1997): *Islam: A Very Short Introduction*, Oxford, p. 21.
12 Brown JAC (2018): *Hadith: Muhammad's Legacy in the Medieval and Modern World*, revised edn, Oneworld Publications, chapter 1, p. 3.
13 Musay AI (2015): 'The Sunnifacion of Hadith and the Hadithication of Sunna', in *The Sunna and its Status in Islamic Law: The Search for a Sound*, ed. Duderrija A, chapter 4, pp. 75–96, Palgrave Macmillan.
14 Brown JAC (2018): *Hadith: Muhammad's Legacy in the Medieval and Modern World*, revised edn, Oneworld Publications, chapter 4, p. 180.
15 Duderija A (2015): 'The Concept of Sunna and its Status in Islamic Law', in *The Sunna and its Status in Islamic Law: The Search for a Sound*, ed. Duderrija A, introduction, pp. 1–12, Palgrave Macmillan.
16 Haleem MA (2011): *Understanding the Quran*, I.B.Tauris, pp. 3–4.
17 Brown JAC (2018): *Hadith: Muhammad's Legacy in the Medieval and Modern World*, revised edn, Oneworld Publications, chapters 9 and 10.
18 Ruthven M (1997): *Islam: A Very Short Introduction*, Oxford University Press, p. 47.
19 *Ibid.*, pp. 39–41.
20 For a discussion of jihad, see Ruthven M (1997): *Islam: A Very Short Introduction*, Oxford University Press, chapter 6, 'The Two Jihads', pp. 116–142.
21 Brown JAC (2018): *Hadith: Muhammad's Legacy in the Medieval and Modern World*, revised edn, Oneworld Publications, chapter 4, p. 135.
22 *Ibid.*
23 Ruthven M (1997): *Islam: A Very Short Introduction*, Oxford University Press, pp. 52, 55.
24 Brown JAC (2018): *Hadith: Muhammad's Legacy in the Medieval and Modern World*, revised edn, Oneworld Publications, chapter 4, p. 136.
25 *Ibid.*, pp. 138–140.
26 Ruthven M (1997): *Islam: A Very Short Introduction*, Oxford University Press, pp. 68–69.
27 DK (2013): *The Religions Book*, UK edn, Dorling Kindersley, p. 341.
28 Ruthven M (1997): *Islam: A Very Short Introduction*, Oxford University Press, pp. 62–66.

29 Hegedus U (2003): 'Islam', in *World Religions*, ed. Gill D, Harper Collins, p. 124.
30 Ruthven M (1997): *Islam: A Very Short Introduction*, Oxford University Press, p. XIII.
31 Qur'an 2:157.
32 For a discussion of these issues, see Haleem MA (2011): *Understanding the Quran*, I.B.Tauris, chapter 7, 'Life and Beyond', pp. 84–95.
33 Qur'an 4:35.
34 Ruthven M (1997): *Islam: A Very Short Introduction*, Oxford University Press, chapter 5, 'Women and Family in Islam', pp. 91–115.
35 Qur'an 2:173.

Chapter 19

Jainism

Description of the religion

Numbers practising the religion

Jains constitute less than 1% of India's population (approximately 4 million people), with the rest living in an international diaspora (estimated at approximately 3 million). The Jain community in the UK numbers around 30,000. Although small in number, the influence of Jainism on Indian life has been such that it is one of India's major religious traditions.[1] Also, Jain thinking on the sacredness of life has contributed to ecology, the vegetarian movement and the doctrine of non-violence that influenced Mahatma Ghandi and Martin Luther King.[2]

Origins and beliefs

Jainism is a religion that is conventionally said to have emerged from Hinduism, but some Jains dispute this and believe their religion to be much older.[3] The usual account is that they had 24 *tīrthaṅkara* (a saviour and spiritual leader of the righteous path), but that it was the 24th, called Mahavira, who firmly set the faith on its independent path distinct from Hinduism and Buddhism.[4] The texts containing the teachings of Mahavira are called the *Agamas*.[5] Jainism is the most ascetic of the Eastern faiths but the majority of those who call themselves Jains are laypersons whose religious life is not monastic.[6] After the death of Mahavira in 527 BCE, divisions occurred, particularly the *Digambara–Shvetambara* schism. The former maintained that an ascetic who had renounced the world should renounce clothing and would not admit women to monastic vows until they had been reborn as men; the latter disagreed and allowed the wearing of simple white clothes and the admission of women to monastic vows.[7] The dispute for fundamentalists continues today.

The cosmology of Jainism, based on reincarnation, is complex. They finesse the problem of evil by not believing in a single Supreme Being but they do believe in divine (or at least perfect) beings who are worthy of devotion.[8] They venerate multiple deities of the distinguished dead (*Jinas*) who, having attained spiritual liberation, are free from re-birth and live eternally as *siddahs* on their way to *moksha* in the uppermost reaches of the universe in innate perfection.[9] The lack of any recognisable deity who is responsible for the universe places full responsibility on the actions and conduct of the individual.[10]

The concept is that animals and plants, as well as human beings, contain living souls. Nothing that exists now was ever created, nor will it be destroyed. The world is made up of *jivas* (the living beings that have souls), and *ajivas* (non-living objects). The material *ajivas* often prevent *jivas* realizing their true immortal nature. Each of these *jivas* is the part that lives on after death and should be treated with respect and compassion. The four arms of the swastika (an important religious symbol) represent the four places where a soul could be reborn: divine, human, netherworld and as an animal or vegetable. *Karma* is believed to attach itself to the soul and soul can only achieve liberation by getting rid of all the *Karma* attached to it.[11] *Karma* or the moral quality of the actions in the previous lives determines the quality and happiness of the present lives.

Worship and lifestyle

The essence of Jainism is concern for the welfare of every being (and thing) in the universe and for the health of the universe itself. The supreme principle of living is non-violence and non-injury (*ahimsa*). In many ways they were eco-warriors before the concept evolved. Jains hope to achieve a path of non-violence by overcoming their innermost feelings of hate, greed and selfishness and place full responsibility on themselves for their actions. They are strict vegetarians and live in a way that minimizes their use of the world's resources.[12] The three guiding principles of Jainism, 'the three jewels', are:[13]

- the right belief
- the right knowledge
- the right conduct.

Jainism has no priests. Its professional religious people are monks and nuns who lead strict and ascetic lives, having taken what are known as the five great vows:[14]

- non-violence
- speaking the truth
- sexual restraint (with celibacy as the ideal)
- not stealing
- detachment from people, places and things.

They practise self-denial. Lay Jains do not take the five great vows but do take lesser but similar vows, practise self-denial and self-discipline and vow to not do work that involves harm to life.[15]

Jains practise their religion communally and personally. Worship (following ritual washing) in the temple is still largely individual but it does bind the community together for mutual strength. It has been called a religion of action rather than one of adoration. Many Jains in India worship at their temple every day, and join forces for community worship on festival days. Worship enhances personal spirituality and removes bad Karma. The religious practices of Jains have remained almost unchanged across the centuries of the faith's existence.[16]

Fasting is very common in Jainism and a Jain may take it upon him or herself to fast at any time. Most Jains fast at special festivals and holy days during the year. Fasts may be done as a penance, especially for monks and nuns. It purifies body and mind, and reminds the practitioner of *Mahavira*'s emphasis on renunciation and asceticism, because he spent a great deal of time fasting.[17]

Care of the dying

When approaching death, Jains believe that possessions are an obstacle to liberation and may relinquish all of them (*Aparigraha*).[18] As patients, their cleanliness and dietary habits (strict vegetarianism) need to be respected, including their wish to undertake a fast. When being treated, a Jain may ask for some peace and quiet for meditation. These days many adopt current medical practices and opt for aggressive treatment to prolong life and/or accept conventional palliative care. Partly because they are a minority group, it is often helpful to both the patient and the staff to encourage the patient and their relatives to be open about their faith and what their wishes are.

Any Jain faced with a serious illness can approach their guru and express a wish to take the vow of *Sallekhana* (which cannot be rescinded) to have a ritual death by fasting. This is a powerful sign of a Jain's dedication to the conquest of material existence by renunciation.[19] The vow is as follows.

Please instruct me sir. I have come forward to seek the vow of Sallekhana which will remain in force as long as I live. I am free of all doubts and anxieties in this matter. I renounce from now until the moment of my last breath, food and drink of all kinds.

Assuming that this is agreed, the person consults with their physician the likely time of remaining life and plans a programme of fasting. On accepting the vow a lay Jain gives up all personal relationships and possessions. Those who succeed in carrying the vow to death are considered to be superior spiritually. When operative, *Sallekhana* is usually completed in the family home,[20] so transfer out of hospital may be needed, even though the patient is seriously ill.

The vow of *Sallekhana* raises a number of important issues related to free will, self-autonomy, depression and mental capacity. Jains do not regard it as suicide. Even under human rights legislation, a person has a right to life, but not a right to death. However, if a competent patient rejects all medical intervention, not to respect their wishes constitutes assault and battery. For others not to accept the patient's decision may, it is believed, create a wounded soul and deprive a Jain of the chance to move further towards *Moska*. It is nevertheless important to be clear with a Jain and their family what treatment options are available and allow them to change their mind. Deliberate starvation in hospital may lead to referral to the coroner or court.

Otherwise, within aspects of their faith particular to them, normal individualized care is appropriate.

Management of death

Family members may or may not want to wash the body. If not, last offices by the healthcare staff are appropriate. Once washed the body will be dressed in new clothes. The body will be taken home by relatives and friends to pray for its soul and for a final view of the deceased.

Jains are normally cremated as soon as possible after death, so the efficient issuing of death-related documentation is important.

On the day of the deceased's death, a service will usually take place in the temple.

Sometimes flowers are placed on the coffin but removed before cremation so as to symbolize that all life is precious.

Unlike other religions, Jains will try not to cry for the deceased as this is believed to prevent the dead from rising. Most Jains do not observe the Hindu post-funeral rites to encourage the transfer of the deceased's soul from one existence to the next.[21]

Autopsy and organ transplantation

These are not usually objected to because Jains believe it is good to enhance the lives of others.

Further reading

- Rutty J: 'Jainism', in *E-Learning for Health*, Royal College of Pathologists, 'Faith Considerations Part 2: Dharmic Faiths', published on the web by Health Education England NHS (undated), available at; www.e-lfh.org.uk/programmes/medical-examiner/.
- Folkert KW, Cort JE (2010): 'Jainism', in *The Penguin Handbook of the World's Living Religions*, ed. Hinnells JR, chapter 7, pp. 342–370.
- BBC (2009): 'Jain Worship'. See: www.bbc.co.uk/religion/religions/jainism/.
- DK (2013): *The Religions Book*, UK edn, Dorling Kindersley, 'The Five Great Vows', pp. 68–71.

Notes

1 Folkert KW, Cort JE (2010): 'Jainism', in *The Penguin Handbook of the World's Living Religions*, ed. Hinnells JR, chapter 7, p. 342.
2 Holloway R (2016): *A Little History of Religion*, Yale University Press, chapter 6, 'Do No Harm', p. 35.
3 DK (2013): *The Religions Book*, UK edn, Dorling Kindersley, 'The Five Great Vows', p. 68; and Folkert KW, Cort JE (2010): 'Jainism', in *The Penguin Handbook of the World's Living Religions*, ed. Hinnells JR, chapter 7, pp. 342–343.
4 *Ibid.*, pp. 343–344.
5 BBC (2009): 'Jainism At a Glance'. See: www.bbc.co.uk/religion/religions/jainism/ataglance/glance.shtml.
6 DK (2013): *The Religions Book*, UK edn, Dorling Kindersley, 'The Five Great Vows', p. 68.
7 Folkert KW, Cort JE (2010): 'Jainism', in *The Penguin Handbook of the World's Living Religions*, ed. Hinnells JR, chapter 7, p. 345.
8 BBC (2009): 'God'. See: www.bbc.co.uk/religion/religions/jainism/beliefs/god.shtml.
9 Folkert KW, Cort JE (2010): 'Jainism', in *The Penguin Handbook of the World's Living Religions*, ed. Hinnells JR, chapter 7, p. 349 and figure 7.2, p. 350.
10 DK (2013): *The Religions Book*, UK edn, Dorling Kindersley, 'The Five Great Vows', p. 69.
11 Folkert KW, Cort JE (2010): 'Jainism', in *The Penguin Handbook of the World's Living Religions*, ed. Hinnells JR, chapter 7, p. 349 and figure 7.2, p. 350.
12 BBC (2009): 'Literal Meaning of Ahimsa'. See: www.bbc.co.uk/religion/religions/jainism/living/ahimsa_1.shtml.
13 BBC (2009): 'The Three Jewels'. See: www.bbc.co.uk/religion/religions/jainism/beliefs/threejewels.shtml.
14 Folkert KW, Cort JE (2010): 'Jainism', in *The Penguin Handbook of the World's Living Religions*, ed. Hinnells JR, chapter 7, p. 353.

15 *Ibid.*, p. 355.
16 BBC (2009): 'Jain Worship'. See: www.bbc.co.uk/religion/religions/jainism/worship/worship_1.shtml.
17 BBC (2009): 'Fasting'. See: www.bbc.co.uk/religion/religions/jainism/customs/fasting_1.shtml.
18 BBC (2009): 'Aparigraha'. See: www.bbc.co.uk/religion/religions/jainism/living/aparigraha.shtml.
19 Folkert KW, Cort JE (2010): 'Jainism', in *The Penguin Handbook of the World's Living Religions*, ed. Hinnells JR, chapter 7, pp. 344–345.
20 Braun W (2017): *Jainism in World Religions for Healthcare Professionals*, Routledge, chapter 6, p. 89.
21 Folkert KW, Cort JE (2010): 'Jainism', in *The Penguin Handbook of the World's Living Religions*, ed. Hinnells JR, chapter 7, p. 360.

Chapter 20

Judaism

Description of the religion

Numbers practising the religion

At present, in terms of practising Jews, there are approximately 6 million in Israel,[1] 5.5 million in the USA and 300,000 in the UK.[2] Outside of Israel, Jews do not form more than 2% of any one country's population.[3] On a looser definition of Jewishness, including secular Judaism, the figures may be 50% higher.[4]

Origins and beliefs

Expressions of the faith

Judaism is the oldest monotheistic (or Abrahamic) religion and has undergone many developments over 3,500 years of existence. Its history is characterized by certain chosen people called prophets,[5] having divine revelations in the form of covenants. A covenant is a *quid pro quo* agreement in which God promises certain things to a chosen person or people in return for carrying out his wishes. Attempts to define Judaism in the 21st century are fraught with difficulty. As a religious group, Jews themselves vary in defining who they are and exactly what they believe in.

It is a religion that people are born into that determines a way of living. Jewish lineage follows the maternal line. Family and inter-family ties are strong. There are few converts. At times, throughout history, easy identification as a distinct group has resulted in unwarranted alienation and demonization.

For simplicity, Judaism can be grouped into its main practising schools (Orthodox, Reform, Conservative, Liberal and Reconstructionist), with the addition of secular Judaism (see later for more details). There can be great tensions between these different movements. 'Marrying out' is increasing *pari passu* with the growth of secular Judaism and there have been estimates of up to 50% of younger Jews doing this in Western societies. There are also substantial differences in attitudes to the status of Israel. Israel approximates to the geographical area of Canaan (the 'Promised Land' of the Hebrew Bible) gifted to the Jews by God before the creation of Christianity and Islam, whose adherents also have claims of occupation.

The overall result is great variation in individual Jews and Jewish families; their exact views and wishes cannot be assumed. The approach here will be to describe briefly the Hebrew Bible and Jewish law, the key historical timelines, the branches of Judaism, Jewish life and then important aspects of death and interment.

The Hebrew Bible and Jewish law

The Hebrew Bible is called the Tanakh. It has the same content as the Christian Old Testament but arranged differently. The first five books of Genesis, Exodus, Leviticus, Numbers and Deuteronomy are called the Torah (the Five Books of Moses or Pentateuch). Orthodoxy maintains that the Torah shows how God wants Jews to live. It contains 613 commandments and Jews refer to the ten best-known of these as the Ten Commandments or Decalogue.[6] Traditional belief is that God dictated the Torah to Moses on Mount Sinai and it was then transferred verbally until its written form emerged. However, problems with logistical datelines and comparison of literary styles has led scholars to the conclusion that there was no single author and that various sources had been brought together over time. Recently this conclusion has been challenged but there seems general agreement that the Torah as we know it dates from 400 BCE[7] and not the time of Moses.

In addition to the written Torah it is also traditionally believed that God revealed an additional 'oral Torah' to Moses that was also passed down by word of mouth until it was first written down in the 2nd century CE.[8] This is known as the Talmud, which is regarded as 'the heart of Judaism'.[9] In medieval times Moses Maimonides (1138–1204) produced his *Mishneh Torah* as a unifying systematic digest of Jewish law and liturgy to clarify the differences with Christianity and Islam.[10]

The Jewish books, as well as the biblical messages of faith in one God and being a chosen people, are essentially manuals of how to live. Although belief in life after death has been accepted by both Orthodox and Reform theologians,[11] the ultimate fate of individuals is left vague and the details are ambiguous and debatable.

Key timelines in the story of Judaism

The early history of the Jews is described in the Hebrew Bible. Abraham (ca 1750 BCE and the tenth-generational descendant of Noah[12]) is regarded as the father of the Jewish nation who professed a belief in a single omnipotent God. This contrasted strongly with the relaxed prevailing polytheism. God said to Abraham 'I promise to give your descendants all this land from the border of Egypt to the River Euphrates'[13] and 'The whole land of Canaan will belong to your descendants for ever and I will be their God'.[14] This is the original source of the Jewish claim to the 'promised land'. For this, God, to guarantee his covenant, required that 'From now on you must circumcise every baby boy when he is 8 days old . . . this will be a physical sign to show that my covenant with you is everlasting.[15]

Abraham's descendants were Isaac and Jacob (later called Israel) and the latter's 12 sons.[16] They ended up in Egypt because of a famine in Canaan and after approximately 140 years began to be persecuted.[17] Led by Moses after a revelation[18] they had a miraculous escape (celebrated by the Passover festival) across the Red Sea back to Canaan. Moses led the Israelites to Mount Sinai where he received more revelations from God who delivered the Ten Commandments (the Decalogue),[19] and additional laws on how to live. He reaffirmed His help to invade and recapture the land promised to Abraham[20] approximately 400 years earlier from those currently living there.[21]

Solomon (970–931 BCE) was the builder of the First Temple in Jerusalem but in the 6th century BCE Judah came under the rule of the Mesopotamian Nebuchadnezzar, who destroyed the First Temple of Solomon and deported around 10,000 wealthy Jewish professionals and craftsmen to his capital in Babylon. The first Jewish Exile had begun. This exilic period saw the emergence of the Hebrew language in its current form, the setting-down in print of sacred texts and the recognition of the Rabbi as a spiritual and educational leader. In 538 BCE Cyrus the Great gave the Jews permission to return to Jerusalem. The construction of a Second Temple began on the site of the First.

The Second Temple period extended for nearly 600 years and the land was sequentially under Persian, Greek, Hasmonean and Roman control. The authority of scripture, the refinement of Jewish law and the establishment of synagogues all developed, as did the emergence of Christianity. The Second Temple was destroyed by the Romans in 70 CE following a Jewish uprising and more Jews went into exile.

Interspersed with Christian crusades, later Islamic conquests built a Muslim shrine, the Dome of the Rock, on the site of the Second Temple in 691 CE, claiming Judaism's most sacred site for their own worship. The Jews regard all that was left from the Second Temple, the base of the Western Wall (the Wailing Wall), as the holiest place at which they can pray.

As Judaism entered the Middle Ages it had to cope with a more and more powerful and monolithic Papacy. Translations of the Jews' sacred books from Hebrew into European languages emphasized doctrinal differences.[22] Over time many religious persuasions and dissenting sects have suffered exclusion and persecution, but some anti-Jewish actions are particularly notable.[23]. Jews became stereotyped as crooked and greedy (e.g., Shylock in Shakespeare's *The Merchant of Venice*) and they were blamed for the 'Black Death' and the death of Christian children.[24] Moses Mendelssohn, the German Jewish Enlightenment Philosopher (1729–1786), believed that Jewish persecution was largely a result of their separateness from the societies in which they lived.[25]

Unfortunately, when the Reformation reduced the power of the Papacy, the Jews fared no better with the Protestants. Martin Luther, in his treatise *On the Jews and Their Lies* (1543), wrote, 'with their accursed usury they hold us and our property captive', 'wherever they have their synagogues nothing is found but a den of devils' and 'I advise that their houses also be razed and destroyed'.[26] Analogous anti-Jewish events increasingly involved the Muslim world.[27] It is argued that Luther's publication in the 16th century became a driver for Nazism in the 20th. In Germany from 1935 to 1945 there was persecution by the Nazis, limiting the Jews' civil rights, containing them in ghettos and ultimately attempting to exterminate them in what is now known as the Shoah (Holocaust), with approximately 6 million deaths; 90% of the Jewish populations of Germany, Poland and the Baltic States died.[28]

Theodore Herzl (1860–1904) believed in Jewish assimilation until he experienced extreme anti-Semitism in Austria. In 1896, he wrote *The Jewish State*, setting out the arguments for establishing a Jewish homeland; the First Zionist Conference was held in Basel, Switzerland, in 1897.[29] The aspiration to re-occupy Canaan as promised to the Jews by God through Abraham around 1750 BCE had been rekindled. Not all Jews welcomed Zionism and many still do not.

Following the end of the Second World War and the Holocaust, sympathy for the Jewish peoples was substantial and in 1947, the United Nations adopted a Partition Plan for Palestine recommending the creation of independent Arab and Jewish states with an internationalized Jerusalem. This was accepted by the Jews but not by the Arabs, and an immediate war followed. Among the continuing hostilities, two notable events are the Six-Day War in 1967 and the Yom Kippur War in 1973. There are Palestinian refugee camps in neighbouring states, with 80% of the Arabs in what became

Israel having been displaced. Their exodus was matched by an influx of Jews from other countries. The conflict continues to this day, with no peaceful resolution in sight.

Worship and lifestyle

Individual Jews' lives vary enormously. A summary of orthodoxy is given here. In a Jewish home, education is paramount, as is the role of the mother. There are strict rules for food – the Kosher diet.[30] Jewish life has a rhythm determined by the lunar months and between the sunsets of Friday and Saturday is the Sabbath. During the Sabbath there are prohibitions of certain types and attendance at the synagogue is usual.

The year has religious days, of which the most important are:

- the festival of the Passover, commemorating the exodus of Israelites from Egypt
- the festival of Pentecost, commemorating God's covenant with Moses on Mount Sinai
- Yom Kippur, the Day of Atonement, with a 25-hour fast on the theme of penitence.

Life has its stages through childhood, adolescence, adulthood and eventually death. Examples are as follows.

- *Brit milah*. Boys are circumcized on the eighth day of life to confirm the ongoing covenant between God and Abraham. Some liberal Jews no longer insist on this.
- *Bat mitzvah*. A ceremony (principally in Reform Judaism) for 12-year-old girls as an equivalent to the bar mitzvah for boys.
- *Bar mitzvah*. A ceremony for 13-year-old boys to celebrate their coming-of-age and adoption of adult responsibilities.

The branches of Judaism[31]

Defining the sub-divisions of Judaism, what exactly they believe in and what they stand for is very difficult – it's a changing landscape with many variations and much overlap. The general pattern is set out in Figure 20.1.

Orthodox Judaism. The majority of Jews in the UK belong to an Orthodox synagogue, although they themselves may not practise strict Orthodoxy, perhaps preferring the term 'traditional'. Orthodoxy is the only officially recognized Judaism in Israel. It implies adherence to the traditional Torah, the Talmud and Rabbinic writings, but 'modern Orthodoxy' attempts a practical and intellectual synthesis between tradition and culture.

A sub-section of Orthodoxy, now sometimes termed 'ultra-Orthodox' are the Heredi, and Hasidism is a sub-group within Heredi Judaism noted for its religious conservatism and social seclusion. The men wear distinctive dress (black overcoats and hats), and often have Payot (hair curls over the temples).

Reform Judaism emerged following the Enlightenment and questioned existing theological dogma. It seeks to adapt religious practice to modern times, carries out services in the vernacular and stresses the ethical and spiritual dimension of a Jewish life rather than strict adherence to the scriptures.

Conservative Judaism is a form of traditional Judaism that falls halfway between Orthodox Judaism and Reform Judaism but is separate from both. It is strong in the USA.

Liberal Judaism was founded in 1902 and is organized as a national union of autonomous communities. Judaism's religious and cultural traditions are applied within the framework of modern thinking and morality. It believes that Jewish texts should be reinterpreted in the light of modern scholarship and Jewish laws reassessed by their suitability for contemporary conditions.

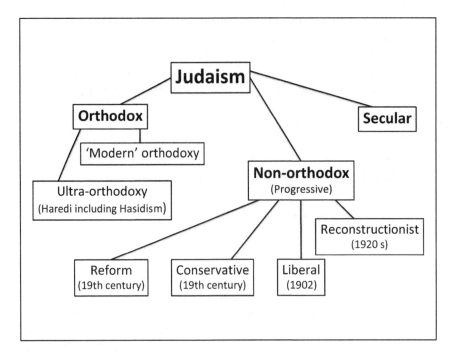

FIGURE 20.1 The main branches of Judaism

Reconstructionist Judaism was founded in the USA calling for a reappraisal of Judaism, including fundamental elements such as God, Israel and the Torah. In its practice it is more liberal than Reform Judaism and rejects the concept of the Jews as a 'chosen people'.

Secular Judaism describes the modern emergence of the 'non-religious' or 'cultural' Jew, who engages in cultural practices and family customs but is not religious, and may not even believe in a God. The majority of them admit to the influence of Jewish descent in their lives without the need or volition to practice it.

Care of the dying

As can be seen from the above, there is huge variety in the forms of Judaism practised and the belief systems followed. This means that patient- and family-oriented care can range from what is essentially the management of an agnostic through to care as set down in the Torah and Talmud. Therefore, establishing individual wishes at the outset is the key to best practice. Death is thought of as being natural, just as our lives are, and it has great meaning as part of God's overall plan. A common quotation from the Mishnah[32] is 'Against your will you live, and against your will you die'. What follows is an account of what would be appropriate for those of Orthodox practice. Non-Orthodox Jews may still follow these practices but many might not.

Judaism professes values for the sanctity of life and respect for the body, the body being a vessel which is a gift from God and must not be violated. One of the principal commandments in Judaism is visiting the sick (*bikur cholim*). To honour the dead and comfort the mourner are also important directives within Judaism, so deep religious meaning is devoted to death and dying, centred around the concepts of ritual, community and memory.

When ill, patients accept almost all forms of treatment and in life-threatening situations, non-Kosher food and omission of the duties of the Sabbath are permitted.

Judaism recognises passive and active euthanasia, and the latter, since it has connotations of suicide, is forbidden, but active palliative care is permitted. Great care needs to be taken in terms of the withdrawal of treatment and opinions vary very widely within the Jewish community. Although there is now genetic counselling, another aspect of Jewish illnesses are genetic diseases such as Tay-Sachs disease, Gaucher type-1 disease, familial dysautonomia, cystic fibrosis and breast and ovarian cancer as a result of intra-faith marriage. There can be a distressing poignancy of family members witnessing deaths of relatives from the same cause.

Hospital staff need to remember that Kosher food is likely to be required subject to the patient's wishes, and some ultra-Orthodox Jews may only accept Kosher medication. Even though in hospital, the patient, accompanied by a friend or relative, may still wish to celebrate the Sabbath, observe festivals and fasts. If these requirements are counter to clinical care, most Jews will accept medical advice.

Orthodox Jewish women prefer to have their bodies and limbs covered and might keep their head covered with a scarf. Orthodox men also keep their head partially covered with a hat or skullcap (Kappel).

The patient may wish to meet with their Rabbi (with or without the presence of relatives), or hear psalms and prayers (particularly Psalm 23, 'The Lord is my Shepherd'), and may appreciate being able to hold onto the page on which it is written. Prayers may also be said by the relatives.

Management of death

Once death has been verified, the eyes and mouth of the body should be closed by a child, relative or close friend. It is customary for Jews to be buried as soon as possible after death, and preferably within 24 hours. Delay in funeral arrangements can be distressing to the relatives, hence certification concerning death should be completed expeditiously. Exceptions allowing delay would be the Sabbath or a major festival. Orthodox Judaism requires that after death the body should not be left alone until the funeral is over since it is believed to be vulnerable until placed in its final resting place in the grave. Somebody known as 'a watcher' may be appointed to stay with the body until its removal from hospital.

The body should be handled as little as possible by healthcare staff with only the minimum of laying out. To prevent causing offence, it is traditional when referring to the deceased to add 'Alav Hashalom' (may peace be upon him). After death the *chevra kedisha* (or holy society) are sent for. They are authorized to clean and ritually purify bodies of the same sex as themselves. Afterwards the body can be covered with a white sheet or dressed in white clothes.

Non-Orthodox Jews would accept the last offices being performed by healthcare staff if the family were not available or did not want to do it themselves. Some non-Orthodox Jews allow cremation, but this is not the norm.

The immediate mourning period, known as the *shiva* (sitting), lasts for seven days. Close relatives (spouses, parents, siblings, children), rend an outer garment, remove their shoes and sit at home on the floor or on a low stool. People who know the deceased visit the bereaved to offer condolences and to pray for the deceased. A further period of less intensive mourning continues for the remainder of 30 days and children mourn for one year for parents.

Autopsy and organ transplantation

Jewish law requires that after death, the body should be buried in its entirety. The belief is that man is created in God's image and mutilation of the body is forbidden.

Autopsy examinations are not allowed under religious rules, but a coroner's decision can overrule this.

There has been a change in the law concerning autopsies. In the High Court in 2015 an application was made by a Jewish family to prevent a conventional autopsy being done on an 86-year-old lady who had already had a post-mortem MRI. Article 9(2) of the Human Rights' Act (the right to freedom of thought, conscience and religion) was cited and the ruling was that religious beliefs should be considered before a coroner makes their decision.[33] This does not negate the ultimate authority of the coroner, but it does change working practices. If there is a post-mortem examination of the body, the ritual cleansing and clothing of the body will begin afterwards.

Preservation of life is important in Judaism, so there is usually no fundamental objection to organ donation. Some Orthodox Jews may be less willing and there remains uncertainty about the concept of brain death in some sects who cannot accept brain death as the death of the individual.

Further reading

- Rutty J: 'Judaism', in *E-Learning for Health*, Royal College of Pathologists, 'Faith Considerations Part 1: Abrahamic Faiths', published on the web by Health Education England NHS (undated), available at; www.e-lfh.org.uk/programmes/medical-examiner/.
- Solomon N (2014): *Judaism: A Very Short Introduction*, Oxford University Press.
- DK (2013): 'Judaism', in *The Religions Book*, UK edn, Dorling Kindersley, pp. 166–199.
- Kahn-Harris K (2012): *Judaism: All that Matters*, Hodder Education.

Notes

1 70% of the population.
2 Solomon N (2014): *Judaism: A Very Short Introduction*, Oxford University Press, p. 17.
3 Kahn-Harris K (2012): *Judaism: All That Matters*, Hodder Education, p. 2.
4 Solomon N (2014): *Judaism: A Very Short Introduction*, Oxford University Press, p. 17.
5 There are generally accepted to be 48 male and 7 female prophets, key figures being Abraham, Isaac, Jacob, Moses and David. Jewish prophets also feature in Christianity and Islam.

6 Most commonly referred to as the Ten Commandments by Christians and non-Jews.
7 Kaminsky JS, Lohr JN (2011): *The Torah*, Oneworld Publications, chapter 3, 'Modern Approaches to the Torah', pp. 42–69 and figure 6, p. 49.
8 Solomon N (2014): *Judaism: A Very Short Introduction*, Oxford University Press, chapter 3, p. 33.
9 *Ibid.*, p. 35.
10 *Ibid.*, pp. 31–54.
11 *Ibid.*, chapter 6, pp. 97–98.
12 Genesis 11:10–26 traces the familial descent from Noah's son Shem to Abram (later called Abraham), through nine generations. All were very long-lived with lifetimes of between 148 and 950 years.
13 Genesis 15:18.
14 Genesis 17:8.
15 Genesis 17:13.
16 The ancestors of the 12 Tribes of Israel.
17 Exodus 1:13–22.
18 Exodus 3:2–12. This is the famous story of the burning bush.
19 Exodus 20:1–18.
20 Exodus 23:20–27.
21 Exodus 33:1–2.
22 Smart N (2002): *The World's Religions*, Cambridge University Press, pp. 269–272.
23 Here, anti-Semitism will be taken to mean an illogical, uninformed and bigoted dislike of Jews, both individually and collectively.
24 Kahn-Harris K (2012): *Judaism: All That Matters*, Hodder Education, pp. 75–76.
25 DK (2013): *The Religions Book*, UK edn, Dorling Kindersley, p. 189.
26 Luther M (1543): *On the Jews and Their Lies*, trans. D'Abrusso D (2015), CreateSpace Independent Publishing Platform, pp. 162, 39 and 168.
27 Kahn-Harris K (2012): *Judaism: All That Matters*, Hodder Education, pp. 78–79.
28 *Ibid.*, p. 87.
29 DK (2013): *The Religions Book*, UK edn, Dorling Kindersley, p. 197.
30 Only animals with a cloven hoof, those who chew their cud, fish with scales and fins and poultry are permitted. The animals must be slaughtered by rapid blood loss (*shechita*), and there will be two sets of cutlery for meat and dairy products.
31 This section is a meld from Charing D (1996): 'Judaism', in *Six World Faiths*, ed. Owen Cole W, Cassell, pp. 62–63; Solomon N (2014): *Judaism: A Very Short Introduction*, Oxford University Press, chapter 7; DK (2013): *The Religions Book*, UK edn, Dorling Kindersley, 'Progressive Judaism', pp. 190–195; Kahn-Harris K (2012): *Judaism: All That Matters*, Hodder Education, chapter 6, 'Divisions'; and the BBC religion/Judaism website: www.bbc.co.uk/religion/religions/judaism.
32 Pirkei Avot 4:22.
33 Neutral Citation Number: [2015] EWHC 2764 (Admin) in the High Court of Justice Queen's Bench Division, the Administrative Court.

Chapter 21

Rastafarianism

Description of the religion

Numbers practising the religion

There are approximately 1 million worldwide adherents of Rastafarianism as a faith, with 5,000 living in England and Wales.[1] They are known by a variety of names (some resented) such as Rastafarians, Rastas, Sufferers, Locksmen, Dreads or Dreadlocks.[2]

Origins and development

Rastafarianism is a political, social and religious movement which emerged in Jamaica during a period of increasing awareness of the 'African-ness' of the black population of the new world in the late 19th century. People descended from African slaves were forced to adopt the slave-owners' mainly protestant Christianity, whilst their traditional beliefs were devalued.[3] A specifically Jamaican interpretation of the scriptures emerged. The Holy Piby, published in the 1920s, became the written basis of what grew to be Rastafarianism, and identified the Old Testament's Zion as being in Africa, probably in Ethiopia – a future home for émigré black people.[4] Following the work of the Jamaican leader Marcus Garvey (who formed the Universal Negro Improvement Association in 1914), and other early activists such as Howells, Dunkley, Hibbert and Henry,[5] by the 1950s the movement was strongly anti-white.[6] This is now no longer the case. The Rastafari were identified as a new force countering oppression and exploitation by 'Babylon', their name for corrupt Europeans who had initiated and maintained the profit-making slave trade from the 1500s to the 1800s.[7] A key objective of Rastafarianism is 'to deligitimise and destroy, or 'chant-down', Babylon, restoring black people to their African selves and their status as human beings endowed with divine consciousness'.[8]

Garvey directed his criticism at white supremacy and those blacks who accepted their inferiority.[9] This position has since been significantly modified accepting that God is in all men, with a deep respect for nature and justice for all.[10,11] There are an increasing number of white adherents,[12] emphasis on racial issues has greatly abated and it is now considered a global movement.[13]

The old texts prophesied that a saviour from the family of Judah would come to Zion (Africa) to free them from oppression. The savior appeared as Ras (Prince) Tafari (God's chosen king on earth), who became Emperor Haile Selassie of Ethiopia, the Conquering Lion of the Tribe of Judah. The new Holy Land for the Rastafari had arrived in the Horn of Africa, and many saw Haile Selassie as the second coming of Jesus.[14]

In the 1950s the religion spread as Caribbean migrants left to seek work in Britain and America. It became associated with Jamaican culture and music. Through the latter medium of reggae, the movement was greatly popularized by the pop star Bob Marley.

Haile Selassie's death in 1975 was described by his followers as his 'disappearance', and some of them refused to believe he had died. Following his death and the increased acceptance of Jamaican culture in other societies, many Rastafarian beliefs have been modified since their inception.[15] There is no formal Rastafari creed and there are differences in the views of different groups, represented by three main 'Houses' or 'Mansions'.[16] There is no ruling body and the membership is best described as a loose association.[17]

Beliefs, worship and lifestyle

It is difficult to describe precisely what the exact belief paradigm is because of its variability amongst different groups. The following are accepted features.[18]

- There is a single Judeo-Christian God (Jah). Rastafarian beliefs are based in Judaism and Christianity, with an emphasis on Old Testament laws and prophecies and the Book of Revelation. Jah was first manifested on earth as Jesus, and second by Emperor Haile Selassie. The temple is within each individual.
- Most believe that reincarnation follows death and that life is eternal. Salvation can be an earthly rather than heavenly state. Some believe in the resurrection of the soul after death, but not the flesh.
- Eating natural vegetarian food (I-tal) and being as close to nature as possible by avoiding processed foods and meat is important. There is abstinence from most or all meat, scavengers, shellfish, artificial foods and alcohol.

- Rastafari don't have specific religious buildings set aside for worship. They usually meet weekly, either in a believer's home or in a community centre. The meetings are referred to as Reasoning Sessions. They provide a time for chants, prayers and singing, and for communal issues to be discussed. The chanting, drumming and meditating is to reach a state of heightened spirituality, sometimes with the ritual use of marijuana (ganja) to increase spiritual awareness.
- Many Rasta men uphold patriarchal values; there is a separate code of religious practice for women and the movement has been charged with sexism.
- Rastafarians are forbidden to cut their hair; instead, they grow it and twist it into dreadlocks.
- Most Rastafari are opposed to abortion and contraception.
- There is no formal marriage structure. A Rastafari man and woman who live together are regarded as husband and wife. If marriage does take place it is regarded as a social occasion rather than a religious event.
- Anyone who takes a life, including their own, is assumed to be condemned forever.

Care of the dying

Usually there are no specifically religious requirements so normal care is appropriate. However, some believers have an antipathy towards Western medicine and may have tried, or prefer, alternative therapies such as herbalism. Some are proud of their flag colours (red for the spilt blood, yellow for the riches of their homeland and green for the beauty of Ethiopia), and may incorporate them into clothing. There is individual variability on the management of their hair for both men and women. Misgivings concerning second-hand clothing may necessitate the use of disposable gowns.

Management of death

There are no formal last rites. Routine last offices with no cutting of the hair is appropriate. The funeral is plain and simple and attended only by family and friends. Burial is preferred, but cremation is permitted. The body may be flown back to the country of origin.

There are no official mourning rituals, but family and friends are very supportive of the bereaved.

Autopsy and organ transplantation

Organ donation and autopsy are traditionally considered distasteful, but many individuals will grant permission.

Further reading

- See BBC website (2009): www.bbc.co.uk/religion/religions/rastafari/.
- Edmonds EB (2012): *Rastafari: A Very Short Introduction*, Oxford University Press.
- Stuart O (2010): 'Africa Diaspora Religion', in *The Penguin Handbook of the World's Living Religions*, ed. Hinnells JR, chapter 20, pp. 717–719.
- DK (2013): *The Religions Book*, UK edn, Dorling Kindersley, 'The Lion of Judah Has Arisen', pp. 314–315.

Notes

1 See BBC (2009): 'Rastafari at a Glance'. Available at: www.bbc.co.uk/religion/religions/rastafari/.
2 *Ibid.*
3 DK (2013): *The Religions Book*, UK edn, Dorling Kindersley, 'The Lion of Judah Has Arisen', p. 315.
4 Rogers AR (1924–1928): The Holy Piby, Global Grey (2017). This is now only available as a pdf download available at: www.globalgreyebooks.com/holy-piby-ebook/; at times it has been a banned book and there are very few original texts left.
5 Stuart O (2010): 'Africa Diaspora Religion', in *The Penguin Handbook of the World's Living Religions*, ed. Hinnells JR, chapter 20, p. 718.
6 Smart N (1998): *The World's Religions*, 2nd edn, Cambridge University Press, 'Latin America and the Caribbean', p. 569.
7 DK (2013): *The Religions Book*, UK edn, Dorling Kindersley, 'The Lion of Judah Has Arisen', p. 315.
8 Edmonds EB (2012): *Rastafari: A Very Short Introduction*, Oxford University Press, chapter 2, p. 42.
9 Stuart O (2010): 'Africa Diaspora Religion', in *The Penguin Handbook of the World's Living Religions*, ed. Hinnells JR, chapter 20, p. 717.
10 See BBC (2009): 'Modern Rastafari Beliefs'. Available at: www.bbc.co.uk/religion/religions/rastafari/.
11 Anbessa-Ebanks KB (2003): *Rastafarianism in World Religions*, ed. Gill D, Collins, chapter 10, p. 156.
12 See BBC (2009): 'Beliefs about Race'. Available at: www.bbc.co.uk/religion/religions/rastafari/.
13 Edmonds EB (2012): *Rastafari: A Very Short Introduction*, Oxford University Press, chapter 4, 'Rastafari International: The Making of a Global Movement', p. 71.
14 DK (2013): *The Religions Book*, UK edn, Dorling Kindersley, 'The Lion of Judah Has Arisen', pp. 314–315.
15 See BBC (2009): 'Modern Rastafarian Beliefs'. Available at: www.bbc.co.uk/religion/religions/rastafari/.
16 Edmonds EB (2012): *Rastafari: A Very Short Introduction*, Oxford University Press, chapter 3, 'Grounding, Houses, and Mansions: Social Formation of Rastafari', p. 52.
17 Stuart O (2010): 'Africa Diaspora Religion', in *The Penguin Handbook of the World's Living Religions*, ed. Hinnells JR, chapter 20, p. 718.
18 This list is a meld taken from www.bbc.co.uk/religion/religions/rastafari/ and Edmonds EB (2012): *Rastafari: A Very Short Introduction*, Oxford. The responsibility for the selection of the list rests with the authors.

Chapter 22

Secular philosophies and other belief systems

Description of secular philosophies and other belief systems

The numbers of followers and the classification of secular philosophies and other belief systems

As can be seen from Chapter 12, the UK estimates for the numbers of the population unassociated with any conventional religion can range from 25% to 50% and the numbers vary across the world. This does not imply that these people will be aligned to another particular alternative spiritual or non-religious philosophy; they may just get on with life without any thought for its meaning or the need for religion. Hence, although the membership of certain organizations (e.g., Humanists UK[1] claim over 65,000 members) can be ascertained, there are little hard data available on the numbers adhering to self-determined secular philosophies or other beliefs. For information, interested readers are advised to consult the many websites available.

Categorizing secular philosophies and belief systems is very difficult because of syncretism, i.e., the variable overlap with conventional religious beliefs and the detail of individual doctrines. There are very many separate sects and movements but here we will consider atheism, agnosticism, humanism, spirituality, New Age movements, paganism and Scientology.

As elsewhere, there are also problems with the interpretation of words, e.g., some 'secularists' do not believe in God; others mean it to imply a separation of Church and State. Consequently, this chapter focuses on those areas where there is general agreement on what the terms mean and what the basic principles are.

Atheism and agnosticism[2]

Atheism

The term 'atheism' comes from the Greek word *atheos* meaning 'without gods'. It is a term often associated with the challenges to religion during the Enlightenment of the 17th and 18th centuries, but atheism has in fact been around for thousands of years.[3] In philosophical discussions atheism can be further sub-categorized by terms such as 'implicit' and 'explicit' and 'strong' and 'weak' atheism, together with the assertion that until children are educated in religion they will have no belief in a God or gods and are hence at least agnostic. For the purposes of this book we will accept the definition given recently by Gray[4] that 'an atheist is anyone with no use for the idea of a divine mind that has fashioned the world'.

Some atheists are criticized that their aggressive dogma is a form of religion because it has no absolute proof; others simply assert that the chances in favour of there being a supernatural being are so small as to be immeasurable. The definition we are using sidesteps these opinions since it is based on the usefulness and relevance of a God (or gods) to everyday life rather than to the details of their existence. As such it is not dissimilar in some ways to deism (see Chapter 4), where God is an absent landlord. Grey describes seven types of atheism and compares them with monotheistic faiths, concluding that 'If you can see how theologies that affirm the ineffability of God and some types of atheism are not so far apart, you will learn something about the limits of human understanding'.[5]

Agnosticism

Agnosticism (Greek prefix *a-*, meaning 'not', combined with *gnostos*, 'known') is, strictly speaking, the doctrine that humans cannot know of the existence of anything beyond the phenomena of their experience. As it is commonly understood today, its usage was introduced by the evolutionary biologist T.H. Huxley in the 19th century[6] to describe his own position in relation to evidential objections to belief. However, even in antiquity Protagoras of Abdera (486–411 BCE) stated (perhaps to defend himself from persecution), that 'Concerning the gods, I have no means of knowing whether they exist or not or of what sort they may be. Many things prevent knowledge including the obscurity of the subject and the brevity of human life'.[7]

Thereby he established himself traditionally as the original agnostic. An agnostic is nowadays regarded as anyone who doesn't claim to know whether any gods exist or not and asserts the position that 'a Creator, creative cause and an unseen world are things unknown and unknowable'.[8]

Current practice

There continue to be discussions about the minutiae of atheism and agnosticism because both deal with questions related to the existence of God or gods. Although not universally accepted, the following two are probably reasonable summary statements.

- Atheism involves what a person does or does not *believe*; agnosticism involves what a person does or does not *know*. Although belief and knowledge are related but separate issues that have occupied many pages in epistemology, the essence of this statement is clear in the context used.
- To further complicate matters, an *agnostic atheist* doesn't believe in any gods while an *agnostic theist* believes in the existence of at least one god but neither make the claim to have the knowledge to back up these beliefs.

All atheists and most agnostics recognize that life has a beginning and an end. There is a cycle and limitation to life with death bringing about the end of an individual's existence. Any significance in life lies in the contribution a person makes to others and the experiences and satisfactions that are achieved. Managing death is a personal matter for the patient and their relatives.

People who follow the social and ethical lifestyle of a religion but no longer believe its supernatural credos often link the name of their family religion with another word to indicate the lack of worship and belief. Examples of this are Christian atheism, humanistic Judaism and those classing themselves as secular Sikhs.[9]

Humanism

Humanism[10] is a belief in human-based morality. It is a system of thought that is based on the values, characteristics and behaviour that are believed to be best in human beings, rather than on any supernatural authority. Its principles have existed in one form or another for thousands of years in the works of Aristotle, Seneca, Marcus Aurelius etc., but the word humanism is a descriptor dating from the 19th century.

Although its boundaries vary, humanism is distinguished by the following (in no specific order of importance).

- Living one's life by a commitment to an ethical framework and rational moral values, with no adherence to imposed dogmas, illogical authority or divine scriptures.

- Life has meaning without the need for a supernatural being. There is no necessity for a belief in God, gods, angels, demons and other supernatural beings.
- A belief that this life is the only one we have; there is no anticipation of an afterlife or reincarnation.
- An emphasis on each person having moral autonomy and being responsible for their own actions to promote the flourishing of themselves and others.
- An acceptance of all types of persons as valuable and a respect for animals and the environment.
- A conviction of the importance of reason (and the scientific viewpoint), and applying it to all areas of life, with no 'no-go' areas. Nothing should be excluded from scrutiny.
- A wish for individual freedom within an open democratic society with the state protecting the rights and freedoms of all of its people and not supporting any particular religion or grouping. Humanists are opposed to coercion into any belief system, whether it be religious or an atheist totalitarianism.

Whilst it is legally necessary to obtain conventional birth, marriage and death certificates, humanists do have ceremonies with humanist celebrants to mark and celebrate the rights of passage through life.

Baby-naming ceremonies do not dedicate a child to follow a religion but instead focus on parents, friends and relations being allowed to express their commitment to help this new life to flourish and in time to develop its own beliefs and moral judgements. Similarly, humanist weddings follow no set menu but instead allow the couple to congregate with their family and friends to celebrate their discovery of each other and to commit to a long-term partnership of mutual respect, understanding and support.

Humanist funerals are becoming increasingly popular. They are non-religious but there is provision within them for religious-based readings. The emphasis is on the marking of an end to an individual's life. The service allows family and friends in their own preferred way to celebrate and grieve for a life with honesty, dignity, sadness and joy without the involvement of a numinous being.

Spirituality

Spirituality is a difficult and variable concept that defies exact definition. This is partly because it has passed from its traditional place in religious scriptures into the parlance of secular lifestyle philosophies. Whatever the reason, there is no doubt that its use as the descriptor of an ideology with links to a respect for ecology and New Age movements is increasing.

The desire to achieve spirituality in some form or another is a feature of almost all religions and is described in the accompanying chapters. In the 19th and early 20th centuries, intellectual questioning of the evidence for the existence of spirituality or of the worthwhileness of its pursuit as a religious concept became more frequent. Although he strongly defended the right to believe and be religious, prominent in this regard was William James with his two books *The Varieties of Religious Experience: A Study in Human Nature*[11] and *The Will to Believe; and Other Essays in Popular Philosophy and Human Immortality*.[12] A regular trickle of similar publications continued but in the 20th century one of the most controversial Christian books emerged with the publication in 1963 of Bishop Robinson's *Honest to God*,[13] which challenged the nature of true belief and was described as 'probably the most talked about theological work of the twentieth century' by a *Guardian* newspaper reviewer.

Although *Honest to God* related to Christianity, it could just have easily been written about any established religion, so its contributions have universal application. As time has passed, science has advanced and society has changed; the views he expressed over 50 years ago now seem prescient, relevant and realistic. *Honest to God* questioned the traditional image of God as an anthropomorphic supernatural being substituting instead a loving immaterial universality around the New Testament's indefinable concept of 'grace'.[14]

For some people these concepts were too radical, but for many they chimed with their experience of life and the need to move on from the fairy-tale elements of traditional scriptures revealed by new discoveries in science, medicine and modern living with its national and international inequalities. Accordingly, profane or non-theistic religions emerged with the concept of 'Religion without God'.[15] Ray Billington, the author, was dismissed from his living as a Methodist minister because of his unconventional views. He said[16] 'it has become engrained in the human psyche that "religion" involves certain specific acts, places, people, lifestyles and beliefs, so that where these are absent from a person's life, he or she is generally viewed as not being religious'; he continued, 'on the one hand religion is real and universal and, on the other God is unreal but has localised aficionados'.

To make the point real he gives examples from music, art and nature (including sexual pleasure), where humans feel an experience beyond and deeper than the norm. This he equates with a form of religious understanding and participation as part of a total universal significance.

Perhaps Wordsworth, as he was musing in July 1798, put the wonder of the mystical aspects of life as well as anybody.

> And I have felt
> A presence that disturbs me with the joy
> Of elevated thoughts; a sense sublime
> Of something far more deeply interfused,
> Whose dwelling is the light of setting suns,
> And the round ocean and the living air,
> And the blue sky, and in the mind of man:
> A motion and a spirit, that impels
> All thinking things, all objects of all thought,
> And rolls through all things. Therefore am I still
> A lover of the meadows and the woods
> And mountains; and of all that we behold
> From this green earth; of all the mighty world
> Of eye, and ear – both what they half create,
> And what perceive; well pleased to recognise
> In nature and the language of the sense
> The anchor of my purest thoughts, the nurse,
> The guide, the guardian of my heart, and soul
> Of all my moral being.[17]

Out of such sentiments arise the elements of spirituality without a religious dependency and the quotation is offered as an insight into the modern understanding of 'spirituality'. Although it defies exact definition, spirituality includes the following dimensions.[18]

- It embodies a vision of human existence and of how the human spirit is to achieve its full potential.
- It expresses a sense that human life involves more than biology.
- It finds an expression in social science, education, business studies, the arts and sport.
- Attention to an individual's spirituality is increasingly seen as important in all aspects of healthcare and has been emphasized as an important factor in psychological illness.[19]
- It can help in the quest to understand the personal meaning of life.
- It promotes a self-reflective existence as opposed to an unexamined life.

New Age movements

New Age movements are very difficult to define and characterize and few have any sort of established creed. They developed in the 1970s and 1980s in Western nations as part of counter-culture, with a significant representation in the UK. The groups typically adopt a belief in a holistic spirit that pervades the whole universe, including human beings themselves. There is a strong emphasis on the spiritual authority of the self, accompanied by beliefs in a wide variety of semi-divine non-human entities, astrology and artefacts such as Tarot cards. They are decentralized social and spiritual movements that seek universal truths and the attainment of the highest individual human potential. As with aspects of spirituality, in various ways they explore the idea that this life and this world is not the totality of existence.

Examples of New Age movements are set within monism, pantheism, and panentheism.[20] There may be involvement of astrology and spiritualism, with common derivatives associated with these belief systems, such as reincarnation, Karma, and auras.[21] Included are personal transformations through mystical experience and mediumship and some very clear ideas about the fate of the human spirit in the first few minutes and hours after death. A focus on ecological responsibility or the possibility of a universal religion is also common.

Spiritualism – also thousands of years old but made famous in the UK after the national grief and bereavement associated with the First World War (see Chapter 6) – asserts a belief in an afterlife where the deceased are contactable through a medium or technologies such as scrying,[22] ouija boards,[23] or electronic voice phenomena[24] (EVP).

These concepts are all also advocated by many in popular literature, and lend support to the idea of an afterlife and afterlife communication, which to some of this persuasion feel to be just in the 'next room'. Sometimes these experiences are accompanied by quite specific associated practices around death, e.g., not cremating the dead for at least three days. These beliefs also complicate and challenge medical ideas about 'brain death' as death of the whole personality. Some New Agers may not be consciously aware that they have incorporated these kinds of beliefs because such ideas and arguments are secreted into today's informal popular writings. A whole raft of this literature and countless authors advocating these ideas are easily found in today's New Age or theosophical book shops where people buy their Tarot cards, healing crystals or inspirational literature while getting their fortunes told or contacting their dead by appointment.

Paganism

Paganism[25] is a word initially used by the early Christian Church to label other, non-Christian practices. Gradually, along with terms such as 'heathen' it came to describe a vast array of belief systems characterized by links with natural forces, iconography and idol worship, often in a derogatory manner. It is therefore necessary to clearly state that pagan practices do not involve harming people or animals. This short section will focus on the expression of paganism in the modern world, often termed neo-paganism.

Pagan practices encompass a diverse community that usually celebrates festivals based on 'the wheel of the year', with the most important dates being the solstices and the equinoxes. Most pagans share an ecological vision that comes from the pagan belief in the organic vitality and spirituality of the natural world. Wiccans, druids, shamans, sacred ecologists, odinists and heathens are all represented within the pagan community. There is a general emphasis on making the most of the present life although there may be a belief in an afterlife.

Probably the best known of the 20th century movements is Wicca, which was founded in England in the 1950s by Gerald Gardiner (1884–1964). He wove an account of how he had been initiated into a witches' coven in the New Forest that practised pre-Christian traditions that had been kept alive in a manuscript known as *The Book of Shadows*. From this story Gardiner created a vibrant pagan revival under the umbrella of 'witchcraft' that spread internationally.

Although there is great variation in pagan expression, a unifying inter-national theme is respect for the environment that can be associated with secular traditions, monotheism and polytheism. Davies concludes[26] that 'As a concept, it (paganism) is no less relevant than when it was redefined by Christians nearly two millennia ago. It has retained its ability to stimulate intellectual curiosity and spiritual exploration'.

Scientology

Scientology was invented in 1954 by L. Ron Hubbard, a science-fiction writer, and he published a creed as to how Scientology should guide its followers. Of note are the first two statements:

- that all men of whatever race, color or creed were created with equal rights;
- that all men have inalienable rights to their own religious practices and their performance.[27]

So, a person can be a Scientologist whilst retaining membership of another faith group. The goal of Scientology is making the individual capable of liv-ing a better life in his own estimation and that of his fellows and the playing of a better game (of life).[28] The movement has the equivalent of religious services, promotes education and counselling and is now international.

The number of followers is estimated in the millions, some of whom are celebrity names, e.g., Tom Cruise and John Travolta. It is accepted in some countries, but not the UK as a religion for the purposes of tax law.

Scientology teaches that man's true spiritual nature is constantly reborn as an eternal spirit called a Thetan, which separates from the body on death.[29] There is a process of counselling known as 'auditing' to assist adherents to free the unconscious mind and return to a true spiritual identity, the effectiveness of which is measured using an E-meter to detect the body's electrical currents. Progressing through various levels of auditing they eventually reach the level of 'Operating Thetan', and re-discover their original potential.[30]

Although Scientology has its supporters, it has also been accused of exploitation, intimidation and the ruination of lives.[31] Readers can weigh the evidence and make their own minds up about this.

Summary

This chapter has described a selection of secular philosophies and alternative belief systems. All demonstrate that it seems inherent in man for him to question his existence and create supports that help with life and death. There are many other sects and groupings that are not covered here and when they present in the clinical situation it becomes necessary for the healthcare worker to sympathetically establish what is important to the individual and how they can best manage their treatment, both physically and psychologically.

Care of the dying

There is so much variation within the groups considered that individual management is required after sympathetic and careful discussion.

Management of death

Again, there are no absolute rules, but with most of the groups considered in this section, last offices by healthcare staff are usually acceptable. Funeral arrangements need to follow individual preferences.

Autopsy and organ transplantation

With atheism, agnosticism and humanism there are usually no objections. For other groups, individual wishes need to be followed.

Further reading

- Rutty J: 'Christianity', in *E-Learning for Health*, Royal College of Pathologists, 'Faith Considerations Part 4: Other Traditions', published on the web by Health Education England NHS (undated), available at; www.e-lfh.org.uk/programmes/medical-examiner/.
- Law S (2011): *Humanism: A Very Short Introduction*, Oxford University Press.
- Sheldrake P (2012): *Spirituality: A Very Short Introduction*, Oxford University Press.
- Billington R (2002): *Religion without God*, Routledge.
- Davies O (2011): *Paganism: A Very Short Introduction*, Oxford University Press.
- Hubbard LR (2007): *Scientology – The Fundamentals of Thought*, New Era Publications International ApS.

Notes

1 https://humanism.org.uk.
2 The origins of these philosophies are traditionally taken to have been dated from Cârvâka (atheism; 600 BCE) and Protagoras (agnosticism; 500 BCE).
3 Whitmarsh T (2016): *Battling the Gods: Atheism in the Ancient World*, Faber & Faber.
4 Gray J (2018): *Seven Types of Atheism*, Allen Lane, p. 2.
5 *Ibid.*, p. 158.
6 Huxley TH (1889): *Collected Essays*, Vol. V, Project Guttenberg e-book, available at: www.gutenberg.org/cache/epub/15905/pg15905.txt, chapters VII, VIII and IX. Huxley used the term verbally before this in 1869, but this is where he discusses its meaning in detail.
7 See the Internet Encyclopedia of Philosophy: 'Protagoras'; Sec 3.c. Available at www.iep.utm.edu/protagor/#SH3c.
8 Anon. (2014): *Chambers Dictionary*, 13th edn, Chambers Harrap Publishers.
9 Singh T (2007): 'Living as a Secular Sikh: A Personal View'. Available at: www.shapworkingparty.org.uk/journals/articles_0708/singh.pdf.
10 This section is taken from Law S (2011): *Humanism: A Very Short Introduction*, Oxford University Press, pp. 1–3, 88–90 and 135–141. The responsibility for the presented text remains with the authors.
11 James W (originally published in 1902, this edition 2009): *The Varieties of Religious Experience: A Study in Human Nature*, Seven Treasures Publications.
12 James W (originally published 1912): *The Will to Believe; and Other Essays in Popular Philosophy and Human Immortality*, published in facsimile by Pantianos Classics.
13 Robinson J (1963): *Honest to God*, SCM Press, reissued 50th-anniversary edition (2013).
14 *Ibid.*, p. 53.
15 Billington R (2002): *Religion without God*, Routledge, chapters 9, 10 and 11.
16 *Ibid.*, p. 92.
17 Wordsworth W (2004): *Selected Poems*, ed. Gill S, Penguin Classics, p. 64.

18 Sheldrake P (2012): *Spirituality: A Very Short Introduction*, Oxford University Press, introduction and chapter 1.
19 RCPsych (2013): 'Recommendations for Psychiatrists on Spirituality and Religion'. Available at: www.rcpsych.ac.uk/pdf/Recommendations%20for%20 Psychiatrists%20on%20Spirituality%20and%20Religion%20Revised.x.pdf.
20 A supreme being is all that exists and transcends the universe.
21 An aura is an energy field radiated by the body invisible to most people.
22 Moody R (1993): *Reunions: Visionary Encounters with Departed Loved Ones*, New York, Villard Books. Scrying is the use of crystal balls and other symbols.
23 Dahlman KA (2013): *The Spirits of Ouija: Four Decades of Communication*, Creative Visions Pub. A ouija board is a board with letters, numbers and other signs around its edge, to which a planchette, movable pointer or upturned glass moves, supposedly in answer to questions from people at a seance.
24 Raudive K (1971): *Breakthrough: An Amazing Experiment in Electronic Communication with the Dead*, Colin Smythe.
25 This section is taken from: Davies O (2011): *Paganism: A Very Short Introduction*, Oxford; BBC (2006): 'Paganism'. Available at: www.bbc.co.uk/religion/religions/ paganism/; and DK (2013): *The Religions Book*, UK edn, Dorling Kindersley, 'Spirits Rest between Lives in Summerland', p. 319.
26 Davies O (2011): *Paganism: A Very Short Introduction*, Oxford University Press, p. 127.
27 See www.scientologyreligion.org/background-and-beliefs/the-creed-of-the-church-of-scientology.html.
28 Hubbard LR (2007): *Scientology: The Fundamentals of Thought*, New Era Publications International ApS, p. 107.
29 *Ibid.*, p. 77.
30 DK (2013): *The Religions Book*, UK edn, Dorling Kindersley, 'We Have Forgotten Our True Nature', p. 317.
31 Sweeney J (2013): *The Church of Fear*, Silvertail Books.

Chapter 23

Shintoism

Description of the religion

Numbers practising the religion

Shintoism is quintessentially the lifestyle religion of Japan and its relevance is largely within Japan's geographical boundaries. Approximately 80% of the Japanese population identify with Shintoism and nearly 70% with Buddhism. These are usually the same people, since dual belief is common.[1] The commonest current form of Buddhism in Japan is Zen. As with other ancient religions, Shintoism's practices and beliefs were passed down verbally before a literature was established. Japanese people don't usually think of Shintoism specifically as a religion – it's more an aspect (and often an important one) of Japanese personal and public life. Shintoism, as an ethnic religion, is little interested in missionary work, and rarely practised outside its country of origin, except by emigrants.[2] There are about 100 million followers worldwide.[3] Its evolution continues to the present day.[4]

Origins and development

Shintoism is an articulation of its Chinese translation – *shen* (spirit) and *dao* (the way)) or 'the way of the gods'. It is the name given to a collection of myths, rites and 'kami' or spirits which have guided Japanese life since pre-history. Originally the rites were performed in beautiful pastoral places but are now held in shrines,[5] the entrances of which characteristically have two uprights topped by a crossbar and are often painted red. It is misleading to regard it as always being an organized tradition and it was only gradually that a centralizing ideology arose.[6]

Pure Shintoism has no known founder, was originally intensely local in its practice and required the subordination of the individual to the group ('the nail that sticks up will be hammered down').[7] Shintoism has no original sacred books but emphasizes the importance of harmony between people and with nature. There is veneration of ancestral spirits, family solidarity, personal and group purity is important, as is the need to maintain 'face'. Wise men are revered[8] and respect for elders became, and still is, one of the main characteristics of the Japanese people. It does not codify good and evil or any proportional rewards after death. It does not define a future state beyond the eternal existence of spirits and it knows neither a heaven nor a hell.[9] There is no absolute dichotomy between good and evil.[10] Human beings are basically seen as good.[11] Trying to closely define Shintoism has always been a problem and at a meeting of the Japanese Society of Science held in Tokyo in 1890, it was agreed that 'it should by no means be regarded as a religion, although it is the most important element in our national thought and feeling'.[12]

Since travellers arrived in Japan from the 6th century CE, the genius of Shintoism has been the ability to accommodate and become syncretic with other religions, particularly Mahayana and 'Pure-Land' Buddhism (see Chapter 14). These promised a fast-track to enlightenment for all classes of society, and Buddhist and Shinto priests shared the same temples. The mixture of Buddhism (with Confucianism) and Shintoism was termed Reigobu (Ryobu) Shintoism, which was, and is, represented everywhere in the shape of gaily decorated lacquer temples, swarming with highly coloured deities.[13,14]

It was the competitive aspect of formalized religions that caused Empress Gemmei in the 8th century CE to identify Japan's native beliefs, and commission documentation of its core values. This resulted in the compilation of texts such as the *Kojiki* (Record of Ancient Matters) and the *Nihon Shoki* (Continuing Chronicles of Japan), so that traditions were identified and preserved, and a superior status was given to the Japanese people.[15] Buddhism and Confucianism continued their happy relationships with Shintoism but Christianity did not enjoy similar success. The didactic preaching of the Jesuits was interpreted as redirecting devotion away from the Japanese emperor towards the 'foreigner' Jesus and therefore Christianity was banned in Japan from 1639 to 1817.[16]

Worship, lifestyle and sovereingty

Shintoism's most ancient and fundamental belief is that energy-bearing spirit-beings known as *kami* govern the natural world and destiny.[17] Some *kami* are great creative beings, some are natural forces and some are the souls of ancestors. Rituals honouring the *kami* link the present to the past. In Shinto, a person's soul (*tama*) is believed to become a kami 33 years[18] after the death of the mortal 'host' and the *kami* of a family's ancestors are venerated at household shrines. Many *kami* live in the sky and return to earth periodically to visit sacred places and shrines and they can take part in festivals. Not all *kami* are good or benign; some are demonic and vengeful spirits responsible for a variety of earthly troubles.[19]

To keep the relationship between the *kami* and humankind harmonious the adherents undergo ritual cleansing (*harai*) and pray and make offerings at shrines and temples. A purification ritual is routine before entering a temple. The most revered and pure Shinto temple is that of Amaterasu, the Sun Goddess, at Ise on the Japanese island of Honsu, and a Japanese person is encouraged to visit at least once. It is traditionally believed that the Emperors of Japan are descendants of Amaterasu.[20]

There are millions of gods and *kami* in a hierarchical structure with some regarded as more eminent than others[21] and prayed to in over 100,000 registered shrines.[22] Each location has its own special god and each god has his/her annual festival. The festival days of the gods are occasions of rejoicing with splendour, gaiety, costumes and street processions. Shrines range from the size of a village through to small domestic shrines known as *kami-dona*[23] (god–shelf), on which a miniature wooden temple contains tablets and papers with the names of the gods in whom the family places its trust. There are also tablets with the posthumous names of ancestors.[24] Public shrines are known characteristically for the benefits they offer with blessings on business, education, marriage, sporting events, new factories and new buildings.[25],[26]

Whilst most religious systems are distinct from political regimes, on the contrary, Shintoism has at times embraced the imperial dynasty of Japan as a sort of godhead. This amalgamation became critical at the end of the Second World War. In the years up to then, generations of Japanese grew up with 'state Shinto' presented as the pure and indigenous religion of their country. When the war ended, 'state Shinto' was dis-established by the Allied Occupation powers and Emperor Hirohito declared that he was not an *akitsumikami* (a deity in human form).[27]

Modern Shintoism is continuing to evolve[28] but has reverted to its more traditional position as a traditional religion which is culturally ingrained, rather than enforced. Shinto priests continue as they used to, to celebrate birth, perform marriages and visit local businesses, new buildings etc., and to perform purifying rituals. In practice Buddhism and Shintoism continue as an entwined social system with toleration for other faiths such as Confucianism and Christianity and new branches of Shintoism are emerging.

Care of the dying

Shinto regards death as the ultimate impurity; death is considered to be an evil. It is accepted to be inevitable, irreversible and heart-breaking for everyone involved. A person's spirit continues after death as a *tama* and is part of the social family group upon whom you must not bring shame.

Traditionally, Japanese patients wish to die at home and some may be taken home once death is inevitable. The hospice movement is growing and gaining acceptance. Whatever the location, it is important that family members are present at the death.

Normal clinical care is appropriate. Most Japanese in the UK understand Western norms, but for those who are more traditional there are some cultural aspects to be aware of in both patients and relatives. Some Japanese avoid eye contact and it is not uncommon for them not to be 'up-front' in their initial answers and wishes as a form of politeness. A Japanese person may, out of respect, say 'no' several times before giving you their genuine reply; this should be taken into particular consideration concerning care after death. Do not presume that a nod or a smile means agreement; ask for confirmation of their intention, and if possible check in the context of other family members.

In contrast to many faiths, there is an old culture that regards suicide as an honourable act (especially in wartime) and an acceptable outcome to atone for failure. Although the rate is now dropping, during the last global recession suicide was the sixth-largest cause of death in Japan, the majority being men.[29]

Management of death

When discussing the deceased, flattery is the conversational norm, especially if they died in a tragic accident. Incense or a candle may be placed next to the deceased's bed.

Last offices by hospital staff are not always considered appropriate within Shintoism and hence should be approached with care. Usually the relatives or professional *nokansha* will bathe the body and perform purification rites before wrapping them in a white kimono (right over left). Family and friends will traditionally visit the deceased for up to two days whilst in their coffin. The coffin may have a window to reveal the face.

Almost all funerals (91%) are held using Buddhist rites, with cremation (99.8%) being preferred to burial and the ashes interred in a Buddhist cemetery. For this, please refer to Chapter 14 for details. The bodies of all but the most elite Japanese are cremated.

Traditional Shinto funerals are normally held only for Shinto priests, important devotees and the emperor and his relatives. There are very few Shinto cemeteries to receive the ashes of the cremated. Funeral rituals within Shintoism provide the dead with a means of escape from decay and corruption, enabling them to grow into exalted beings in order to become part of the world of *kami*.

Bunkotsu is the ritual of allowing close relatives to have some of the ashes for their family shrines at home. The remaining ashes are put in the urn with any bones and are to be kept within an above-ground mausoleum. The priest also gives the deceased a new name that the person uses in Heaven, which is called *Tengoku*. After the funeral, each person who goes back to the deceased's house throws salt over his shoulder to ward off evil spirits. Although post-cremation customs are very local, in many traditions, the urn containing the ashes is interred in a ceremony called *nōkotsu* on the forty-ninth day, and the family stays in mourning until this time.

Autopsy and organ transplantation

The topics of autopsy and organ donation create certain culture-specific problems for many Japanese people. First, there is a widespread belief about the survival of the human spirit and its staged journeys after death. Second, 'brain death' is not widely accepted by the public as decisive for the death of personality or spirit. Therefore, for these two reasons alone, caution must be exercised in any discussions about these topics. That said, post-mortem examination, if required for a good reason, is acceptable except where there is belief that an intact physical body is necessary for transmission to the spirit world. To try to help with transplantation, in 1997, the Japanese Parliament voted to accept brain death to allow organ donation.[30]

As a general interpersonal rule, older people are more likely to be ambivalent or opposed to these procedures than younger generations. More certain ground and impressions are best gained in 'family discussions' rather than discussions with single individuals. This strategy optimizes trust and rapport on both sides and carefully considers the group nature of decision-making in most Japanese circles. The practice of ensuring that important decisions are made by families rather than individuals also optimizes and respects age-related differences to do with tradition, authority and social change among the Japanese.

Further reading

- Rutty J: 'Shintoism', in *E-Learning for Health*, Royal College of Pathologists, 'Faith Considerations Part 3: Eastern Faiths', published on the web by Health Education England NHS (undated), available at; www.e-lfh.org.uk/programmes/medical-examiner/.
- Littleton CS (2005): 'Shinto', in *Eastern Religions*, ed. Coogan MD, Duncan Baird Publishers, part 5, pp. 417–517.

- DK (2013): *The Religions Book*, UK edn, Dorling Kindersley, 'Ritual Links Us to Our Past', pp. 84–85.
- Reid D (2010): 'Japanese Religions', in *The Penguin Handbook of the World's Living Religions*, ed. Hinnells JR, Penguin, chapter 10, pp. 481–515.

Notes

1 Statistics Japan; Ministry of Internal Affairs and Communications (2015): Statistical Yearbook of Japan. Available at: https://en.wikipedia.org/wiki/Ministry_of_Internal_Affairs_and_Communications.
2 BBC (2011): 'Shinto At a Glance'. Available at: www.bbc.co.uk/religion/religions/shinto/ataglance/glance.shtml.
3 Bocking B (2003): 'Shinto' in *World Religions*, ed. Gill D, Collins, p. 157.
4 Reid D (2010): 'Japanese Religions', in *The Penguin Handbook of the World's Living Religions*, ed. Hinnells JR, Penguin, chapter 10, pp. 495–510.
5 Smart N (1999): 'Japanese Philosophies', in *World Philosophies*, Routledge, p. 116.
6 Smart N (1998): 'Japan', in *The World's Religions*, 2nd edn, Cambridge University Press, chapter 4, pp. 134–137.
7 Littleton CS (2005): 'Shinto', in *Eastern Religions*, ed. Coogan MD, Duncan Baird Publishers, part 5, pp. 419, 422, 423.
8 Reid D (2010): 'Japanese Religions', in *The Penguin Handbook of the World's Living Religions*, ed. Hinnells JR, Penguin, chapter 10, pp. 470–478.
9 Bishop IB (1911): 'Shintoism (2)', in *Religious Systems of the World*, eds Sheowring WM and Thies CW, 10th edn, George Allen & Unwin, pp. 109, 110.
10 Littleton CS (2005): 'Shinto', in *Eastern Religions*, ed. Coogan MD, Duncan Baird Publishers, part 5, p. 438.
11 BBC (2011): 'Shinto At a Glance'. Available at: www.bbc.co.uk/religion/religions/shinto/ataglance/glance.shtml.
12 Goh D (1911): 'Shintoism (1)', in *Religious Systems of the World*, eds Sheowring WM and Thies CW, 10th edn, George Allen & Unwin, pp. 101.
13 Bishop IB (1911): 'Shintoism (2)', in *Religious Systems of the World*, eds Sheowring WM and Thies CW, 10th edn, George Allen & Unwin, pp. 102, 103.
14 Littleton CS (2005): 'Shinto', in *Eastern Religions*, ed. Coogan MD, Duncan Baird Publishers, part 5, p. 429.
15 DK (2013): *The Religions Book*, UK edn, Dorling Kindersley, 'Ritual Links Us to Our Past', p. 83.
16 Reid D (2010): 'Japanese Religions', in *The Penguin Handbook of the World's Living Religions*, ed. Hinnells JR, Penguin, chapter 10, pp 485–486.
17 DK (2013): *The Religions Book*, UK edn, Dorling Kindersley, 'Ritual Links Us to Our Past', p. 83.
18 Littleton CS (2005): 'Shinto', in *Eastern Religions*, ed. Coogan MD, Duncan Baird Publishers, part 5, p. 503.
19 *Ibid.*, p. 447.
20 DK (2013): *The Religions Book*, UK edn, Dorling Kindersley, 'Ritual Links Us to Our Past', pp. 84–85.
21 Littleton CS (2005): 'Shinto', in *Eastern Religions*, ed. Coogan MD, Duncan Baird Publishers, part 5, pp. 436–447.
22 Bocking B (2003): 'Shinto', in *World Religions*, ed. Gill D, Collins, p. 162.
23 DK (2013): *The Religions Book*, UK edn, Dorling Kindersley, 'Ritual Links Us to Our Past', pp. 84–85.

24 Littleton CS (2005): 'Shinto', in *Eastern Religions*, ed. Coogan MD, Duncan Baird Publishers, part 5, p. 493.
25 DK (2013): *The Religions Book*, UK edn, Dorling Kindersley, 'Ritual Links Us to Our Past', p. 83.
26 Bocking B (2003): 'Shinto', in *World Religions*, ed. Gill D, Collins, p. 162.
27 Littleton CS (2005): 'Shinto', in *Eastern Religions*, ed. Coogan MD, Duncan Baird Publishers, part 5, pp. 418–423.
28 Reid D (2010): 'Japanese Religions', in *The Penguin Handbook of the World's Living Religions*, ed. Hinnells JR, Penguin, chapter 10, pp. 495–498.
29 Motohashi Y, Kaneko Y, Sasaki H (2005): 'Lowering Suicide Rates in Rural Japan', *Akita Journal of Public Health*, Vol. 2, 105–106.
30 Wise J (1997): 'Japan to Allow Organ Transplants', *British Medical Journal*, Vol. 314, 1298.

Chapter 24

Sikhism

Description of the religion

Numbers practising the religion

Worldwide Sikhs number 24 million, with the large majority of 15.6 million being in the current Punjab. There are approximately 450,00 in Canada, 400,000 in the UK and 300,000 in the USA.

Origins and beliefs

Sikhism was founded in the Punjab (in northern India), by Guru Nanak (1469–1539 CE) at a time when the indigenous religion was Hinduism but there were Islamic Mogul overlords. His home town was Nankana Sahib, which, through boundary changes, is now in Pakistan (see Figure 24.1). These boundary changes, caused by politics, ethnic and religious issues, have created a diaspora of displaced Sikhs in many other countries, but the emotional link with the Punjab remains strong. The word 'Sikh' means 'disciple' in the Punjabi language.[1]

At the age of 30, Nanak, content with neither Hinduism nor Islam, had a mystical revelation when he felt swept into the presence of a single God. After this revelation he pronounced:

> There is neither Hindu nor Muslim . . . God is neither Hindu nor Muslim and the path I shall follow is God's.[2]

He then gave away all his possessions, became a travelling preacher and formed a settled community on the western bank of the River Ravi at Kartarpur (see Figure 24.1) that combined work and worship. He preached that true inner spirituality transcends all religions, that there is equality of men and women and of all people regardless of their background[3] and that man has a body and a soul.[4] Whilst believing in one God (as Islam does), he did not challenge the Hindu belief that the soul passes through many lives, but also believed that it was possible to be liberated from the cycle of rebirth (possibly within one lifetime[5]), to enter a blissful state representing the union of man and God (*mukti*).[6] He accepted the karmic law that we reap what we sow, with our deeds determining whether or how we will be born again.[7] Death is a stage in spiritual development and the body is a clothing for the soul which is discarded on death.

Sikhism stresses that the importance of what we do is more important than ritual.[8] The priesthood was abolished because he felt it had become corrupt and self-serving[9] and encouraged formality.[10] Before Guru Nanak

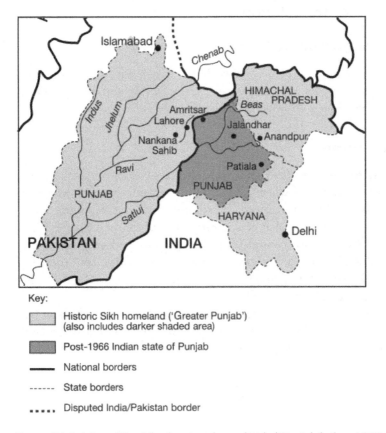

Key:

▨ Historic Sikh homeland ('Greater Punjab') (also includes darker shaded area)

▨ Post-1966 Indian state of Punjab

— National borders

------ State borders

▪▪▪▪▪ Disputed India/Pakistan border

FIGURE 24.1 Map of Punjab, showing the undivided Punjab before 1947, its division between the new state of Pakistan and the sub-division of India's post-partition state of Punjab in 1966. Reproduced under license from Nesbitt E (2016): *Sikhism: A Very Short Introduction*, Oxford University Press, p. 10.

died in 1539, he appointed one of his disciples to succeed him as Guru. This process of re-appointment continued until the death of the Tenth Guru in 1708. During this period all the religious sayings and texts were integrated into a Sikh scripture known as the *Guru Granth Sahib*. The Tenth Guru, *Guru Gobind Singh*, was the man who gave Sikhism the identity it possesses today principally by doing two things.

- He bestowed the Guruship forevermore to the *Guru Granth Sahib* (i.e., to the Holy Book) as the eternal teacher for all time. Every Sikh place of worship (the Gurdwara) has a copy of the *Guru Granth Sahib*, where it is duly venerated.[11]
- He created a community of believers called the *Khalsa* who were formally committed to and admitted into it by the ceremony of *Amrit Pahul*.[12]

The primary purpose of the *Khalsa* is not active aggression, but it is committed to religious freedom. *Amrit* initiation can be taken at any age but the initiate must comprehend its meaning and subsequently abide by the Sikh code of conduct. The order encompasses both men and women who by convention wear the five signs of their faith, otherwise known as the Five Ks.[13]

- Kesh: uncut hair.
- Kanga: a comb to hold the hair in place.
- Kara: a steel or iron bangle.
- Kirpan: a small sword or dagger.
- Kacchera: short trousers or breeches.

It is surprising that the most outward sign of being a male Sikh, the wearing of a turban, is not on this list despite its great importance and being confirmed by the Tenth Guru as obligatory for men. In Britain, the UK Deregulation Act 2015[14] effectively established the turban as part of a male Sikh's religious dress. There are also other groups who wear turbans (e.g., some Moslems, Christians and Kurds) who can be mistaken for Sikhs. There are also modern female turbans in a variety of styles and colours but they do not have formal religious significance.

Worship and lifestyle

At religious services (Sikhs have adopted Sunday as their holy day), which are essentially congregational with no priests,[15] both men and women read from the *Guru Granth Sahib*. Great reverence is shown to the holy book, which is kept in a special room. Whilst the scripture is being read a *chauri* (a special fan made of yak hairs or nylon) is waved over the book as a sign of respect. There are no altars or statues. Sikhs are expected to meditate and say personal devotional prayers daily. A congregational service starts with readings from the scriptures, then the singing of *kirtan* (devotional songs), and concludes with lectures or speeches.[16] The Gurdwara is a socio-political and educational institution[17] as well as a place of worship above which flies the traditional yellow flag with the *khanda* symbol on it. Community service in the form of voluntary work is also usually centered on the Gurdwara. Attached to the Gurdwara is a free kitchen (*Guru ka langar*) with mingling of all social classes during the meal following services. This is prepared in the *langar* where all people are welcome to a free meal regardless of their sex, colour or religion. All the food is vegetarian so that no religious group is offended.[18]

Family life is greatly valued through the threefold disciplines of:[19]

- *Nam Japna*: the conscious remembrance that keeps God in our minds and leads to a feeling of His presence and discourages the temptations of evil
- *Dharam di Kirat Karmi*: honest work done according to one's ability and capacity without corruption
- *Wand Chhakna*: the sharing of the product or the profit of one's work with others in the spirit of serving other human beings.

Although change is occurring, two areas where there remain traditional Hindu influences are relationships between the sexes and marriage. All the Gurus and the text of the *Guru Granth Sahib* eschewed the caste system but Sikhs have never entirely freed themselves of it, for example, in marriages,[20] when not only two people are being joined together till one of them dies, but so too are their families.

Sikhs still look to *Amritsar* for guidance from the elders in the *Akal Takhat* (Throne of the Timeless One). Through edicts it issues guidance or clarification on points of Sikh doctrine or practice. On 16 August 2007, it issued the following.[21]

> only Sikh couples can engage in the Anand Karaj Ceremony.[22] If either is not a Sikh, then they *must* embrace the Sikh faith. This includes that they *must* change their second name to Singh or Kaur in their official documents *before* the Marriage Ceremony.

This caused both joy and despair in equal measure to Sikh communities around the world, and is an example of the problems that all religions face as society moves forwards in its unpredictable ways. Like Pope Paul VI's encyclical *Humanae Vitae* of 1968 rejecting birth control, the centre produced satisfaction and frustration in equal measure in the peripheries. However, these traditions are changing in today's world and the situation is very fluid, as is the response of the Sikh community to those who choose to 'marry out', or co-habit as a married couple.[23]

Food can be a contentious subject.[24] Traditionally, the choice of food was dictated by what was available in a particular region. Hence the diet in the Punjab homeland was predominantly cereals, fresh vegetables and milk products. Many Sikhs are vegetarians. Eating meat and other foods is essentially left to the discretion and conscience of the individual, but it must never be Halal.[25] Tobacco, alcohol, social drugs and other intoxicants are banned by the scriptures but used freely by a number of adherents.[26]

Care of the dying

In the traditional teachings of the Gurus, health and disease are causally connected because body and mind are in a continuum, so for some older and devout patients, the modern conception of system-based disease may be rather narrow. Disease can result from the ebbs and flows of life's vicissitudes and when managing dying patients, the psychological elements are important. In their records, most Sikhs have three names, a first name, a religious middle name and a family name. The middle name for men is 'Singh' and for women is 'Kaur', and many Sikhs use these as surnames, so the husband of Mrs Kaur is Mr Singh. This is important to remember in telephone conversations and so that there is not confusion between different families.

For many seriously ill patients it is important to keep the Five Ks undisturbed, so staff should try to manage this: if they have to be moved, this needs to be explained sensitively. When caring for a Sikh, cleanliness is paramount. If possible, a shower is preferred and if there isn't one, jugs and a bath may be offered (rather than sitting in the water). Many Sikhs are vegetarian, others are not, so there needs to be attention to diet. Although not permitted in the holy book, a number of Sikhs do drink alcohol.

The family should be informed if death is likely to ensure so that they have time to be with the patient. As death approaches, the dying person is encouraged to say *Wahe Guru, Wahe Guru* (wonderful lord) a few times and one of those present will recite *Sukhmai* (the hymn of peace) or some other text from the scripture. The relatives are dissuaded from weeping and wailing by quoting suitably reassuring scriptures to them, e.g., 'He who is born shall die. It is God's will. We must abide by His will'. After death, a person's behaviour during life is judged by God, with the result of either being in eternal union with God or rebirth. Sikhs believe that those who have the spirit of God are not afraid of death. Suicide is regarded as tragic, rather than as a mortal sin.

Management of death

Cremation is preferred and should occur as soon as possible, so the efficient issuing of documents is important. If there is a need for an autopsy, this needs careful and sensitive explanation. Their belief that the physical body is not needed in rebirth and that the real essence of a person is in their soul helps in this regard.

Full last offices by hospital staff may or may not be necessary because the family might wish to wash and lay out the body themselves and then wrap it in a sheet. After touching the body the family members will probably want to wash before going home. If the deceased was a member of the *Khalsa*, they will be left with the Five Ks intact (no trimming of hair or beards etc.).

If the family is not available the local Gurdwara can be contacted for advice or last offices can be done by healthcare staff of the same gender. In addition to the attention to the Five Ks, close the eyes, support the jaw, straighten the limbs and then cover the body with a white sheet with no religious emblems. The deceased's face may be viewed on many occasions before the funeral, so a peaceful appearance is desirable.

The coffin is usually taken home prior to the funeral and for the last time the face will be viewed and prayers offered before it travels to the Gurdwara and then onto the crematorium. No prayers to, or for, the dead are ordained in the *Guru Granth Sahib*. Traditionally the body is burnt within 24 hours, but in UK this is not always possible. Prayers are said as the corpse is cremated. With a traditional pyre the eldest boy lights the pyre, or these days may accompany the body to the furnace. The ashes are scattered in the Punjab or in a river or at sea. In countries where cremation is not available, the Sikhs bury their dead. It is forbidden to erect a monument in case it becomes an object of worship.

Sikhs hold that it is wrong to mourn excessively for the deceased, as their soul will soon exist in a different body or be in fusion with God. The whole family will mourn for some days, with friends and relatives coming to the home to visit. White is worn as a sign of mourning, as in Hinduism. Some families will refuse to eat until after the cremation. The distribution of *karah prashad* (ceremonial food) after the funeral signifies that social life should continue as normal.

Autopsy and organ transplantation

Autopsy is acceptable if there is a good reason. All wounds should be carefully sutured so that there is no loss during the subsequent ritual proceedings, which will begin after the autopsy. There are no fundamental objections to blood transfusion or the receipt or donation of human organs.

Further reading

- Rutty J: 'Sikhism', in *E-Learning for Health*, Royal College of Pathologists, 'Faith Considerations Part 2: Dharmic Faiths', published on the web by Health Education England NHS (undated), available at; www.e-lfh.org.uk/programmes/medical-examiner/.
- Nesbitt E (2016): *Sikhism: A Very Short Introduction*, Oxford.
- DK (2013): *The Religions Book*, UK edn, Dorling Kindersley, 'We Must Live as Sikh-Soldiers and All May Enter Our Gateway to God', pp. 296–303.
- Cole WO (2010): 'Sikhism', in *The Penguin Handbook of the World's Living Religions*, ed. Hinnells JR, Penguin, chapter 6, pp. 312–341.

Notes

1 Nesbitt E (2016): *Sikhism: A Very Short Introduction*, Oxford University Press, p. 3.
2 Cole WO (2010): 'Sikhism', in *The Penguin Handbook of the World's Living Religions*, ed. Hinnells JR, chapter 6, p. 316.
3 Nesbitt E (2016): *Sikhism: A Very Short Introduction*, Oxford University Press, p. 26.
4 Sambhi PS (1996): 'Sikhism', in *Six World Faiths*, ed. Cole WO, Cassell, p. 289.
5 Nesbitt E (2016): *Sikhism: A Very Short Introduction*, Oxford University Press, p. 26.
6 *Ibid.*
7 Sambhi PS (1996): 'Sikhism', in *Six World Faiths*, ed. Cole WO, Cassell, pp. 289–291.
8 DK (2013): *The Religions Book*, UK edn, Dorling Kindersley, 'The Sikh Code of Conduct', p. 301.
9 DK (2013): *The Religions Book*, UK edn, Dorling Kindersley, 'All May Enter Our Gateway to God', p. 302.
10 Sambhi PS (1996): 'Sikhism', in *Six World Faiths*, ed. Cole WO, Cassell, p. 284.
11 DK (2013): *The Religions Book*, UK edn, Dorling Kindersley, 'All May Enter Our Gateway to God', p. 303.
12 DK (2013): *The Religions Book*, UK edn, Dorling Kindersley, 'The Sikh Code of Conduct', p. 299.
13 Nesbitt E (2016): *Sikhism: A Very Short Introduction*, Oxford University Press, pp. 48–55.
14 www.legislation.gov.uk/ukpga/2015/20/contents.
15 Cole WO (2010): 'Sikhism', in *The Penguin Handbook of the World's Living Religions*, ed. Hinnells JR, chapter 6, p. 335.
16 Sambhi PS (1996): 'Sikhism', in *Six World Faiths*, ed. Cole WO, Cassell, pp. 298–304.
17 Cole WO (2010): 'Sikhism', in *The Penguin Handbook of the World's Living Religions*, ed. Hinnells JR, chapter 6, p. 327.
18 Nesbitt E (2016): *Sikhism: A Very Short Introduction*, Oxford University Press, p. 61.
19 Sambhi PS (1996): 'Sikhism', in *Six World Faiths*, ed. Cole WO, Cassell, pp. 284.
20 Cole WO (2010): 'Sikhism', in *The Penguin Handbook of the World's Living Religions*, ed. Hinnells JR, chapter 6, p. 338.

21 www.sikhphilosophy.net/threads/akal-takhat-hukumnama-regarding-interfaith-marriages.16947/.
22 Sikh marriage.
23 For an in-depth discussion of contemporary attitudes to caste and gender, see Nesbitt E (2016): *Sikhism: A Very Short Introduction*, Oxford University Press, chapter 7, pp. 102–119.
24 Nesbitt E (2016): *Sikhism: A Very Short Introduction*, Oxford University Press, pp. 60–61.
25 Sambhi PS (1996): 'Sikhism', in *Six World Faiths*, ed. Cole WO, Cassell, pp. 314–315.
26 Sambhi PS (1996): 'Sikhism', in *Six World Faiths*, ed. Cole WO, Cassell, p. 316.

Chapter 25

Zoroastrianism

Description of the religion

Numbers practising the religion

The exact number of adherents is not known, but estimates put the world total at 130,000, of whom about half are in India and 4,500 are in the UK, with an emigrant diaspora is across the world.[1] The population of believers in Asia has been in decline for some time,[2] because of endogamy and the reluctance to accept children from mixed marriages. The numbers are, however, growing in Iran and other locations.[3]

Origins and beliefs

Zoroastrianism is an ancient religion founded by the prophet Zoroaster (a Greek adaptation of Zarathustra) around 1200 BCE in ancient Persia[4] (now Iran) that competes with Judaism to be the first monotheistic faith. For 1,000 years Zoroastrianism was one of the most powerful religions in the world, being the official religion of Persia from 600 BCE to 650 CE, but it is now one of the world's smallest. The 'Three Wise Men of the East' who visited the baby Jesus were thought to be Zoroastrians.

In the 10th century CE, Zoroastrians migrated from Persia to India to avoid the compulsory conversion to Islam by Muslim invaders, where they became known as Parsis or Parsees.[5] Zoroaster's teachings are contained in their holy book, the *Avesta*.[6]

Zoroastrians believe there is one God called *Ahura Mazda* (Wise Lord) and He created the world, revealing the truth to the prophet Zoroaster. He wants to rule over a good and just universe. All the time, *Ahura Mazda* is opposed by the corrupting influence of the destructive spirit *Angra Mainyu*. It is important to realize that *Angra Mainyu* is not the equal of God, but ageing, sickness, famine, natural disasters, death and so on are attributed to him.[7] This separation of good and evil is a form of dualism. The path of evil leads to misery and ultimately Hell. The path of Righteousness leads to peace and everlasting happiness in Heaven, but the determinant of what happens is free will: choice is crucial. We are all responsible for our actions.[8] God is revered through the medium of fire, which is present in all temples.

Zoroaster recruited humankind to the fight between good and evil and he taught that at the end of life, humans will be judged twice. The first judgement will address the individual's morality of thought and the second the morality of action. In both cases, moral failings will be punished in Hell, but not for eternity. Punishment ceases when lessons have been learned and insight has been gained; after this the person goes to dwell in Heaven for evermore.[9]

Worship and lifestyle

Children are initiated into the faith between the ages of 7 and 15 years, when they are given a *sudreh* (shirt) and *kusti* (cord). After ritual ablutions, a Zoroastrian has a duty to pray five times per day (sunrise, noon, sunset, midnight and dawn), in the presence of fire (the symbol of righteousness). Prayers are said standing whilst the sacred cord is repeatedly tied and untied.[10] There are seven obligatory festivals.

Zoroastrians consider all food, and the animals and plants it comes from, as sacred, because they all originate from God. Most of them have a mixed meat-vegetarian diet, tending to favour fish and meat that comes from herbivores (chicken, lamb and mutton). Dairy food is greatly appreciated, and there are few absolute 'No's. The killing of animals for food is perceived as a religious act of sacrifice and must be done with great respect. Having said this, many tend to vegetarianism and those in Iran and India may avoid pork and beef. Because food is a gift from God it is precious and waste and excess are unacceptable. Any leftovers are given to animals.[11]

In practice, modern Zoroastrianism has a positive outlook. It teaches that mankind is ultimately good and that this goodness will finally triumph over evil. This could be seen as a retrenchment from the faith's original purity of dualism. Suicide is abhorred and in India bodies are disposed of in different places.

Care of the dying

Of all life's rites of passage, ceremonies at death are important: they aim to isolate the impurity of the dead body and assist the soul.[12] Running water is preferred for washing. Daily prayers are important to those of a traditional inclination. Because there will be individual variations, it is important to establish the wishes of the patient and their family at the outset and establish if there are any sensitive issues. Zoroastrians wish their family to be present at death and they may say prayers. There are no last rites before death, but relatives and friends, and sometimes (but rarely) a Zoroastrian priest, may say prayers.

Management of death

Believers traditionally hold that a soul is allowed three days after death to meditate on its life, during which time priests and relatives pray for it. Before dawn on the fourth day family and friends gather to wish it well on its journey. Following this, the soul will be judged, and if good thoughts, words and deeds outweigh the bad, then the soul is taken into Heaven; alternatively, the soul is led to Hell to be corrected. After death the body is believed to become impure, the cause of death being *Angra Maiynu*, the evil god. The family may supply an attendant or hospital staff can carry out routine last offices. It is important that the body is washed before being wrapped in white garments. Families often bring a *sadra* to be worn under the shroud together with a girdle or *kusti* and they may wish the head to be covered with a hat or scarf.

The body should be disposed of as soon as possible after death (preferably within 24 hours) so efficiency with the necessary documentation is important.

Contaminating the earth and other elements with decaying flesh is considered to be sacrilege, so traditionally Zoroastrians put the body on the top of a mountain or a 'tower of silence' to be open to the elements and to be eaten by carrion. In most countries this is now substituted by cremation whilst some bury a coffin in cement to protect the earth. Memorial ceremonies for the soul are performed monthly for the first year and annually for the next 30 years.[13]

Autopsy and organ transplantation

Autopsies are prohibited by ritual law and will usually be declined.

Orthodox Zoroastrians deem that the body should not be additionally polluted and are also likely to decline organ transplantation.

Further reading

- Rutty J: 'Zoroastrianism', in *E-Learning for Health*, Royal College of Pathologists, 'Faith Considerations Part 4: Other Traditions', published on the web by Health Education England NHS (undated), available at; www.e-lfh.org.uk/programmes/medical-examiner/.

- Boyce M (2010): 'Zoroastrianism', in *The Penguin Handbook of the World's Living Religions*, ed. Hinnells JR, Penguin, chapter 4, pp. 238–262.
- DK (2013): *The Religions Book*, UK edn, Dorling Kindersley, 'The Battle between Good and Evil, pp. 62–65.
- Shahin B (2003): 'Zoroastrianism', in *World Religions*, 2nd edn, ed. Gill D, Collins, pp. 181–188.

Notes

1 Boyce M (2010): 'Zoroastrianism', in *The Penguin Handbook of the World's Living Religions*, ed. Hinnells JR, Penguin, chapter 4, pp. 254–257.
2 *Ibid.*, p. 253.
3 *Ibid.*, pp. 256–257.
4 *Ibid.*, p. 238.
5 Smart N (1998): *The World's Religions*, 2nd edn, Cambridge University Press, chapter 9, 'Persia and Central Asia', pp. 219–229.
6 B Shahin (2003): 'Zoroastrianism', in *World Religions*, 2nd edn, ed. Gill D, Collins, p. 185.
7 DK (2013): *The Religions Book*, UK edn, Dorling Kindersley, 'The Battle between Good and Evil', p. 62.
8 *Ibid.*, p. 64.
9 *Ibid.*, p. 65.
10 Boyce M (2010): 'Zoroastrianism', in *The Penguin Handbook of the World's Living Religions*, ed. Hinnells JR, Penguin, chapter 4, pp. 247–248.
11 Chalo J (2002): 'The Eating Habits of the Parsis', in *A Zoroastrian Tapestry*, eds Godrej PG, Mistree FP, Mapin Publishing, pp. 526, 518; and Stevens P (n.d.): 'Food Faith and the Zoroastrian Community'. Available at: www.shapworking party.org.uk/journals/articles_0910/stevens.pdf.
12 Boyce M (2010): 'Zoroastrianism', in *The Penguin Handbook of the World's Living Religions*, ed. Hinnells JR, Penguin, chapter 4, p. 249.
13 *Ibid.*

Part III

Legal aspects of death in the UK

Chapter 26

Life and death as biological and legal constructs

Introduction

What the words 'life' and 'death' actually mean depend on context,[1] but at a common-sense, everyday level, life and death are easy to define. The people one meets and converses with at work are alive; those whose memorials you visit are dead. On closer inspection, however, the concepts of life and death are much more complex. Are they truly separate or, for example, simply different parts of a continuum of nature?

In this chapter we will not be looking further into this conundrum, nor will we be discussing metaphysical questions such as 'Is death the absence of life or a positive process in its own right?' We will be focusing instead on the life event that Marcus Aurelius, whilst meditating on the River Gran in the 2nd century CE, described as when 'all things of the body stream away like a river' and added 'life is warfare and a visit in a strange land; the only lasting fame is oblivion.'[2] In essence we will be looking at death as the biological irreversibility that precedes the legal certification of the end of a human life.

Consideration of the termination of life can be approached from a number of directions, none of which 'covers all the angles'. The two main approaches, which are also complementary, are firstly an established irreversible loss of cellular function and second an established irreversible loss of the capacity to be conscious. Here we will begin by trying to define what life actually is, both in simple cells and complex humans before linking them again in terms of death. Finally, the ways of actually diagnosing human death as a legal happening will be described.

What is life?

Dictionary definitions of 'life' provide circular arguments and beg the question: none is satisfactory. In 1862 Herbert Spencer, the 19th-century philosopher and polymath had a go at defining life as follows:

Life is definable as the continuous adjustment of internal relations to external relations.[3]

In doing this he was influenced by the prevailing influences of Darwinism, but it does give the basic indication that something that is alive has titratable control over its internal *milieu* and is in some way separated and independent from the environment it occupies. The definition of life also depends upon the position of the organism in the genetic phylum, so it is instructive to compare very simple (single-celled) with complex (mammalian) forms of life. This is especially useful because the latter are constructed from combinations of multiple and specialised cellular modifications of the former.

Simple forms of life

The amoeba shown in Figure 26.1 is a simple, single-celled form of life. It is approximately one quarter of a millimeter in diameter. What makes it, and other 'living creatures', alive? There are two ways of answering this question, one from biology and another from physical science, which are different but mutually supportive.

The first, from biology, is to look at the fundamental processes of living organisms that separate them from inanimate objects. The following list is representative:[4]

- ingestion, or intake of nutritive foods (usually complex molecules)
- digestion of ingested material into smaller molecules, usually by enzymes, and their subsequent rebuilding into cellular components
- respiration, a process extending from the external environment to the intracellular machinery whereby chemical energy from ingestion and digestion is made available for the cell's use, allowing cells to manufacture complex molecules from simple building blocks
- excretion, which allows unwanted materials to be expelled from the cell
- a responsive 'irritability', which enables the organism to detect and respond to changes in its environment
- growth and reproduction, which allow maturation and propagation of the species.

The singled-celled organism *Amoeba proteus* shown in Figure 26.1 possesses all these characteristics necessary for life. It is surrounded by a membrane which insulates it from the environment, it can engulf food particles and digest them, it can make complex molecules to recreate itself, it can excrete waste products and it can reproduce by simple mitosis. When an amoeba can no longer carry out these processes, it dies.

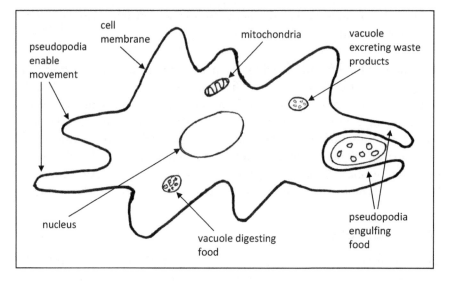

FIGURE 26.1 A single-celled organism, the amoeba

Approaching the problem of life from physical science, i.e., 'how is life different from all other spontaneous processes in the universe?' produces a different concept. The Nobel Prize winner for physics in 1933, Erwin Schrödinger, in his book *What is Life?*,[5] addressed the problems of genetics and looked at the phenomenon of life from the perspective of physics. In particular he explored the consequences of the Second Law of Thermodynamics.[6]

For the purposes of this discussion we can paraphrase this law to say that all natural processes (chemical and physical) lose stored, usable energy and are not spontaneously reversible. Large molecules decay into smaller ones that will not be able to be reassembled unless there is an active synthetic process using energy supplied from elsewhere that promotes it. This gives the important deduction that time, as we know it, has a direction and that ultimately, one day, through spontaneous decay, the universe will die. It is the process of spontaneous decay in the sun that produces the heat essential for keeping the earth warm. Neither humans nor the earth can reverse their existences.

In contrast to these naturally occurring environmental breakdown processes, healthy living organisms reverse the universal tendency to decay. This makes them special. Throughout their lives they are continually reversing the tendency to decay using the list of biological processes given above so that they can construct the complex molecules needed by themselves to ensure their continued life. In thermodynamic parlance (see note 6) an organism interacts with its environment and reduces its own internal entropy at the expense of its surroundings. When this fails, it no longer reverses entropy, its essential processes stop and it dies. In this way the biological and physico-chemical evidences of death are related.

Complex forms of life

A schematic version of a higher mammal (let's assume this is a human) is shown in Figure 26.2. It differs from a simple amoeba in two significant ways.

- The human has a number of specialized organs, each of the cells of which has the same basic components as the amoeba but which are designed to fulfill specialized, defined functions. They are not interchangeable and may replace themselves in more complex ways than by simple mitosis based on growth. If sufficient cells within a single organ fail, that organ will, *pari passu*, functionally fail (e.g., heart failure, liver failure, kidney failure etc.). Because that organ produces unique support to the other organs, they also sequentially fail unless the function of the failing organ can be replaced, e.g., by renal transplantation or dialysis, or therapeutically cured. If there is no replacement or cure possible, the death of the whole human is inevitable; e.g., pneumonia is often termed 'the old man's friend'. Therefore, the bodily life of a human is dependent upon the successful co-operative function of effectively independent organ systems, each having billions of cells.
- As shown in Figure 26.2, in addition to separate, mutually interdependent physical organ systems, the higher mammals, when healthy and not naturally asleep, have the property of consciousness during which time thought is possible. Here we will not consider where on the evolutionary scale consciousness and thinking appeared, but in humans, consciousness and the ability to think are critical components of what it is to be defined as being alive in a meaningful way. The link between a functioning physical brain and consciousness, which clearly exists, still cannot be explained and will not be examined further here.

Human life

Although there is no single, succinct definition of a normal and healthy human life, for the purposes of this text, it can be thought of as having three essentials.

- organ systems that are working as they should in a mutually constructive and co-ordinated manner
- possession of consciousness and the capacity for thought when not asleep
- individual cells and organs constantly working to slow down the chemical disorganization (entropy) of the cells by constructive metabolism utilizing energy and materials from external sources.

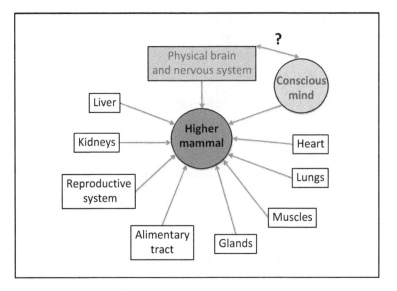

Figure 26.2 Schematic diagram of a higher mammal

There are, however, also people who are clearly alive who do not fully meet all three criteria. It is in fact actually very common for people to only partially meet them. Examples are those who have lost a paired organ or one or more parts or the whole of limbs or those who are maintained by medical care, e.g., patients on organ support (e.g., renal failure), those with non-fatal chronic disease (e.g., arthritis), those with disease that would be fatal if not treated (e.g., insulin-dependent diabetes mellitus) and those who are temporarily unconscious. Another group are many of those receiving chemotherapy whose lives are being extended rather than being cured or managed indefinitely. Although all these are examples of people who are not fully healthy humans (in the elemental biological sense), they are certainly alive and retain full legal, ethical and human rights just like anybody else until the criteria for the pronouncement of death have occurred.

The above arguments, definitions and discussion have been deduced and presented in this manner to subsequently aid the definition of death.

What is death?

Introduction

Like life, death has no easy definition. Considering the amoeba, if something happens to prevent the single cell from functioning normally (e.g., no nutrients, excessive temperature, being crushed etc.), the death of the cell is the total death of the organism. In a human the death of a single cell is not the death of the whole organism. In fact, most of the body's cells have a given cell lifetime, after which they are replaced by new versions. Examples are intestinal cells that last for four days, alveolar cells that last for eight days, red blood cells that last for 120 days, and liver cells that last for a year. So, as time passes the majority of one's tissues is continuously replaced. This means that whole-person death is fundamentally different to individual cell death. In addition, with higher animals and humans, there is the added complication of consciousness and thought.

How does death happen?

There are innumerable ways of dying, but they can largely be categorized into three groups.

- Sudden death from events such as trauma, electrocution, unexpected cardiac arrest and aortic rupture that occur without any warning or prodromal period. This is often termed 'instant death' – a major support system is disabled in a flash. The majority of these deaths occur in a community setting and the person is already dead before medical assistance can be given.
- Death which occurs after a period of illness or failure to recover from an earlier insult such as major trauma, surgery or myocardial infarction. There is some indication of the possibility of dying that can extend from hours to years depending on the circumstances. These types of dying occur in both hospital and community settings, usually with the patient in bed accompanied by a variable number of professional staff and family members. The mode of actual death is commonly a sequence of the eyes glazing with jaw laxity and gradual loss of consciousness followed by respiratory arrest.
- Death diagnosed whilst the person is ventilated with a beating heart and is having their vital functions supported artificially. This has to occur in a 'high-tech' setting, most commonly in a critical care unit or during transfer; it is termed 'brain death' and is dealt with in detail in Chapter 34. This diagnosis of death, above all others, demonstrates that the death of the person is not the death of all the cells in the body.

What happens to the body after death?

There is much speculation about the continuity of individual cell life occurring after death of the complete human has been diagnosed, especially in the horror genre. Any life that does continue that is more than a few milli-meters from the body's surface would have to do so anaerobically – without oxygen. The subject was considered by a researcher in the journal *Scientific American*,[7] who wrote the following.

> As best as anyone can gauge, cell metabolism likely continues for roughly four to 10 minutes after death (taken to be the cessation of circulation), depending on the ambient temperature around the body.
>
> During this time period, oxygenated blood, which normally exchanges carbon dioxide with oxygen, is not circulating. Thus, cell respiration—which uses oxygen to make cellular energy while creat-ing carbon dioxide as a by-product—creates carbon dioxide that is not transported out of the cell. This lowers the pH of the cell, resulting in an acidic intracellular environment. This acidic environment causes intracellular membranes to rupture—including those around the cell's (internal) lysosomes, which contain enzymes for digesting everything from proteins to fats and nucleic acids. Once the membranes have burst, these enzymes are released and begin to digest the cell from the inside out. This process is known as autolysis (or self-digestion) . . . Autolytic spread is most intimately tied to environmental temperature. In cold surroundings, the autolytic process slows down, while warm conditions speed up the progression.

Autolysis[8] rapidly progresses to putrefaction, which is the process whereby microbiological organisms (in the body, on the body and in the environ-ment) feed on the nutrient-rich fluids produced during autolysis.

From the point of what it is to be human, death, or immediately impend-ing death, can be categorized in two ways, one related to cognition and consciousness, the other related to the failure of life to reverse the processes of thermodynamic equilibrium.

- The first of these is the recognition that the person is dead or dying because they are unconscious and their brain is irreversibly damaged, either directly through trauma or disease, or indirectly through loss of circulating oxygenated blood.
- The second is the recognition that enough cells, through disease in one or more organs, are failing to maintain their internal environment such that the whole organism subsequently fails.

Clearly there are overlaps between these two concepts, but when autol-ysis and putrefaction supervene, it demonstrates a complete loss of the vital functions of life to use energy and nutrients from the environment to maintain the necessary internal *milieu*. At this stage, the second law of thermodynamics is fully active in irreversibly breaking down all the body's complex constituents to their basic molecular level with maximum molecular disorder and maximum entropy. What were previously the atomic components of the human are now ready to re-enter the well-known nitrogen and carbon cycles etc. Although the recycling of many things from bottles to nuclear fuels is a key strategy of today's 'green' policies, it has been occurring in nature for eons. Whilst the statistics are open to challenge, it has even been calculated that over the space of a few hours we will all breathe in at least one of the atoms of carbon that was exhaled in Julius Caesar's last breath,[9] which produced the famous words 'Et tu, Brute?', on the Ides of March in 44 BCE.[10]

The diagnosis of death

Introduction

In the UK there are no absolute criteria set down in law that can be used to determine death, although there are criteria determined by custom and practice. In legal terms a person is dead when a person qualified or approved to say so confirms that death has occurred – you're dead when we say you're dead! When this has happened, all transactions in that person's name legally cease, e.g., their bank accounts are frozen, their pension payments stop, there can be no further documents sent carrying their signature and any creditors and dues to the taxman are paid from their assets by the executors. Through an anomaly in British law it is not possible to be guilty of either libel or slander against the deceased, and so far efforts to bring cases by relatives under Article 8 of the Human Rights Act[11] have not succeeded.

Declaring a person dead

In this chapter it is assumed that the death is normal. Unnatural deaths and brain death are covered in Chapters 27 and 34, respectively.

The person confirming death does not have to be a registered clinical practitioner (e.g., nurse or doctor), but does have to be a 'competent' adult defined by the Care Quality Commission[12] as 'an individual with the knowledge, skills and competencies required to be able to confirm death'. This has obvious application in situations with expected deaths in care homes or other community settings. English law is surprisingly silent on many issues; for example, it:

- does not require a doctor to confirm death has occurred or that 'life is extinct'
- does not require a doctor to view the body of a deceased person
- does not require a doctor to report the fact that death has occurred.

However, it:

- does require the doctor who attended the deceased during their last illness to issue a certificate detailing the cause of death.

Guidance on defining and diagnosing human death

There have been a number of guidance documents on the diagnosis of death, such as those published by the Academy of Medical Royal Colleges[13] and the Royal College of Nursing[14]. In the USA in 2008, the US President's Council on Bioethics[15] explored the possibilities of defining what is life and what is death. They reasoned as follows.

> All organisms have a needy mode of being. Unlike inanimate objects, which continue to exist through inertia and without effort, every organism persists only thanks to its own exertions. To preserve themselves, organisms must—and can and do—engage in commerce with the surrounding world. Their constant need for oxygenated air and nutrients is matched by their ability to satisfy that need, by engaging in certain activities, reaching out into the surrounding environment to secure the required sustenance. This is the definitive work of the organism as an organism. It is what an organism 'does' and what distinguishes every organism from non-living things. And it is what distinguishes a living organism from the dead body that it becomes when it dies.

In offering this definition, the President's Council was equating life with the concepts of Erwin Schrödinger and life's ability to reverse the second law of thermodynamics as described above. They then continued to examine the consequences of this for the whole, sentient human. In so doing they introduced the importance of consciousness and human characteristics and concluded as follows.[16]

> If there are no signs of consciousness and if spontaneous breathing is absent and if the best clinical judgment is that these neurophysiological facts cannot be reversed . . . it . . . would lead us to conclude that a once-living patient has now died. Thus, on this account, total brain failure

can continue to serve as a criterion for declaring death—not because it necessarily indicates complete loss of integrated somatic functioning, but because it is a sign that this organism can no longer engage in the essential work that defines living things.

In stating this they unified the link between individual 'thermodynamic' cell death and death of the whole organism that is a recognizable human being. Thus, the death of the human occurs at a time not when all the cells of the body are necessarily definitively dead, but when what makes them human has irreversibly died. This is of course why a live organ can be harvested from a dead body.

With a 'normal' death, within 15 seconds of absent cerebral circulation consciousness is lost. For many years, 'normal' death meant the sequential onset of apnoea, unconsciousness and circulatory arrest and this was used as the basis for diagnosing death. Diagnosing death in this situation requires confirmation that there has been irreversible damage to the vital centres in the brain-stem due to the length of time in which the circulation to the brain has been absent.

Although there are no 'rules', custom and practice in the UK[17] would, as a minimum, recommend:

- an external examination of the person
- palpation of the major pulses
- auscultation of the heart and breath sounds with adequate exposure of the chest.

for a period of at least five minutes, together with

- confirmation of the absence of pupillary reflexes (and if possible an examination of the retina).

To these, the UK 2008 Code of Practice would add:[18]

- confirmation of the absence of any motor response to supra-orbital pressure
- confirmation that any spontaneous return of cardiac or respiratory activity during this period of observation should prompt a further five minutes observation from the next point of cardiorespiratory arrest.

Meticulous note-keeping of the procedure undertaken to confirm death is paramount and the time of death is recorded as the time at which the criteria are fulfilled (not when the person stopped breathing).

Although common as dramatic events in popular literature, even when applying care, mistakes concerning the diagnosis of death can still occur in clinical practice. It is good advice to wait before pronouncing life extinct in the presence of relatives because of agonal gasps etc., and errors can be made with hypothermia,[19] drug overdoses and electric shocks. For many young doctors a particularly stressful time is when they are encouraged to declare death (by those with no responsibility for it) so that a patient does not have to be formally admitted into a hospital (e.g., in an ambulance, arrival at an A&E department). The rule is to be as sure as you can be, through thoroughness and patience: never pronounce life extinct when you just 'think' it might or should be.

International consensus on the diagnosis of death

Over recent years there has been a considerable international effort to harmonize the definition of death and its determination. Although some details differ, there is now a consensus[20] that death requires both:

- the irreversible loss of the capacity for consciousness
- the irreversible loss of the capacity to breathe.

Using this definition, death can be diagnosed using three different sets of criteria:

- somatic
- circulatory
- neurological.

The most appropriate set of criteria to use is determined by the circumstances of death, although in practice, as before, they are commonly used in combination. This scheme is shown in Figure 26.3.

The three sets of criteria in Figure 26.3 are intended to be applied as follows.[21]

Somatic criteria

Somatic criteria are those that can be applied by simple external inspection of the corpse without any need to undertake a detailed clinical examination. They include such things as decapitation, rigor mortis and decomposition. Examples are given below.

1   massive cranial and cerebral destruction
2   hemicorporectomy

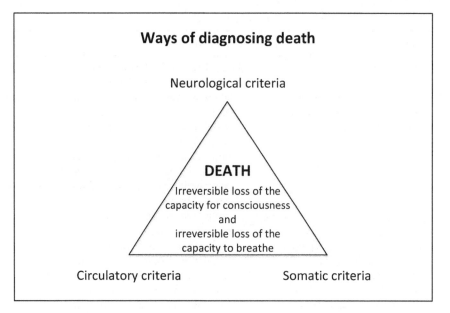

Ways of diagnosing death

Neurological criteria

DEATH
Irreversible loss of the
capacity for consciousness
and
irreversible loss of the
capacity to breathe

Circulatory criteria   Somatic criteria

FIGURE **26.3** The three sets of criteria for diagnosing death

3   massive truncal injury incompatible with life including decapitation
4   decomposition/putrefaction (where tissue damage indicates that the
    patient has been dead for some hours)
5   incineration (the presence of full-thickness burns with charring of
    > 95% of the body surface)
6   hypostasis (the pooling of blood in congested vessels in the dependent
    part of the body in the position in which it lies after death)
7   rigor mortis (the stiffness occurring after death from the post-mortem
    breakdown of enzymes in the muscle fibres).

On finding such a deceased person, in the record it is often referred to as
'recognition of life extinct' (ROLE).

Circulatory criteria

The essential components to declare circulatory death and predict irreversible
loss of consciousness and the capacity to breathe are set out in Table 26.1.

The UK has adopted five minutes as the observation period for the
diagnosis of death from the observed time of the loss of circulation. Other
countries have different time criteria and international agreement is hoped
to evolve.

217

TABLE 26.1 The essential criteria for diagnosing circulatory death

Component	Explanation
1 A clear intention not to attempt cardiopulmonary resuscitation (CPR) in order to restore circulatory, and therefore cerebral, function	An exclusion of indications to commence or continue CPR. This may be because there has been a decision not to perform CPR, or a decision after unsuccessful CPR that further attempts are futile. Importantly, contributory causes to any cardiorespiratory arrest (e.g., hypothermia ≤ 34°C, endocrine, metabolic or biochemical abnormality) should be considered and treated, if appropriate, before diagnosing death
2 An observation period to confirm continuous apnoea, absent circulation, and unconsciousness, after which the likelihood of spontaneous resumption of cardiac function will have passed	After this observation period the circulation will not spontaneously return and the inevitable anoxic ischaemic injury to the brain that follows the loss of the cerebral circulation will continue unabated. There is international variation in the length of observation period required to establish safe practice.
3 The prohibition at any time of any intervention that might restore cerebral blood flow by any means.	Were cerebral circulation to be re-established, the diagnosis of death using circulatory criteria would be invalidated.

Neurological criteria

These are covered in Chapter 34 on brain-stem death.

Summary on the diagnosis of death

The diagnosis of death can be easy or difficult, depending upon the circumstances. However, there is now widespread acceptance that the death of a human does not require the death of every cell in the body; instead it means the death of what constitutes the essence of what it is to be a human. There are two necessary criteria that need to be present before a person can be declared dead. These are:

• the irreversible loss of the capacity for consciousness
• the irreversible loss of the capacity to breathe.

In most cases in both hospital and community practice, clinical examination and observation can establish when death has occurred but the diagnosis of death must never be rushed. There is an increasing international consensus around the definition of death but there are some details (e.g., time of observation of circulatory death) that continue to vary from country to country.

Notes

1 As discussed in Part I, Chapters 5 and 7.
2 Aurelius M (2006): *Meditations*, trans. Hammond M, Penguin Classics, Book 2, paragraph 17.1.
3 Spencer H (1862): *First Principles*, 6th edn, Williams and Norgate Ltd., section 25, 'The Relativity of All Knowledge', p. 70.
4 Sharp JA (1973): *Cells, Organs and Animals*, Blackwell Scientific Publications, chapter 1, 'Life and the Protozoa', p. 9–12.
5 Schrödinger E (1944): *What is Life?*, republished as *What is Life, Mind and Matter, and Autobiographical Sketches* (1992), Cambridge University Press; see chapters 6 and 7, pp. 67–85.
6 The second law of thermodynamics studies the properties of a derived physical variable known as entropy. Entropy is a measure of the 'disorder' of physical matter, such that a molecule of petrol in the fuel tank would have less entropy than its breakdown products after it is burnt. Furthermore, the petrol molecule could not be spontaneously recreated, i.e., the reaction had a direction which can only be reversed with the further input of external energy. In its usual form the second law is stated as 'In all spontaneous processes, the total entropy always increases and the process is irreversible'.
7 Vass A (2018): 'After a Person's Pulse and Breathing Stop, How Much Later Does All Cellular Metabolism Stop?' *Scientific American* (16 July 2007). www.scientific american.com/article/experts-cell-metabolism-after-death/
8 It should be noted *en passant* that autolytic change in the absence of a supply of oxygen is variable in onset from tissue to tissue. Nervous tissue quickly becomes irreversible damaged within about four minutes whereas muscle is more resistant, without which surgery under tourniquet would not be possible.
9 Kean S (2018): *Caesar's Last Breath*, Transworld Publishers, pp. 4–11.
10 Shakespeare W (ca. 1599): *The Tragedy of Julius Caesar*; there are many publishers. Caesar utters these words in Act III, Scene 1, as he is being stabbed to death, having recognized his friend and protégé Brutus as one of the assassins.
11 Human Rights Act 1998: Schedule 1, Part 1, Article 8 reads 'Everyone has the right to respect for his private and family life, his home and his correspondence'.
12 www.cqc.org.uk/guidance-providers/gps/nigels-surgery-13-who-can-confirm-death.
13 Academy of Medical Royal Colleges (2008): 'A Code of Practice for the Diagnosis and Confirmation of Death'. Available at: http://aomrc.org.uk/wp-content/uploads/2016/04/Code_Practice_Confirmation_Diagnosis_Death_1008-4.pdf.
14 Royal College of Nursing (2018): 'Confirmation or Verification of Death by Registered Nurses'. Available at: www.rcn.org.uk/get-help/rcn-advice/confirma tion-of-death.
15 The President's Council on Bioethics (2008): *Controversies in the Determination of Death: A White Paper by the President's Council on Bioethics*, Washington, DC, p. 60. Available at: https://repository.library.georgetown.edu/bitstream/handle/10822/559343/Controversies%20in%20the%20Determination%20of%20Death%20for%20the%20Web.pdf?sequence=1&isAllowed=y.
16 *Ibid.*, pp. 64–65.
17 Green J, Green M (2006): *Dealing with Death*, 2nd edn, Jessica Kingsley, chapter 1, p. 29.

18 Academy of Medical Royal Colleges (2008): 'A Code of Practice for the Diagnosis and Confirmation of Death'. Available at: http://aomrc.org.uk/wp-content/uploads/2016/04/Code_Practice_Confirmation_Diagnosis_Death_1008-4.pdf.

19 People who have drowned in very cold water and are not recovered for an hour or so can, in some rare circumstances, be completely revived. The cold temperatures slow down the autolytic process to the point that no permanent damage occurs in the tissues.

20 Gardiner D, Shemie S, Manara A, Opdam H (2012): 'International Perspective on the Diagnosis of Death', *British Journal of Anaesthesia*, Vol. 108, i14–i28.

21 *Ibid.*

Chapter 27

Medico-legal issues at the end of life

Introduction

The main aim of this chapter is to address medico-legal considerations that healthcare workers caring for patients at the end of their life need to be aware of. These considerations include matters around confidentiality, consent for examination of the body, advanced directives and powers of attorney. In addition, we will address some other, albeit uncommon, issues around death such as euthanasia, suicide, unnatural deaths and persistent vegetative state.

Confidentiality

The duty of confidentiality does not cease with death and all details of the patient, their condition and any results of tests must be kept confidential just as when they were alive.[1] Information must not be disclosed to a third party, such as a solicitor or a police officer, without the permission of the person concerned, or, after death, the permission of their closest relative. If there was a breach of confidence that led to personal damage of the deceased or their relatives, a civil case for compensation could be brought and the doctor's registration would come under scrutiny. There are a few exceptions to this general rule, as follows.

- Although the courts have some discretion, if the judge requests confidential information in the interests of justice, the doctor is not entitled to refuse to answer.
- If the life of another person is put at risk by strict confidentiality, it is usually regarded as allowable to breach the general rule. This could for instance be for a communicable infectious disease or an inheritable condition the surviving relatives were unaware of.

Consent

When consent is sought to undertake an examination of the whole or a part of a deceased person's body, full weight must be given to any advance directives and living wills they had made (see below).

The law in England and Wales regarding the examination and use of human post-mortem tissues was introduced in the Human Tissue Act 2004, which created the Human Tissue Authority (HTA) as a statutory body. The HTA's regulatory remit is, through its licenses, to regulate the following activities:

a) post-mortem examination
b) anatomical examination
c) public display of tissue from the deceased
d) the removal and storage of human tissue for a range of purposes, including transplantation, research, medical treatment, education and training.

To examine a dead person, in whole or in part, permission has to be sought from the deceased's nominated representative or otherwise from a person in a *qualifying relationship* with the deceased immediately before their death. Consent must be obtained from the person ranked highest in the hierarchy and is only needed from one person in the hierarchy. The listed legal hierarchy of qualifying relationships are ranked in the following descending order:

a) spouse or partner (including civil or same-sex partner)
b) parent or child (in this context a child may be of any age)
c) brother or sister
d) grandparent or grandchild
e) niece or nephew
f) stepfather or stepmother
g) half-brother or half-sister
h) friend of long standing.

The HTA has guidance for relatives and staff on all issues related to dead tissue, including consent[2] and it issues model consent forms. The latter are given in Appendix 27.1 to this chapter.

The doctrine of double effect

The doctrine of double effect is the situation when life is shortened by the therapeutic relief of symptoms. It implies that sedatives and opioids can be given to relieve suffering but cannot be prescribed for the primary effect of hastening death.

The death of a patient under these conditions is commonplace in UK hospitals, although the actual law is not really clear. There have been a number of key test cases that have influenced current practice. Examples are as follows.

- In 1997, Annie Lindsell established that doctors could legally administer potentially life-shortening drugs not only for the relief of physical distress but also for mental distress.
- In 1999, Dr David Moor was found not guilty of murder for administering diamorphine and chlorpromazine to distressed dying patients.

Currently, the last word to date on this situation was from the Director of Public Prosecutions in 2010. He issued guidance to say that it was acceptable to balance compassion against malign intent. The guidance gave no immunity from prosecution but to date there have been no prosecutions, and the liberal use of opioids and sedatives remains frequent in the management of the dying.

There have been several attempts to get the law changed in this area but to date all have failed.

Advance directives and powers of attorney

There have been changes to the law that have modified the landscape of the management of some end-of-life issues particularly with respect to a person's future wishes. The most important are that competence and capacity are covered by the Mental Capacity Act 2005 and the Mental Health Act 2007. The Court of Protection was also created under the Mental Capacity Act 2005. It has jurisdiction over the property, financial affairs and personal welfare of people who lack mental capacity to make decisions for themselves and carries powers of attorney.

There are five core principles relating to capacity. These are as follows.

1 All people over 16 years should be assumed to have capacity unless clearly incapable.
2 A person should be helped to express their capacity (e.g., using an interpreter).
3 Capable patients can make unwise decisions.

4   Incapable patients are to be treated in their best interests, which are not necessarily their medical best interests.
5   The minimum necessary intervention must be used if acting in the patient's best interests.

If a person is deemed not to have capacity when a significant decision has to be made about their future (e.g., when they are ill), then the most important documents to be consulted are 'living wills' and 'powers of attorney' which were signed when the person did have capacity. These count ahead of the wishes of relatives and friends if they are relevant to the situation needing resolution. The documents are different but also related in that they both respect the autonomy of the individual. Not to respect an individual's autonomy and human rights in the 21st century can lead to the charge of assault and battery.

An advance directive, also known as a living will:

- has legal force if relevant to the situation needing resolution
- is not registered with any statutory agency
- is often written so as to be for specific circumstances and may direct particular actions in ambiguous situations
- often tends to reflect what the person thinks could happen and is a reflection of their fears, e.g. surviving in a brain-damaged state
- can sometimes be difficult to apply in practice.

Power of attorney:

- is registered with the Court of Protection on prescribed forms which support sensible statements being made
- requires that one or more people (attorneys) are appointed to act for an individual by the individual as if it were that individual who was making the decision
- grants attornyes wide powers of decision making
- can be applied to any situation
- is usually easier to apply in practice than an advance directive, which is specific only to certain circumstances.

Euthanasia

Euthanasia is the term given to a situation in which another person, e.g., a doctor, nurse or relative, intentionally ends a patient's life. It should be emphasized that this is a deliberate act by a different individual from the patient, and so is distinct from the assisted dying and assisted suicide that are described below. There are two broad categories.

- *Voluntary euthanasia* is usually defined as terminal illness, intolerable suffering or an incurable condition affecting a patient whose life is ended on their request by a clinician administering lethal drugs. This is legal in the Netherlands, Belgium and Luxembourg.
- *Involuntary euthanasia* is when the clinician takes the decision to end their life without the permission of the patient. This is illegal everywhere, but there is evidence from anonymous surveys that it happens on occasions.[3]

Any type of euthanasia is illegal in the UK, and it leads to the charge of murder if a practitioner is accused of it.

Suicide

Suicide is the taking of a person's own life. It ceased to be a crime in England and Wales following the 1961 Suicide Act. However, it remains a crime for a second person to assist a person who wishes or is attempting to die from suicide, and criminal charges can be brought with a maximum penalty of 14 years. This has occurred from time to time in a number of well-intentioned so-called 'mercy killings'. At the time of writing, despite many efforts in the UK Parliament, assisting a suicide remains a crime on the statute book.

If a person who has died from suicide is discovered, then the health professional first on the scene should treat it as an unnatural death (see below), realizing that if it is a suicide there is always an inquest and, second, remembering that other unnatural deaths (e.g., manslaughter, murder), can be arranged to look like suicide.

In some other jurisdictions, taking one's own life when terminally ill or having intolerable suffering is permitted provided that the patient is in a sound mental state. The terminology of this area is difficult, but an accepted terminology based on the type of intervention would be as follows.

- *Assisted dying* is usually defined as a terminal prognosis of less than six months; the patient takes the prescribed lethal drugs. In the USA it is permitted in Oregon, Vermont, Montana and Washington.
- *Assisted suicide* is usually defined as intolerable suffering or an incurable condition without necessarily being terminally ill; the patient takes the prescribed lethal drugs. It is permitted in Switzerland.

The best known of these options is in Switzerland to where terminally ill patients and their families travel for the patient to receive self-administered treatment leading to their death at the Dignitas Clinic. Dignitas describe themselves as:

> a not-for-profit members' society which advocates, educates and supports for improving care and choice in life and at life's end.

The details of their principles and facilities can be found on their web page.[4]

Elective ventilation of potential organ donors

The management of brain dead potential organ donors in an intensive-care setting is described in Chapter 34. This section covers the situation where an intervention is needed to electively ventilate someone to provide organs for others after their death. It is an ethical quagmire.

The nub of the problem is that in many instances the potential donor is incompetent, the relatives cannot give consent to remove organs as long as the patient is alive and the only justification for interventions is the best interests of another patient. On the other hand, the patient may have made an advance directive wishing others to benefit from their death. Elective ventilation may be of benefit for the future recipients, but it is not in the best interests of the patient because the intervention is futile.

Following efforts to intervene with elective ventilation in the early 1990s, it was effectively declared illegal in 1994. Since then there has been renewed interest in it and guidance has been published by the Academy of Medical Royal Colleges. Their summary of the position is as follows.

> The UK faces a continuing shortage of organ donors and many people who wished to donate die in circumstances that do not allow them to do so. NTEV (non-therapeutic elective ventilation) has been reported as a technique that, for some patients, can make donation possible and can increase the number of organs available. It has not been used in the UK for over two decades because it was thought to be unlawful, but major changes in the law since then may suggest that NTEV is lawful in some cases. Clinical practice has also changed so that we no longer know when NTEV would be possible or suitable, or for how many patients. There is existing generic guidance on non-therapeutic interventions, and if the law allowed it then the principles of this guidance could be applied to NTEV to help determine its suitability.

The debate about the use of NTEV has become unproductive because of the perception that it is unlawful. That perception is driven by legal advice that is no longer reliable because the legal context has changed. The barriers to the use of NTEV are so large that it could not yet be readily recommended, but its potential use needs to be re- examined.[5]

Watch this space.

Persistent vegetative state

The persistent vegetative state is a difficult and contentious area of practice which has recently received guidance from a court judgement.

The vegetative state is one where a patient with clearly demonstrable brain injury has sufficient brainstem and hypothalamic function to allow breathing and neuroendocrine function but shows no signs of awareness of either self or environment for a prolonged period of time. The diagnosis of vegetative state is untenable if there is any degree of voluntary movement, or evidence of sight, hearing or protective reflexes. The person needs to be fed to keep them alive. If the condition persists for over a year it is known as a 'persistent vegetative state' (PVS).

The condition came to public prominence with the Tony Bland case. He was injured in a disaster at a football stadium in 1989 and in 1992, with the permission of his parents, Airedale Trust (where he was being cared for) applied to the High Court for permission to remove his feeding tube; this was granted. We will not here consider the often rather philosophical arguments as to what was in his best interests or whether ethical calisthenics could distinguish between the active ending of life (as in murder), or the (passive) double effect of removing his nutrition

Since that time individual cases have been dealt with through the Court of Protection system. However, on 30 July 2018, following an application by an NHS Trust and a patient's relatives it was ruled that in the majority of cases there was no longer a need to refer decisions on withdrawal of support in cases of PSV.[6] The ruling put in place safeguards that have to be followed before any decision can be taken, but if these are satisfied and both the medical team and the relatives are in favour of the cessation of nutrition, then it can be withdrawn.

Unnatural death

If a doctor suspects that there has been an unnatural death (e.g., body lying at the bottom of the stairs, lividity incompatible with the position in which the body was found), the law, and custom and practice is clear. Once death has been confirmed, the doctor must ensure that no further changes are made to the scene of death and immediately inform the police. From that moment on they will process the case.

Appendix 27.1 Model consent form from the Human Tissue Authority

This model consent form is available at: www.hta.gov.uk/policies/post-mortem-model-consent-forms.

Post-mortem examination consent form

Introduction

This model consent form provides a suggested format for NHS Trusts obtaining consent for post-mortem (PM) examination of adults, in line with the requirements of the Human Tissue Act 2004. The form may be adapted, providing it complies with the Act and follows the Human Tissue Authority's (HTA) codes of practice on consent, post-mortem examination and disposal of human tissue found at: www.hta.gov.uk/legislationpoliciesandcodesof practice/codesofpractice.cfm. It could be used for older paediatric cases, but is not recommended for stillbirths, neonatal deaths, fetal tissue or non-fetal products of conception.

Staff seeking consent for PM examination must ensure that they have appropriate consent, in line with the Human Tissue Act 2004. Staff must ensure that consent is given by the person concerned whilst alive, their nominated representative or (in the absence of either of these) someone in a qualifying relationship with the deceased immediately before they died. See Guidance Note 6 at the end of this form for more information.

The consent form is important as a record of consent given. The completion of the form is just one part of the consent process. Full explanation of the PM examination procedure along with discussion and time for reflection by those consenting are equally important. Individuals and relatives should be able to discuss this process fully and ask any questions. Staff seeking consent for PM examination must be trained in how to obtain valid consent.

Consent is only valid if proper communication has taken place. Consideration should be given to the needs of individuals and families whose first language is not English.

The consent form covers consent for the PM examination itself as well as for the retention and use of organs and tissue following the PM examination.

Format of the form

Please note that there are three sections to this form.

This form is produced as a Word file. You can edit the sections to make them appropriate for your Trust. *Guidance notes*, available at the end of this form, are also indicated by yellow shaded sections. They offer extra guidance and some suggest text that you might like to consider inserting, according to local practices.

If you are having the form printed professionally, you may wish to consider producing it as a three-page booklet with duplicate copies.

Consent for post-mortem examination of an adult

Name of deceased:

Date of birth: Date of death:

Consultant / GP in charge of the patient:

Hospital number for deceased:

This form enables you to consent to a post-mortem examination of the body of the person named above. Please read it carefully with the person obtaining consent from you. For each section tick the relevant box to indicate your decisions and sign beneath each section.

☐ I confirm that I have had the opportunity to read and understand the *[insert name of information leaflet]*.

☐ I confirm that my questions about the post-mortem examination have been answered to my satisfaction and understanding.

Signed by.................................Name..

Part 1: Post-mortem examination

A post-mortem examination may be full or limited. The benefits and disadvantages of each will be explained to you. Please choose **one** of the following options.

Option 1: Consent to a full post-mortem examination

☐ I consent to a **full** post-mortem examination of the body of the person named above. I am not aware that he / she objected to this. I understand that the reason for the examination is to further explain the cause of death and study the effects of disease and treatment.

Option 2: Consent to a limited post-mortem examination

☐ I consent to a **limited** post-mortem examination of the body of the person named above. I am not aware that he / she objected to this. I understand that this may limit the information about the cause of death and effects of treatment.

I wish to limit the examination to (please specify) ....

[See guidance note 1]

[See guidance note 2]

Signed by.....................................Name..

Part 2: Retention and future use of tissue samples

As part of a full or limited post-mortem examination tissue samples and small amounts of bodily fluids may be taken and used to determine the diagnosis and extent of the disease. Bodily fluids will usually be disposed of following a diagnosis. However, the tissue samples removed during a post-mortem examination can be stored for use in the future. The storage of the tissue samples and their later use require your consent. These samples can be valuable for the education and training of healthcare professionals, research and other purposes. Please indicate whether you consent to this:

☐ I consent to the tissue samples being stored for future use, and

☐ I consent to the tissue samples being used for the purpose of evaluating the efficacy of any drug or treatment administered to the deceased, or for review on behalf of the family if a need arises

☐ I consent to tissue samples being used for education and training relating to human health, quality assurance, public health monitoring or clinical audit

☐ I consent to the tissue samples being used for research that has been approved by an appropriate ethics committee

If you decide tissue samples should <u>not</u> be kept after the post-mortem examination, further diagnosis will not be possible and the tissue samples will be disposed of.

[See guidance note 3]

Signed by.................................Name.......................................

Part 3: Retention of organs for more detailed examination

As part of a full or limited post-mortem examination, it may be necessary to retain some organs for more detailed examination. The person explaining about the post-mortem examination will tell you what may be required. The retention of organs for more detailed examination requires your consent. Please indicate whether you consent to this:

☐ I consent to the retention, for more detailed examination, of the following organ(s):

....
....

Disposal of retained organs

After more detailed examination of organs removed during a post-mortem examination, they must be either stored for specified uses or disposed of in a lawful manner. You have the option of donating retained organs for research or medical education. Please indicate your wishes by choosing **one** of the following options:

☐ I wish to donate retained organ(s) for research into related diseases, after which they will be disposed of lawfully

☐ I wish to donate retained organ(s) for education, after which they will be disposed of lawfully

☐ I wish the hospital to lawfully dispose of any retained organ(s), without them being used for research and/or education

☐ I will make my own arrangements for lawful disposal of any retained organ(s) *[See guidance note 4]*

Signed by.................................Name.......................................

Other requirements of the post-mortem examination

In some cases there may be further requirements of the post-mortem examination, such as genetic testing of tissue samples. The person explaining about the post-mortem examination will explain these to you. Other requests or conditions which you would like to make:

....

....

Thank you for consenting to a post-mortem examination. You can change your mind about any of the decisions you have made, although there may be a short time limit for some of these. If you wish to make changes to anything you have consented to, or wish to withdraw your consent, please telephone *[insert contact details]* as soon as possible and not later than.................................... *[See guidance note 5]*. Please do not hesitate to contact the *[insert contact details]* if you have any questions.

Signed..Name ....

Address...

....Tel no..

Relationship to the deceased ....Date ....

[See guidance note 6]

Details of person obtaining consent

Name ....Job title ....

Contact details...

Notes for person(s) obtaining consent

- I confirm that the person consenting has a full understanding of the post-mortem examination procedure.
- I confirm that I have checked that the person consenting is the appropriate person for the purposes of the Human Tissue Act 2004 *[See guidance note 6]*.
- I have discussed tissue samples being retained for future use and the potential uses for the tissue that is retained.
- Consent is indicated by boxes which are ticked and signature of the person giving consent.
- I have discussed any special requests or conditions concerning the post-mortem examination procedure.

- Where appropriate, I have discussed the requirements of the post-mortem examination.

with.. *[insert name of pathologist]*

Signed...Date...............................

- I have offered a photocopy of this form to the person giving consent
- If consent is subsequently withdrawn, either for the entire post-mortem examination, or for specific sections of it, each page of each copy of the form (or the relevant section(s)) should be clearly struck through. The person taking the withdrawal should also sign and date the form clearly, and note action taken to inform the mortuary (the date and time and member of mortuary staff informed).

Guidance notes

Guidance notes are indicated by sections in this form. They offer extra guidance and some suggest text that you might like to consider inserting, according to local practices.

Guidance note 1

You may wish to add more detail about what will be included in a limited post-mortem examination and replace 'Option 2: Consent to a limited post-mortem examination', with the below:

Option 2: Consent to a limited post-mortem examination

☐ I consent to a limited post-mortem examination of the body of the person named above. I am not aware that he / she objected to this. I understand that this may limit the information about the cause of death and effects of treatment.

I wish to limit the examination to:

☐ The head and mouth cavity, including the brain
☐ The chest and neck
☐ The abdomen and pelvis
☐ Other (please specify) ....

....

Signed by...............................Name.......................................

Guidance note 2

You may wish to add this option if it is applicable to your Trust:

Option 3: Consent to a non-invasive post-mortem examination

☐ I consent to a non-invasive post-mortem examination of the body of the person named above. I am not aware that he / she objected to this. I understand that this may limit the information about the cause of death and effects of treatment.

Guidance note 3

You may wish to add here:

If you decide tissue samples should <u>not</u> be kept after the post-mortem examination, further diagnosis will not be possible. Please indicate one of the options below for the disposal of tissue samples:

☐ I wish the hospital to dispose of any retained tissue samples
☐ I will make my own arrangements for lawful disposal of any retained tissue samples *[See guidance note 4]*

Guidance note 4

If the wishes of the relatives are to reunite organs and tissue with the body before burial or cremation, the establishment should have a system of checking that any retained tissue is accounted for before the body is released to the family. If there is tissue not accounted for, the establishment should have a clear procedure for the course of action to be followed. Efforts should be made to keep the relatives informed throughout the process.

Tissue blocks and glass slides should not be placed inside the body for the purpose of reuniting tissues with the deceased, and this should be discussed with the relatives during the consenting process. Blocks and slides should be placed in a suitable container and transported with the body should the family wish to delay the funeral until they are returned.

If retained tissue cannot be reunited with the body before it is released for burial or cremation, the establishment should have a procedure that ensures the relatives are informed and that there is prompt and appropriate disposal in accordance with the Code of practice on Disposal of human tissue.

Guidance note 5

Once a decision has been made to proceed with the PM examination and consent has been given, the family should be given the opportunity to change their minds or to change the scope of the PM examination. The time relatives have to reflect on their decision and the point up to which they may withdraw their consent should be clearly stated and should not be less than 12 hours. The HTA recommends 24 hours.

Guidance note 6

Staff seeking consent must ensure that they have appropriate consent, in line with the Human Tissue Act 2004. Staff must ensure that consent is obtained from, **in this order:**

1 **the person concerned**- where an adult has, whilst alive, given valid consent for a post-mortem examination to take place after their death, this consent is sufficient
2 their **nominated representative**- the Human Tissue Act 2004 sets out the terms for valid appointment of a nominated representative. See the code of practice on Consent for more information www.hta.gov. uk/legislationpoliciesandcodesofpractice/codesofpractice.cfm **or**, in the absence of either of the above,
3 a person in a **qualifying relationship** with the deceased immediately before their death. Consent must be obtained from the person ranked highest in the hierarchy and is only needed from one person in the hierarchy:

Hierarchy of qualifying relationships Persons are ranked in the following descending order:

i) spouse or partner (including civil or same sex partner)
j) parent or child (in this context a child may be of any age)
k) brother or sister
l) grandparent or grandchild
m) niece or nephew
n) stepfather or stepmother
o) half-brother or half-sister
p) friend of long standing.

Notes

1 This is stated in the GMC's Good Medical Practice, para 50; General Medical Council (2013): 'Good Medical Practice'. Available at: www.gmc-uk.org/-/media/documents/Good_medical_practice___English_1215.pdf_51527435.pdf.
2 HTA (2017): 'Guiding Principles and the Fundamental Principle of Consent'. Available at: www.hta.gov.uk/sites/default/files/files/HTA%20Code%20A_0.pdf.

3 See: Searle C (2009): 'End of Life Decisions in the UK Involving Medical Practitioners'. *Palliative Medicine*, Vol. 23, 198–204.
4 Available at: www.dignitas.ch/?lang=en.
5 Academy of Medical Royal Colleges (2016): 'Nontherapeutic Elective Ventilation'. Available at: www.aomrc.org.uk/wp-content/uploads/2016/07/Nontherapeutic_elective_ventilation_0416-2.pdf.
6 Available at: www.supremecourt.uk/cases/docs/uksc-2017-0202-judgment.pdf.

Chapter 28

The responses of professionals and relatives around death

Introduction

During and soon after the end-of-life period, a number of relatives and healthcare workers become involved in various roles. Funeral directors also have an essential part to play. It is important that all involved are clear regarding their own responsibilities, and the responsibilities of others, during this extremely sensitive time. Also, certain formalities and etiquettes must be observed. The present chapter aims to bring clarification regarding the roles of relatives, healthcare professionals and funeral directors.

The health professionals' role

All health professionals get instruction in the management of death and there is little point in reiterating that which is commonly taught. The GMC issues good advice for doctors,[1] and the NMC for nurses.[2] In 2014 a collaboration of both these bodies and several others published a document, 'One Chance To Get It Right',[3] which is full of sound advice. Extracts from this publication are below.

The priorities for care are that, when it is thought that a person may die within the next few days or hours:[4]

- this possibility is recognized and communicated clearly, decisions made and actions taken in accordance with the person's needs and wishes and these are regularly reviewed and decisions revised accordingly
- sensitive communication takes place between staff and the dying person, and those identified as important to them
- the dying person, and those identified as important to them, are involved in decisions about treatment and care to the extent that the dying person wants

- the needs of families and others identified as important to the dying person are actively explored, respected and met as far as possible
- an individual plan of care, which includes food and drink, symptom control and psychological, social and spiritual support, is agreed, co-ordinated and delivered with compassion.

They set out the collective and individual commitment to ensuring that all care given to people in the last days and hours of life:[5]

- is compassionate
- is based on and tailored to the needs, wishes and preferences of the dying person and, as appropriate, their family and those identified as important to them
- includes regular and effective communication between the dying person and their family and health and care staff, and between health and care staff and themselves
- involves assessment of the person's condition whenever that condition changes and timely and appropriate responses to those changes
- is led by a senior responsible doctor and a lead responsible nurse, who can access support from specialist palliative care services when needed
- is delivered by doctors, nurses, carers and others who have high professional standards and the skills, knowledge and experience needed to care for dying people and their families properly.

Every death is different, as is every patient and every set of relatives. Skilled care means tailoring and adapting to do what is best in any particular set of circumstances. There are no magic solutions and this is where experience and anticipation of individual needs counts. Much of what is best may be determined from the cultural norms of the patient and their relatives, and at the end of life it is important for the health professional to adapt to them, rather than the other way round. Respect for the patient and relatives is clearly paramount, but there are problems that can arise. Examples of dilemmas with no right or wrong answer are as follows.

- What words should be used when breaking bad news or speaking to a bereaved person?
- What should one's policy be on touching – is it alright to squeeze a hand or even put an arm round a shoulder?
- Can the person's pets be allowed in whilst they are dying?

- How does one deal with relatives who have genuine or misplaced aggression?
- What limitations should be put on the relatives' wishes that disturb other patients?

Compassionate and thoughtful care are clear professional duties to the dying and bereaved. However, what is often forgotten is that health professionals also have a duty towards their own welfare as well. This is obvious in terms of preventing cross-infection and analogous risks. However, protecting the psyche is not – yet it is very important to do this, if only to allow the health professional to continue to provide care to other patients in the future.

No health professional, if they have to care for dying patients, will escape experiencing at least some deaths that cause them considerable psychological upset. On occasions, having actually seen a dying person, a dead body or the pain some relatives suffer, some may find their resilience and beliefs (either religious or secular) suddenly challenged. Importantly, these disturbances are often not present at the time of providing the care during the so-called 'heat and burden of the day', but creep up later in quiet moments, sometimes when the person is alone. Guilt can also arise from taking part when a decision is made to withdraw futile life-prolonging treatment.

There are little hard data in this area, but in general these upsets are more frequent in the trainee or young professional. It is not uncommon for them to be bottled up within a false bravado. More senior staff have a duty to look out for unhappiness in junior colleagues and, if they suspect it, to tackle it promptly in confidence. If there has been a particularly upsetting death it is good practice for the team to have a reflective 'debriefing' session where everybody 'can tell it as it was for them'. This does much to alleviate feelings of loneliness and alienation and both spreads and alleviates the burden of responsibility.

The relatives' tasks, bereavement and grief

Tasks

In current clinical practice the role of relatives has been considerably increased from what it used to be, and this has been recognized in GMC guidance. In issues surrounding death it is particularly important because is allows clarity on the objectives of care, better decision making and aids the resolution of bereavement.

Guidance from the GMC is as follows.

> The people close to a patient can play a significant role in ensuring that the patient receives high-quality care as they near the end of life, in both community and hospital settings. Many close relatives and partners, as well as paid and unpaid carers, will be involved in discussing issues with a patient, enabling them to make choices, supporting them to communicate their wishes, or participating directly in their treatment and care. In some cases, they may have been granted legal power by the patient, or the court, to make healthcare decisions when the patient lacks capacity to make their own choices.
>
> It is important that doctors and other members of the healthcare team acknowledge the role and responsibilities of people close to the patient. They should make sure, as far as possible, that their needs for support are met and their feelings respected, although the focus of care must remain on the patient.
>
> Those close to a patient may want or need information about the patient's diagnosis and about the likely progression of the condition or disease, in order to help them provide care and recognise and respond to changes in the patient's condition. If a patient has capacity to make decisions, healthcare staff should check that they agree to you sharing this information. If a patient lacks capacity to make a decision about sharing information, it is reasonable to assume that, unless they indicate otherwise, they would want those closest to them to be kept informed of relevant information about their general condition and prognosis.
>
> When discussing the issues with people who do not have legal authority to make decisions on behalf of a patient who lacks capacity, it should be made clear that their role is to advise the healthcare team about the patient's known or likely wishes, preferences, feelings, beliefs and values. They must not be given the impression they are being asked to make the decision.[6]

Finally, after the patient has died, one of the relatives needs to adopt the role of the informant (see Chapter 30), and the hospital bereavement service should give them every assistance in arranging the registration of death and disposal of the body.

Bereavement and grief

Any discussion about death and dying eventually leads us all into the realm of grief. Dying people grieve for the life and relationships that they will leave behind. Family and friends will grieve for the loss of their dying loved one. Bereavement invariably leaves an impact that reverberates into wider circles associated with the deceased and their social networks – their workplaces, schools, places of play or worship. Clinicians too will inevitably form attachments to those under their care and will naturally grieve for their dying patients and feel for their grieving families.

Grief is the natural emotional and social consequences of attachment and loss, whether this is loss of a limb, one's country, one's employment or marriage, or other crucial relationships important to identity and personal aspiration. Although there are many sources of personal loss, the term 'bereavement' refers specifically to the loss of an important relationship through death. The grief associated with loss after bereavement is widely acknowledged to be associated with a number of serious co-morbidities and mortalities. These consequences can be medical (e.g., arrhythmias, gastrointestinal disorders, insomnia), psychological (e.g., anxiety, depression, sexual acting out) and social (e.g., lost work or school days, social isolation and loneliness, increased use of health services).[7] The more serious consequences can follow, for example, the sudden death of a surviving spouse/ partner, or suicide.[8]

The psychological literature about grief is intimidatingly large, and largely problem-focused. There have been serious professional and academic concerns over the 'pathologizing' of human sorrow – unnecessarily making sadness into a psychological 'condition' and blurring the boundaries between 'complicated' or 'abnormal' grief and normal grief[9,10] Some of this criticism is based largely on the ever-shrinking time period that is considered 'usual' for adaptation.[11] This body of professional opinion and research too often portrays grief as largely a negative, destructive force.[12] But although some people do encounter serious problems and challenges during the course of their grief, the most important public health insight is to acknowledge that the overwhelming majority of people more or less come to terms with their loss over time. The experience of a significant loss lasts forever. And the potency of that loss changes over time, as do our personal ways of dealing with these changes over the years. Many of these changes elicit constructive and positive (albeit under-recognized) responses to both character and to society – from greater compassion, meaning-making or personal insight to contributions to reform agendas and legacies in medicine, science or the arts.

For those whose grief takes them from the initial periods of unrelenting distress towards further physical, psychological or social decline, the debates about which therapeutic interventions are most effective, and when, are ongoing. Initial presentations of grief can vary widely – from highly demonstrative and persistent weeping and wailing to somber stoicism to apparent indifference. These differences are encouraged or moderated by different social conventions, but they do vary even within the same ethnic or religious communities. As such, these early expressions cannot in and of themselves, be used to predict long-term outcomes from bereavement. In this context, most clinicians dealing with the impact of dying or death will adapt their approach to the patient or family in their initial phases of grief.

Much of the current literature suggests that encouraging people into counseling in their initial period of bereavement is neither a particularly helpful nor an effective solution to this early experience of personal loss.[13,14] In the first days and weeks of grief after bereavement, friends and family should be encouraged to come together and support each other for the longer term, in the ways they know best, employing the intimate knowledge they have of each others' needs. Clinicians can also play an important role in offering comfort and support within their workplace environments – for patients, family and – just as importantly – for other colleagues. This should involve prioritizing listening over talking and awareness raising about support services. However, the epidemiological reality is that most people do cope with loss in the longer term with little to no professional assistance. Most people find their own social networks to be satisfactory, or even superior, to professional interventions from the health services.[15]

These above comments notwithstanding, it is important to recognize that sometimes there are patients with little or no family. There are also many instances of surviving family members with little or no extended social supports beyond themselves. This is particularly the case for some migrant families, older patients, international visitors or for the homeless and imprisoned. For these and other similar examples, a counselor or a spiritual advisor (such as a hospital chaplain) can be a very useful referral or additional colleague in support. It may also be useful to ensure that people in these particular circumstances are made aware of the support services that the hospital, hospice or care home can provide for them after death. It is common for patients and families not to be aware of the support services that are available to them in matters to do with dying, death and bereavement. This type of information is a sound first-order response to experiences of grief in patients and their families.

It is important to re-emphasize here that grief is not the sole province of surviving family and friends, and that dying people and many of our own colleagues grieve too. Many patients (and colleagues) will try to 'be strong' for family (or for other colleagues) and may more conveniently find comfort and support from a 'stranger' such as a chaplain. Supervision arrangements for colleagues should always explicitly create a space for the experience of loss and grief during the course of professional practice. On the other hand, many individuals, families and colleagues can feel embarrassed or vulnerable if the extent of their grief is made known to others. In the UK there are many ways that patients and their families can seek confidential, even anonymous, support.[16]

In the final analysis – sociologically and psychiatrically – religions can, and have, supplied comfort and support during life's most important transitions, including death. Many grieving people for whom religion remains important can and do seek meaning and solace from these sources. For others for whom religion is an unsteady or uncertain support, and still others for whom religion has no meaning, the company of family and friends remain an important comfort. In all the spaces where such supports fail, even momentarily, professional help can be a useful adjunct or alternative. Encouragement to use what supports exist, and accessible information about what supports are available when more is needed or the existing ones fail – these strategies remain our most important companions in our work among the dying and dead.

The funeral director's role

The role of the funeral director tends to get forgotten but it is critical to the legal and humanitarian management of bodies. In a multi-cultural society, they need knowledge of funeral practices across different faiths and different countries and of course must deal sympathetically with the bereaved. They may both embalm and cosmetically improve the appearance of bodies for viewing and have a range of coffins, furnishings and environmental styles available to match the needs of religious and secular groups.

Basic funeral procedures vary little between burial and cremation. In hospital practice they will collect the body from the mortuary once they have the certificate of disposal from the registrar or coroner. When a natural death occurs at home and the doctor completes an MCCD (medical certification of the cause of death; see Chapter 29), the funeral director usually removes the body to their premises, where it is laid out before rigor mortis sets in. Only rarely these days do relatives keep the body at home. The authority to dispose is obtained from the registrar by the informant in the usual way. Funeral directors often assist the relatives with the necessary paperwork and help with registration and completion of cremation certificates.

The role of the funeral director in the actual disposal process is tailored to the faith and needs of the relatives, as well as their means and what they can afford, extending to things such as memorial cards, press notices, floral tributes and refreshments. Burial authorities normally require several days' notice of intended internment, although in Judaism and Islam it is important to try to get the deceased buried within 24 hours.

Notes

1 GMC (2018): 'Ethical Guidance for Doctors; Treatment and Care towards the End of Life'. Available at: www.gmc-uk.org/ethical-guidance/ethical-guidance-for-doctors/treatment-and-care-towards-the-end-of-life.

2 NMC (2018): www.nmc.org.uk/about-us/policy/position-statements/end-of-life-care/.

3 Leadership Alliance for the Care of Dying People (2014): 'One Chance to Get it Right: Improving People's Experience of Care in the Last Few Days and Hours of Life'. Available at: https://assets.publishing.service.gov.uk/government/uploads/system/uploads/attachment_data/file/323188/One_chance_to_get_it_right.pdf.

4 *Ibid.*, p. 7.

5 *Ibid.*, p. 8.

6 GMC (2018): 'Ethical Guidance for Doctors; Treatment and Care towards the End of Life', paragraphs 18–21 and 28–30. Available at: www.gmc-uk.org/ethical-guidance/ethical-guidance-for-doctors/treatment-and-care-towards-the-end-of-life/working-with-the-principles-and-decision-making-models#paragraph-17.

7 Abel J, Kellehear A, Karapliagou A (2018): 'Palliative Care: The New Essentials'. *Annals of Palliative Medicine*, Vol. 7, No. 2, S3–S14.

8 Raphael B (1983): *The Anatomy of Bereavement*, Basic Books.

9 Walter T (1999): *On Bereavement: The Culture of Grief*, Open University Press.

10 Howarth G (2007): *Death & Dying: A Sociological Introduction*, Polity Press.

11 Horwitz AV, Wakefield, JC (2007): *The Loss of Sadness: How Psychiatry Transformed Normal Sorrow into Depressive Disorder*, Oxford University Press.

12 Kellehear A (2002): 'Grief and Loss: Past, Present, and Future'. *Medical Journal of Australia*, Vol. 177, No. 4, 176–177.

13 Stroebe W, Schut H, Stroebe MS (2005): 'Grief Work, Disclosure and Counseling: Do They Help the Bereaved?' *Clinical Psychology Review*, Vol. 25, 395–414.

14 Neimeyer R (2010): 'Grief Counseling and Therapy: The Case for Humility'. *Bereavement Care*, Vol. 29, No. 1, 4–7.

15 Aoun S, Breen LJ, White I, Rumbold B, Kellehear A (2018): 'What Sources of Bereavement Support do the Bereaved Perceive to be Helpful and Why? Empirical Evidence for the Compassionate Community Approach'. *Palliative Medicine*. DOI: 10.1177/0269216318774995.

16 See, for example, Cruse Bereavement Care. Available at: www.cruse.org.uk/bereavement-services/get-help). The NHS also have useful information sites for both advice and action; see www.nhs.uk/conditions/stress-anxiety-depression/coping-with-bereavement/#stages-of-bereavement-or-grief.

Chapter 29

Medical certification of the cause of death (MCCD)

Introduction

After death, a medical practitioner who has attended the deceased is required to record the cause of death to her/his best belief and understanding on a 'medical certification of the cause of death' (MCCD) form. Only doctors on the GMC register can do this. This subsequently allows the registration and certification of death by the Registrar. These are important formal procedures with far reaching implications. This chapter describes why medical certification of the cause of death matters and what the required procedures are. The procedures are similar but differ in detail in Scotland and Northern Ireland and are described in Chapter 37.

Why the MCCD matters

The requirement for the formal recording of the event of death was introduced in 1836 by an Act of Parliament requiring registration of births, deaths and marriages in England.[1] It established the General Register Office (headed by a Registrar General) and divided England into registration districts. It had three main aims:

- to establish legal proof of death
- to prevent concealment of crime
- to produce accurate population statistics.

Paradoxically, at first there were no penalties for failing to comply with the legislation. It also introduced the position of 'the informant', who was the person (usually a relative) who registered the death with the local Registrar. At first, doctors did not have to provide information as to the cause of death. Over the intervening years the legislation experienced many updates which have been incorporated into present practice.

There are a number of important reasons why the cause of death should be accurately recorded.[2] These include:

- trend data for public health metrics to plan health services for the future
- detection of geographical differences in the survival of given diseases
- assessing the success or otherwise of control measures and environmental policies in reducing occupational and environmental deaths
- detecting changes in the incidence and virulence of a disease
- assessing the impact of inequality and poverty
- reviewing targeted interventions
- research
- providing information for the surviving relatives in case there are implications for them.

It is increasingly becoming clearer that certain kinds of genetic drivers may be associated with particular conditions or illnesses that can make significant contributions to the disease pathway leading to death. As this knowledge base increases, the genetic code of the dead will become increasingly more important for medical advice to the living. Hence, historically, there has never been a period when the accuracy of the cause of death becomes more important to those who remain.

Superimposed on all these 'medical reasons', there is a general trend in society demanding transparency and accountability in public services combined with a 'decline in deference' to authoritarian organizations.

Procedure and description of the forms

When a person dies under normal circumstances, life is pronounced extinct by a person qualified to do so, and later a medical practitioner on the UK Medical Register completes a medical certificate of the cause of death (an MCCD). Books of numbered MCCDs are issued by the local Registrar to hospitals and general practitioners. The front and back sides of an MCCD are shown in Figures 29.1 and 29.2. The doctor who completes an MCCD must have been in attendance during the deceased's last illness and feel they are sufficiently confident of the cause of death and that the death was natural to complete the form.[3] There is no actual legal requirement for the doctor to see the body after death but this is now accepted practice. If they do not feel able to complete it, the death is reported to the coroner. In hospitals, the doctor completing the MCCD is often a junior member of the healthcare team that has looked after the patient. It is best practice for them to discuss what is actually written with a senior colleague first.

The MCCD is *not* the official death certificate, a common misapprehension of the public. The doctor who fills it in is charged with the responsibility of the duty of delivery to the Registrar. This can be done by registered post, but it is custom and practice for the certificate to be put in an envelope and handed to the informant (see immediately below) to take it with them to the Registrar when they register the death.

The function of 'the informant', defined in the original 1836 legislation, is retained in current practice. Their defined responsibility is to take the tear-off slip on the MCCD to the Registrar when it is handed to them by the doctor or bereavement officer. The Registrar enters the death in their register and gives one or more copies of the official death certificate, which includes information from the MCCD, to the informant. In the rare instance that there is no informant, the complete MCCD is taken or posted to the Registrar, or in other circumstances they receive it directly from the coroner. The role of the Registrar and the coroner are described in Chapters 30 and 31.

The front of an MCCD (Figure 29.1) is divided into three sections with perforated divisions for ease of tearing, each of which carries the same serial number for subsequent cross-referencing.

- At the left-hand end is a narrow section labeled 'counterfoil'. This is bound into the spine of the book of MCCDs, and the books must be retained by the hospital or the general practice for a minimum of ten years. It is a statutory duty for the doctor to fill it in and not to do so constitutes an actionable offence. As can be seen in Figure 29.1, it contains a summary of what is written on the main part of the MCCD.
- The middle section is the largest and it is this that carries details of the cause of death. The required information is self-evident and the manner of describing the 'cause of death' is described below in this chapter. Two points to note are that if the death is due to an industrial disease there is a box to tick, and it is now expected that the doctor signing will include their GMC number as well as their registered qualifications.
- The narrow right-hand section becomes the note which the informant must take to the Registrar and is headed as such. It contains information on who died but nothing else. Beneath the written entry of death the 'duties of the informant' are set out and on the reverse side (see Figure 29.2) the list of persons able to act as an informant are listed.

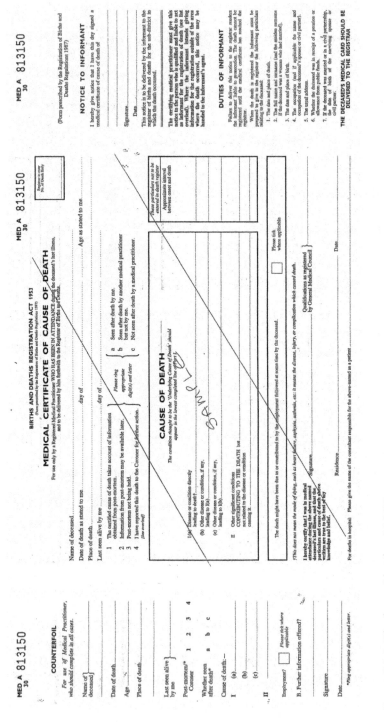

FIGURE 29.1 The front side of an MCCD

Complete where applicable

The following persons are designated by the Births and Deaths Registration Act 1953 as qualified to give information concerning a death; in order of preference they are:

DEATHS IN HOUSES AND PUBLIC INSTITUTIONS

(1) A relative of the deceased, present at the death.
(2) A relative of the deceased, in attendance during the last illness.
(3) A relative of the deceased, residing or being in the sub-district where the death occurred.
(4) A person present at the death.
(5) The occupier* if he knew of the happening of the death.
(6) Any inmate if he knew of the happening of the death.
(7) The person causing the disposal of the body.

DEATHS NOT IN HOUSES OR DEAD BODIES FOUND

(1) Any relative of the deceased having knowledge of any of the particulars required to be registered.
(2) Any person present at the death.
(3) Any person who found the body.
(4) Any person in charge of the body.
(5) The person causing the disposal of the body.

*"Occupier" in relation to a public institution includes the governor, keeper, master, matron, superintendent, or other chief resident officer.

A

I have reported this death to the Coroner for further action.

Initials of certifying medical practitioner. _____

The death should be referred to the coroner if:
• the cause of death is unknown
• the deceased was not seen by the certifying doctor *either* after death *or* within the 14 days before death
• the death was violent or unnatural or was suspicious
• the death may be due to an accident (whenever it occurred)
• the death may be due to self-neglect or neglect by others

B

I may be in a position later to give, on application by the Registrar General, additional information as to the cause of death for the purpose of more precise statistical classification.

Initials of certifying medical practitioner. _____

• the death may be due to an industrial disease or related to the deceased's employment
• the death may be due to an abortion
• the death occurred during an operation or before recovery from the effects of an anaesthetic
• the death may be a suicide
• the death occurred during or shortly after detention in police or prison custody

LIST OF SOME OF THE CATEGORIES OF DEATH WHICH MAY BE OF INDUSTRIAL ORIGIN

MALIGNANT DISEASES — Causes include:

(a) Skin — radiation and sunlight — pitch or tar — mineral oils
(b) Nasal — wood or leather work — nickel
(c) Lung — asbestos — chromates — nickel — radiation
(d) Pleura and peritoneum — asbestos
(e) Urinary tract — benzidine — dyestuff manufacture — rubber manufacture
(f) Liver — PVC manufacture
(g) Bone — radiation
(h) Lymphatics and haematopoietic — radiation — benzene

POISONING

(a) Metals — e.g. arsenic, cadmium, lead
(b) Chemicals — e.g. chlorine, benzene
(c) Solvents — e.g. trichlorethylene

INFECTIOUS DISEASES — Causes include:

(a) Anthrax — imported bone, bonemeal hide or fur
(b) Brucellosis — farming or veterinary
(c) Tuberculosis — contact at work
(d) Leptospirosis — farming, sewer or under-ground workers
(e) Tetanus — farming or gardening
(f) Rabies — animal handling
(g) Viral hepatitis — contact at work

CHRONIC LUNG DISEASES

(a) Occupational asthma — sensitising agent at work
(b) Allergic alveolitis — farming
(c) Pneumoconiosis — mining and quarrying — potteries — asbestos
(d) Chronic bronchitis and emphysema — underground coal mining

NOTE.—The Practitioner, on signing the certificate, should complete, sign and date the Notice to the Informant, which should be detached and handed to the Informant. Where the informant intends giving information for the registration outside of the area where the death occurred, the notice may be handed to the informant's agent. The Practitioner should then, without delay, deliver the certificate itself to the Registrar of Births and Deaths for the sub-district in which the death occurred. Envelopes for enclosing the certificates are supplied by the Registrar.

FIGURE 29.2 The back side of an MCCD

On the back side (Figure 29.2), there are again three sub-divisions reflecting those on the front. The counterfoil section is blank. The informant section is described above. The central section carries the following.

- Two rectangular boxes relating to the coroner. That on the left indicates whether or not the death had been reported to the coroner, and the right-hand side says that further information may be available later (e.g., after the results of tests are back or if there might be a post-mortem investigation). If there is further information later, this is sent to the Registrar and s/he enters it into the Register, but the death certificates already issued are mot modified.
- The lists below the two rectangular boxes are an aide-memoire of what needs to be reported to the coroner.
- Below this is a large section listing industrial diseases that need to be indicated as such on the front of the MCCD.

Filling in an MCCD

Completing an MCCD is not an exact science and on occasions where there has been a natural death but the actual final cause of death is not clear (e.g., was it pneumonia, was it left-ventricular failure, was it simply the frailty of old age (if over 80)?), common sense is needed. It is, however, important that the entry is as accurate as it can be so that correct statistical data can be collected, e.g., use 'glomerulonephritis' rather than 'renal failure' and 'hepatocellular cancer' rather than 'liver failure'. As a general rule, abbreviations are not allowed

The format of the entry is as follows. There is an upper set of three lines, part 1, labeled a, b and c; these sequentially describe the conditions leading directly to death in a sequential manner. The legend on each of the lines is:

I (a) Disease or condition directly leading to death

....

(b) Disease or condition, if any, leading to (a)

....

(c) Other disease, if any, leading to (b)

....

Below this there is a part 2, in which can be recorded indirectly contributing conditions. The exact wording is:

II: Other significant conditions CONTRIBUTING TO THE DEATH but not related to the disease or condition causing it ....

Examples of satisfactory entries are given below.

Example 1

> I (a) Disease or condition directly leading to death
>
> left-ventricular failure
>
> (b) Disease or condition, if any, leading to (a)
>
> ischaemic heart disease
>
> (c) Other disease, if any, leading to (b)
>
> II: Other significant conditions contributing to the death but not related to the disease or condition causing it
>
> Hypertension, Type 3 hyperlipidaemia

Example 2

> I (a) Disease or condition directly leading to death
>
> Sub-arachnoid haemorrhage
>
> (b) Disease or condition, if any, leading to (a)
>
> ....
>
> (c) Other disease, if any, leading to (b)
>
> ....
>
> II: Other significant conditions contributing to the death but not related to the disease or condition causing it
>
> ....

Example 3

An example of an unsatisfactory entry would be:

> I (a) Disease or condition directly leading to death
>
> diabetes mellitus
>
> (b) Disease or condition, if any, leading to (a)
>
> (c) Other disease, if any, leading to (b)

II: Other significant conditions contributing to the death but not related to the disease or condition causing it

rheumatoid arthritis

The Office of National Statistics and the Home Office have published guidance for doctors completing an MCCD.[4]

Notes

1 Available at: http://freepages.rootsweb.com/~framland/genealogy/acts/1836Act.htm.
2 Minister of State for Crime Prevention (2015): 'Hutton Report'. Available at: https://assets.publishing.service.gov.uk/government/uploads/system/uploads/attachment_data/file/477013/Hutton_Review_2015__2_.pdf.
3 It is customary to have a time within which the doctor must have seen the patient before death, e.g., two or four weeks, but this is not in the primary legislation and in practice varies with coronial jurisdiction and the exact circumstances.
4 www.gro.gov.uk/Images/medcert_July_2010.pdf.

Chapter 30

The registration of death

Introduction

The General Register Office was created in 1836 by the Births and Deaths Registration Act and is headed by the Registrar General, who is a crown servant rather than a member of the civil service. The Office has, over the years, been housed in different government departments but at present is part of Her Majesty's Passport Office. It is responsible for the civil registration of births (including still births), adoptions, marriages, civil partnerships and deaths in England and Wales and maintains the national archive of all births, marriages and deaths dating back to 1837. It does not deal with records of such events occurring within the land or territorial waters of Scotland or Northern Ireland (see Chapter 37).

The Registrar General oversees regional and local Register Offices across England and Wales. An informant can go to any Register Office, but if it is not the one in the area where the person died, the documents will be sent to that within whose jurisdiction the death occurred. The death should be registered within five days. If it is done local to the place of death it takes about 30 minutes, and if the papers have to be transferred it usually takes a few days.

The duties of the Registrar are carried out with the 'Guidance for Registration Officers: Births and Deaths' which is issued and updated from time to time under the authority of the Registrar General. This is an official document which at the time of writing is only available by a Freedom of Information Request. It is one of the duties of the Registrar to issue books of MCCDs to the relevant doctors and hospitals within their jurisdiction. Together with these are envelopes of specified design to hold the MCCD in its transmission to the Registrar either by the informant or by the Royal Mail. At the moment in England and Wales there are about 500,000 deaths per year, of which 55% are reported directly to the Registrar without the intervention of the coroner.

The process of registration

When the Registrar receives an MCCD, they are required to check the following things:

- that the appropriate form has been used (this is usually only an issue with still births)
- that the MCCD relates to the person identified by the informant
- that the doctor is registered with the GMC and has attended the deceased during their last illness
- that the deceased was seen after death by a registered medical practitioner
- whether or not the death may in part have been caused by an industrial disease
- whether or not the doctor has informed the coroner of the death, and if so, to confirm the coroner's permission to register the death
- whether or not the cause of death listed should have normally been reported to the coroner (e.g., unnatural death or uncertain cause), and if it hasn't then to inform the coroner and wait for their decision.
- that the cause(s) of death listed do accurately describe the events leading to death. If they do not (e.g., the mode rather than the cause of death has been listed or abbreviations have been used), or the Registrar is unable to accept what is written for other reasons, they make further enquiries to the doctor who signed the MCCD; this delays the registration of death for the relatives.

The entry into the register and the issuing of a copy of the entry proceeds as follows.

- The informant is questioned directly about all the information related to the deceased except the cause of death. If there are any discrepancies, these need to be clarified.
- Provided that there are no reasons to refuse the MCCD (see above), the Registrar then completes a draft certificate with the following information:
  - date and place of death
  - name and surname
  - gender
  - maiden name (if relevant)

o   date and place of birth
o   occupation and address, including the postcode
o   name and qualification of the informant
o   the cause of death; this is recorded precisely as stated on the MCCD, without any omission, addition, abbreviation or alteration, followed by the words 'Certified by' and the name and qualification of the medical practitioner who signed the MCCD.

This information is then entered into the Official Register and a copy of the entry (the form regarded by the public as the death certificate) is handed to the informant. Further copies can be purchased. Figure 30.1 shows such a copy.

If there is subsequent information sent to the Registrar after making the entry the main register is amended but the copies are not.

The informant

The position of the informant was created in the original 1836 Births and Deaths Act. Once a person has accepted the role, although most people do not know, they have adopted the statutory role to register the death and to organize for the disposal of the body. If there is no informant the duty is adopted by the local medical and social services.

The informant's duties to register the death with the Registrar and to furnish them with the details as listed immediately above (apart from the cause of death) are printed on the tear-off slip on the MCCD which was handed to them (see Chapter 29, Figures 29.1 and 29.2). Although it is the duty of the doctor signing the MCCD to transmit it to the Registrar, custom and practice is to give the MCCD in the prescribed envelope to the informant to deliver it.

Persons who can normally act as an informant are listed on the reverse of the tear-off slip. For deaths in houses and public institutions these are:

- a relative of the deceased present at the death
- a relative of the deceased, in attendance during the last illness
- a relative of the deceased living in the local area where the death occurred
- a chief officer of a public institution where the death occurred if s/he knew of the happening of the death
- any inmate of a public institution if s/he knew of the happening of the death
- the person causing disposal of the body
- an executor.

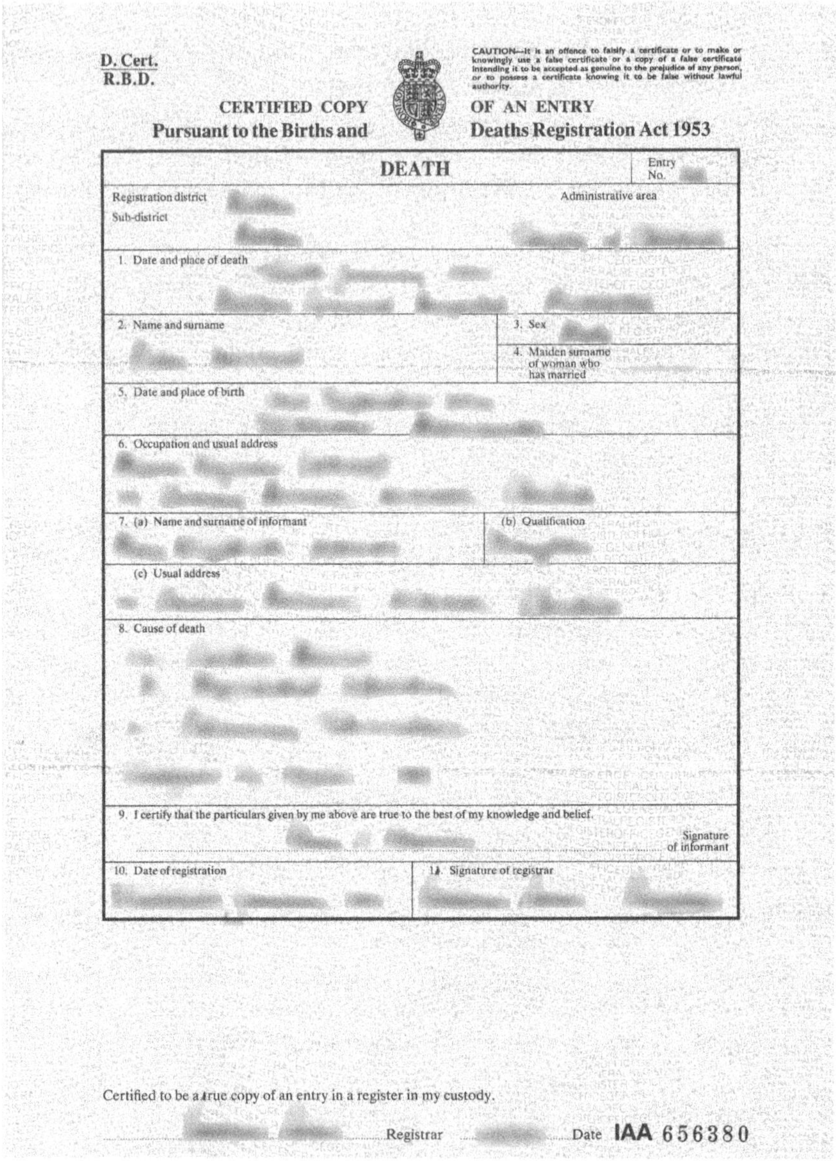

FIGURE 30.1 A completed death certificate

For deaths not in houses or public institutions or if the body is found:

- any relative of the deceased who knows the circumstances of death
- any person present at the death
- any person who found the body

- any person in charge of the body
- the person causing the disposal of the body.

The government issues guidance to informants that can be downloaded from the web.[1] A representative example of guidance available from such a route is in Appendix 30.1.

Appendix 30.1 Typical guidance to relatives available in the public domain

Registering the death

The registration of the death is the formal record of the death. It is done by the Registrar of Births, Deaths and Marriages and you will find the address of the nearest register office on the web or in the telephone directory. When someone dies at home, the death should be registered at the Register Office for the district where they lived. If the death took place in hospital or in a nursing home it must be registered at the Register Office for the district in which the hospital or home is situated. In England and Wales, if it is convenient, you can go to a different office to register the death and the details will be passed on to the correct office. You should check the opening hours of the office you wish to go to. Some offices have an appointments system.

A death should be registered within five days but registration can be delayed for another nine days if the registrar is told that a medical certificate has been issued. If the death has been reported to the coroner you cannot register it until the coroner's investigations are finished.

- It is a criminal offence not to register a death.
- The death should be registered by one of the following (in order of priority):
  - a relative who was present at the death
  - a relative present during the person's last illness
  - a relative living in the district where the death took place
  - anyone else present at the death
  - an owner or occupier of the building where the death took place and who was aware of the death
  - the person arranging the funeral (but not the funeral director).

You cannot delegate responsibility for registering the death to anyone else.

You must take with you the medical certificate of death, since the death cannot be registered until the Registrar has seen this. If possible, you should also take the person's NHS medical card and birth and marriage certificates. The registrar will want from you the following information:

- date and place of death
- the full name of the person (including maiden name) and their last address
- the person's date and place of birth
- the person's occupation and, in the case of a woman who was married or widowed, full name and occupation of her husband
- if the person was still married, the date of birth of their husband or wife
- whether the person was receiving a pension or other social security benefits.

Forms you will be given

When you have registered the death, the Registrar will give you a green certificate (for which there is no charge) to give to the funeral director. This allows either burial or cremation to go ahead. Occasionally the Registrar may be able to issue a certificate for burial only (but never cremation) where no one has yet been able to register the death.

The Registrar will also give you a form to send to the Department for Work and Pensions (DWP) (in Northern Ireland the Social Security Agency). This allows them to deal with the person's pension and other benefits.

Death certificate

The death certificate is a copy of the entry made by the Registrar in the death register. This certificate is needed to deal with money or property left by the person who has died, including dealing with the will. You may need several copies of the certificate, for which there will be a charge.

You can get copies of a death certificate from the General Register Office. Its contact details are on the GOV.UK website at www.gov.uk.

In Northern Ireland details of District Registrars can be found on nidirect's website at www.nidirect.gov.uk.

When a coroner is needed

Anyone who is unhappy about the cause of a death can inform a coroner about it, but in most cases a death will be reported to a coroner by a doctor or the police.

A coroner is a doctor or lawyer appointed by a local authority to investigate certain deaths. In Northern Ireland, the Lord Chancellor appoints a coroner. The coroner is completely independent of authority and has a separate office and staff. You will find the address of your local coroner's office on the web or in the telephone directory.

A coroner can investigate a death if the body is in their district, even though the death took place somewhere else, for example, abroad. A death must always be reported to a coroner in the following situations:

- the person's doctor had not seen them in the 14 days before they died or immediately afterwards (28 days in Northern Ireland)
- a doctor had not looked after, seen or treated the person during their last illness (in other words, death was sudden)
- the cause of death is unknown or uncertain
- the death was violent or unnatural (for example, suicide, accident or drug or alcohol overdose)
- the death was in any way suspicious
- the death took place during surgery or recovery from an anaesthetic
- the death took place in prison or police custody
- the death was caused by an industrial disease.

In some cases, the coroner will need to order a post-mortem, in which case the body will be taken to hospital for this to be carried out. You do not have the right to object to a post-mortem ordered by the coroner, but should tell the coroner if you have religious or other strong objections. In cases where a death is reported to a coroner because the person had not seen a doctor in the previous 14 days (28 in Northern Ireland) the coroner will consult with the person's GP and will usually not need to order a post-mortem.

For more information about post-mortems and your rights to know what happens with organs and tissue, go to the Human Tissue Authority website at www.hta.gov.uk.

A death reported to a coroner cannot be registered until the coroner's investigations are complete and a certificate has been issued allowing registration to take place. This means that the funeral will usually also be delayed. Where a post-mortem has taken place, the coroner must give permission for cremation.

Note

1 www.gov.uk/register-a-death/y/england_wales/at_home_hospital/yes.

Chapter 31

Coroners and autopsies

Introduction

In the previous chapter, we described the need on occasions for a death to be referred to a coroner. There are a number of medico-legal requirements around this process, and healthcare professionals should be familiar with the roles and powers of a coroner, and procedures related to autopsy and retention of tissues.[1]

What is a coroner and what does the coroner do?

The Office of the Area Coroner and the Coroners and Justice Act (2009)

Although in existence earlier, during the reign of Richard I the office of the coroner was recorded in September 1194 by Article 20 of the 'Articles of Ayre' to 'keep the pleas of the Crown' (*custos placitorum coronae*), from which the word 'coroner' is derived. Coroners were introduced into Wales following its military conquest by Edward I of England in 1282 through the Statute of Rhuddlan in 1284. A feature of coroners is that they work within a geographical area known as their jurisdiction; they are embedded in English and Welsh constitutional life as law officers with a community commitment. As such they enjoy considerable autonomy and, as was demonstrated by the *Touche* case in 2001, their decisions can only be challenged by a legal process of appeal to the higher courts.[2]

England and Wales are divided into 98 coroner areas, formerly known as 'districts', and each is a separate legal geographical entity. Each must have a senior coroner in charge. In a few places there are additional coroners who are at a level below the senior coroner. The coroner's area of relevance is (normally) the limit of the senior coroner's jurisdiction, although following the Coroners and Justice Act 2009, bodies may be now moved outside the senior coroner's area and inquests may also be held outside in appropriate circumstances.

The law prescribes that in England and Wales coroners shall investigate the body of a person lying within their jurisdiction where they have reason to suspect that:

- the deceased has died a violent or unnatural death;
- the cause of death is unknown; or,
- the deceased has died while in prison or otherwise in state detention such as an immigration centre or while detained under the Mental Health Act 1983.

The objects of the investigation are to establish the identity of the deceased, and how, when and where they came by their death. This investigation may or may not result in an autopsy.

The value of coroners to the public interest is not in doubt, but their fitness for purpose in the twenty-first century has been repeatedly challenged. New legislation in the form of the Coroners and Justice Act 2009[3] resulted from issues identified in various reviews. A summary of the changes and the secondary legislation subsequent to it can be found in the 'Chief Coroner's Guide' (CCG) published in 2013.[4] Some of the changes relevant to medical practice were as follows.

- All newly appointed coroners must be legally qualified and satisfy the judicial-appointments eligibility condition on a five-year basis. This does not apply to coroners appointed before July 2013. Persons with medical qualifications practicing in a medical capacity are no longer eligible for appointment (Schedule 3, 2009 Act).
- Medical Examiners were to be introduced to examine all deaths not directly dealt with by coroners (Chapter 38; Section 19, 2009 Act). They have at the time of writing still not been officially established and they are only active in a handful of volunteer pilot sites.
- It enabled coroners' districts, now known as 'areas', to be changed to create larger administrative areas (paragraph 13 of CCG).
- It removed the restrictions on where an autopsy could take place, allowing bodies to be moved geographically (Section 15, 2009 Act).
- A coroner is now able to release a body when all the necessary information has been obtained during an investigation without having to first open an inquest (paragraph 86 of CCG).

- If an investigation has been commenced, the coroner may, on request, provide the next of kin or personal representative with a Coroner's Certificate of Fact of Death (paragraph 87 of CCG) to enable legal processes related to the death (e.g., dealing with bank accounts).
- Section 14 of the 2009 Act gives a coroner the power to ask 'a suitable practitioner' to make a post-mortem examination of a body. The coroner is free to select which individual practitioner s/he wishes to undertake the examination of the body.
- Inquests may be heard anywhere in England and Wales (p. 40 of CCG).
- It created the Office of Chief Coroner for England and Wales.

The Office of Chief Coroner

The 2009 Act (paragraph 8 of CCG) created the new Office of Chief Coroner to provide judicial oversight of the coroner system. The Chief Coroner's main responsibilities are to:

- provide support, leadership and guidance for coroners
- set national standards for all coroners
- develop training for coroners and their staff
- approve all future coroner appointments
- keep a register of coroner investigations lasting more than 12 months
- take steps to reduce unnecessary delays
- monitor investigations into deaths of service personnel overseas
- oversee transfers of cases between coroners
- direct coroners to conduct investigations
- provide an annual report on the coroner system to the Lord Chancellor, to be laid before Parliament
- collate, monitor and publish coroners' reports to authorities to prevent other deaths.

Very importantly, the Chief Coroner's position was established to provide leadership and oversight. It is a common misconception that he has day-to-day direct line-management control of individual coroners; he does not. An exception is in relation to complaints, when he may be required by the Judicial Conduct and Investigations Office (JCIO) to provide quasi-line-management functions by giving specific training and advice. The coroners referred to in the Act as 'Senior Coroners' still run the coroners' service in an area of England and Wales in accordance with the law *and are judicially independent in their actions and decisions.*

Referral of a death to the coroner

There is no statutory requirement for a doctor to report any death to the coroner but it is custom and practice that doctors, registrars of births and deaths (see Chapter 30) or the police must report deaths to a coroner in certain circumstances. Not to do so would bring their professional standing and registration into question. These circumstances are listed in the 'Guide to Coroner Services'[5] as deaths where one or more of the following factors apply:

- no doctor saw the deceased during his or her last illness
- although a doctor attended the deceased during the last illness, the doctor is not able or available, for any reason, to certify the death
- the cause of death is unknown
- the death occurred as a result of certain infective diseases
- the death occurred during an operation or before recovery from the effects of an anaesthetic
- the death occurred at work or was due to industrial disease or poisoning
- the death was sudden and unexplained
- the death was unnatural; the death was due to violence or neglect
- the death was in other suspicious circumstances; or the death occurred in prison, police custody or another type of state detention.

If any of these factors are engaged, a coroner may request an autopsy if there are reasonable grounds to suspect that the cause of death is unknown or unnatural, i.e., a medical practitioner does not feel able to provide a natural cause of death, 'to the best of his knowledge and belief' or because they have not seen the patient for more than two weeks. Because of the autonomy of individual coroners, in certain areas, in addition to the above list, there may be additional local 'rules' for the automatic referral of certain cases unique to that jurisdiction, e.g., the death of a child, the death of persons with a transplanted organ.

After having a case referred to her/him the coroner has four ways to respond.

- In practice, in many cases the medical practitioner refers a death to the coroner because although they are comfortable with the cause of death on the balance of probabilities and knows that it was a natural death, they would like the coroner's permission to complete an MCCD. In this case the MCCD will be marked that the case has been referred (see Chapter 29), and once the coroner's permission has been granted, the MCCD will be transmitted to the Registrar in the usual manner and the coroner records that no further action was taken.

- The coroner may assume control of the case and decide, after further discussion with medical staff and others, that an autopsy is not required. He will then issue a Form A to certify that no autopsy is needed and give the cause of death in the normal format (1a, 1b etc.). The informant takes the Form A to the Registrar and a death certificate is issued.
- If a post-mortem examination is undertaken and the death is natural, the coroner issues a Form B, which certifies that after a post-mortem examination, the cause of death was 1a, 1b etc., exactly in the format of the MCCD. If cremation is planned, he also issues a Form E, which substitutes for the usual cremation forms (see Chapter 33).
- If the cause of death cannot be determined easily, or is found to be unnatural, some delay is inevitable and the coroner will usually open an inquest (see below). Depending on the circumstances (e.g., that the pathological findings are clear and that appropriate tissue has been retained), he will issue a disposal order. In different circumstances he may retain the body. The coroner's decision in these matters is final. If a long delay is anticipated, he will issue an interim document confirming the death of the person to allow the family to progress the settlement of the deceased's affairs, but this is not the death certificate.

The coronial autopsy

Strictly speaking, all autopsies, including forensic autopsies, are 'coronial' in the sense that the coroner orders them to occur. Forensic autopsies are described later in this chapter; this section looks at those autopsies in which foul play is not suspected at the outset. There are estimated to be approximately 700–800 pathologists in the UK who perform autopsies for coroners but there is no central register.

When a coroner has decided to hold a post-mortem examination it has to go ahead, irrespective of the wishes of others such as relatives. So-called 'hospital autopsies' which are done to increase the accuracy of the cause of death, for audit, for teaching or for research, are now quite rare. Such an autopsy may not be performed without the written consent of the relatives, nor may any organs or tissues be retained without such consent.

In 2016 (the last year with full statistics at the time of writing), in England and Wales[6] there were:

- 524,371 deaths, of which
- 228,000 (46%) were reported to the coroner
- 86,545 (38%) of the reported deaths (16.5% of the total deaths) had an autopsy, of which

- 38,626 (44.6%) of the autopsies led to an inquest
- 15,962 (41%) of the inquests concluded the death was due to natural causes.

The Chief Coroner in his Annual Report[7] expressed his belief (without quantifying it), that too many autopsies were being undertaken in England and Wales. He encouraged coroners 'to make sufficient well-focused early inquiries to see whether a finding that the death was from natural causes can be made without the need for any post mortem examination'.

It is true that England and Wales carry out more autopsies in proportion to the total annual deaths by a clear margin of up to approximately 40% when compared to other jurisdictions. This is especially surprising when other parts of the UK (Northern Ireland and Scotland) are much more similar to other parts of the world (see Chapter 37). There is no evidence from other jurisdictions that the lower number of referred deaths and autopsy rates reduces the ability to meet the needs of justice or death certification.

This excess of autopsies in England and Wales that could probably be significantly changed:

- through the introduction of the proposed Medical Examiner system
- through closer working between doctors, police and coroners when deaths are reported
- through a greater preparedness of medical practitioners to offer a cause of a natural death on the basis of a high probability.

There has been frequent concern expressed about the accuracy of coronial post-mortem examinations and in 2006 the National Confidential Enquiry into Patient Outcome and Death (NCEPOD) was directed to an audit of the coronial autopsy.[8] It painted a bleak and unsatisfactory picture of the present and (then-)future provision of this service. Since then, in 2014 the Royal College of Pathologists published 'Standards for Coroners' Pathologists in Post-Mortem Examinations of Deaths that Appear Not to be Suspicious'. This document,[9] however, remains advisory, and although it describes clear and appropriate standards, there is no statutory obligation on pathologists to adhere to them or on coroners to insist on them.

The 'Guide to Coroner Services' clearly indicates the rights and expectations of relatives of the deceased and the intent to be sensitive to different religious and ethnic groups.[10] It describes the possibility of the use of imaging and, when possible, of tailoring the autopsy to accommodate relatives' wishes. It is the coroner who will decide if a scanning technique is appropriate (if available), depending on the circumstances of the death. Where a scanning technique is used, the family or other next of kin will usually be required to pay a fee (for this and for any additional tests that the coroner decides are needed).

There has been a legal challenge against performing a conventional autopsy. In the High Court in 2015 an application was made by a Jewish family to prevent a conventional autopsy being done on an 86-year-old lady who had already had a post-mortem MRI. Article 9(2) of the Human Rights' Act (the right to freedom of thought, conscience and religion) was cited and the ruling was that religious beliefs should be considered before a coroner makes their decision.[11] The judgment did not negate the ultimate authority of the coroner, but will influence acceptable working practices.

When a coroner does order an inquest, they, via the Coroner's Officer, must, where relevant, inform the next of kin, the family doctor, the police, the health and safety inspectorate or any other interested party of the time and place of the post-mortem examination so that they can appoint a medical practitioner to be present on their behalf as an observer. In practice, this right is rarely claimed. If the relatives are dissatisfied with the cause of death as given by the pathologist, they can request a second autopsy by an independent pathologist.

Coronial inquests and 'verdicts' or 'findings'

As stated above, the object of the coronial investigation is to establish the answers to four questions:

- the identity of the deceased; and
- how; and
- when; and
- where.

they came by their death. It is not an arena to establish the responsibility for a death, but if evidence emerges suggestive of a relevant crime, the coroner will adjourn the inquest and refer the case to the Director of Public Prosecutions.

Under the terms of the legislation, a coroner can only hold an inquest when a death was unnatural, but this has now been broadened to include other circumstances. A typical list of the reasons for holding an inquest is:

- the person was unlawfully killed
- a post-mortem examination has revealed the death to be unnatural

- human failings or lack of care may have been a factor
- death in custody
- death during arrest by a police officer
- death in a transportation or industrial incident
- death through chronic misuse or neglect
- suspected suicide
- death through alleged negligence.

Instead of simply coming to a decision themself, when the death requires to be reported to a governmental department (e.g., Health and Safety Directorate, the police), the coroner must empanel a jury of 7 to 11 people. This includes all deaths in custody, all deaths resulting from air, sea, road and rail transport accidents and all industrial accidents. The coroner also has the discretion to empanel a jury in any other case they feels it is needed. If not more than two of the jury disagree with the others, they may return a majority verdict.

Prior to undertaking the inquest, the coroner has a duty to inform interested parties such as:

- next of kin and other relatives
- an executor or personal legal representative
- anybody with a life insurance interest in the deceased
- in the case of industrial accidents, a trade union official
- anybody involved in the circumstances of the death
- a representative of the Chief of Police
- anybody who has requested to be present.

If there are witnesses (which is usually the case), the coroner questions them first and they can then be cross-examined by an individual, a lawyer or the jury. When all the evidence has been heard, the coroner either makes his decision on the outcome or, in the case of a jury, sums up and directs the jury as to what verdicts are available to them. After the inquest is over, the coroner and jurors (if present), sign the 'Certificate after Inquisition' that permits registration formalities to be completed and, if not already done so, to allow disposal of the body.

The use of the word 'verdict' is recognized as carrying criminal overtones and some coroners describe their conclusions as 'findings'. Like many aspects of the coronial process there is guidance but little legislation on the exact form of verdicts, there is no definition of either 'accident' or 'misadventure' and there are restrictions on the apportionment of blame. There is no standard appeal process against a coroner's finding and to question it requires a complex procedure leading to a judicial review. Typical verdicts are as follows:

- natural causes
- unlawful killing
- accidental death and misadventure (there is a difficult distinction between these, but misadventure relates to an unintentional form of death from a situation the deceased has put themselves into, e.g., a medical mishap; an accidental death is one in which the deceased has made no contribution, e.g., being fatally injured by another party when s/he fell into the path of a passing vehicle)
- certain industrial diseases
- neglect
- an open verdict is rare and reserved for those circumstances in which the cause of death cannot be satisfactorily determined
- a narrative verdict which simply describes what happened is increasing being used rather than 'shoehorning' the evidence into a specific labelled category.

If the death involves an avoidable circumstance, to try to prevent future deaths, the coroner can report the death as described in 'Guidance No. 5', issued by the Chief Coroner.[12] Section 10(3) states:

> The concern is that circumstances creating a risk of further deaths will occur, or will continue to exist, in the future. It is concern of a risk to life caused by present or future circumstances.

If these risks remain, the coroner, at Section 35 of the Guidance:

> must send the report to 'a person who the coroner believes may have power to take such action'. 'Person' includes an organisation. Where a report is sent to an organisation the coroner should seek to identify a relevant person in the organisation who is sufficiently senior to have the 'power' to take action.

This used to be called the Rule 43 procedure.

The forensic autopsy

A forensic autopsy is undertaken when the death is suspicious, is thought to be unlawful or if concerns arise during a standard coroner's autopsy. Forensic autopsies are performed by pathologists specially trained in the discipline and the Home Office keeps a register of approved practitioners (Home Office Pathologists). At present there are approximately 35 in England and Wales, each with a mean annual workload of about 50 cases.

Because of its importance and the need for a high degree of accuracy and reliability, forensic pathology is strictly controlled, although still under voluntary oversight. In 2012 a collaboration between the Home Office, the Forensic Science Regulator, the Department of Justice and the Royal College of Pathologists resulted in good practice guidance. This has now been updated and is inclusive of Northern Ireland as 'Code of Practice and Performance Standards for Forensic Pathology in England, Wales and Northern Ireland'.[13]

In those cases where someone has been charged with homicide or manslaughter etc., the defence lawyers usually request and obtain a second autopsy by an independent forensic pathologist of their choosing. This is a grey area of legal practice since it is not certain if the coroner has the authority to permit a second autopsy if the death has been satisfactorily explained. Other circumstances in which a coroner may order a second autopsy by a different pathologist is when nobody has yet been charged with the crime. This second report is then confidentially kept on file for future use by the defence when the suspect has finally been found.

Retention of tissues

The Human Tissue Act (2004) created the Human Tissue Authority (HTA), which is charged with the proper and safe management of retained tissues.[14] There are mandatory procedures laid down for obtaining informed consent for the retention of organs and tissues, for their storage, for the time usually deemed acceptable for their retention, for record keeping and for final disposal. Breaching these requirements is a criminal offence. The coroner can only require evidence to be kept for the duration of her/his interest in the case.

When the samples are no longer required, all the organs, tissues and slides have to be offered back to the relatives for disposal in their preferred manner. If they do not want them back, then they are ethically disposed of, taking into account any requests of the relatives.

For further discussion of these issues, see Chapter 27 and its Appendix.

Notes

1 Much of the text here is taken from the Hutton Report; Minister of State for Crime Prevention (2015): 'Hutton Report: A Review of Forensic Pathology Pathology in England and Wales'. Available at: https://assets.publishing.service.gov.uk/government/uploads/system/uploads/attachment_data/file/477013/Hutton_Review_2015__2_.pdf.

2 Court of Appeal (Civil Division): R (Touche) v Inner North London Coroner (2001) QB 1206.
3 Available at: www.legislation.gov.uk/ukpga/2009/25/contents.
4 Available at: www.judiciary.gov.uk/wp-content/uploads/JCO/Documents/coroners/guidance/chief-coroners-guide-to-act-sept2013.pdf.
5 Ministry of Justice (2014): 'Guide to Coroner Services', p. 5. Available at: https://assets.publishing.service.gov.uk/government/uploads/system/uploads/attachment_data/file/363879/guide-to-coroner-service.pdf.
6 Ministry of Justice (2017): 'Coroners Statistics Annual 2016: England and Wales'. Available at: https://assets.publishing.service.gov.uk/government/uploads/system/uploads/attachment_data/file/613556/coroners-statistics-2016.pdf.
7 Ministry of Justice (2013–2014): 'Report of the Chief Coroner: First Annual Report 2013–2014', paragraph 13, p. 10. Available at: www.gov.uk/government/publications/chief-coroners-annual-report-2013-to-2014.
8 NCEPOD (2006): 'The Coroner's Autopsy: Do We Deserve Better?' Available at: www.ncepod.org.uk/2006Report/Downloads/ncepod_2006_report.pdf.
9 www.rcpath.org/search-results.html?q=standards+for+post+mortem.
10 Ministry of Justice (2014): 'Guide to Coroner Services', p. 8. Available at: https://assets.publishing.service.gov.uk/government/uploads/system/uploads/attachment_data/file/363879/guide-to-coroner-service.pdf.
11 Neutral Citation Number: [2015] EWHC 2764 (Admin) in the High Court of Justice Queen's Bench Division the Administrative Court.
12 Chief Coroner (2016): 'Guidance No. 5: Reports to Prevent Future Deaths'. Available at: www.judiciary.uk/wp-content/uploads/2013/09/guidance-no-5-reports-to-prevent-future-deaths.pdf.
13 www.gov.uk/government/publications/standards-for-forensic-pathology-in-england-wales-and-northern-ireland.
14 HTA.gov.uk.

Chapter 32

The body after death

Introduction

After death, and before final disposal, the body undergoes a number of changes which the healthcare workers, and those who may come in contact with or handle the body, should be aware of. In addition, during this period, some other matters, such as removal of implanted items and control of infection, are important considerations for those involved. This chapter addresses these issues.

Changes to the body after death

The three main changes to the body after death[1] are lividity, rigor mortis and signs of decomposition. Decomposition is associated with a considerable time lapse from the moment of death and is obvious when present (see Chapter 26). Although the degree of decomposition is of considerable importance for forensic purposes, it is not considered further here.

Lividity

After death, the body loses temperature, all muscle tone fails and within the blood vessels the blood falls under gravity to the dependent areas.[2] This causes changes in the appearance of the skin. There is a bluish-purplish-red discolouration of the lower parts of the body which starts to become apparent between 30 mins and 3 hours after death and continues to develop for about 12 hours, during which time it blanches under digital pressure. If, after death, the body lies supine, the lividity will be parallel to the coronal plane (i.e., over the back and buttocks), and if it is on its side, it will at right angles to the coronal plane (i.e., along the lower side). After about 18–24 hours the lividity becomes fixed. This may allow recognition that a body has been moved over 18 hours after death. There are a number of exceptions to note.

- Over time there may be a change in the colour of lividity. Also, deaths from carbon monoxide poisioning show cherry-red lividity.
- In some instances, the upper levels of lividity may be mottled and suggest bruising, but the difference is usually clear, especially when the lividity blanches under finger pressure.
- Lividity depends upon sufficient haemoglobin being available to deposit in the dependent areas. If there was severe anaemia before death or if the patient bled out before death, its appearance may not be so evident.
- Lividity may be difficult to identify easily in individuals with highly pigmented skin.

Rigor mortis

At the time of death, a condition called 'primary flaccidity' occurs, followed by rigor mortis. This is the process of muscles stiffening after death because of intracellular changes.[3] Its typical progress is as follows.

- The process starts in small muscles and it becomes observable in, for example, the eyelids, jaw, face and neck. It then progresses to the shoulders and then to the big muscle groups of the limbs.
- Typically, rigidity becomes established in all muscle groups by approximately 6–8 hours and remains until 24–36 hours after death.
- After 24–36 hours after death rigidity starts to diminish with the muscles becoming flaccid again.
- The process is very temperature-dependent. A warm environment accelerates it and a cold environment hinders it.

The use of stages of rigor to assess the time of death is difficult and can be inexact, so should be left to a forensic specialist.

Identification and external examination of a dead body

Identification of a dead person

The identification of a dead body is for one purpose only and that is to confirm who it is. It can be done by the next of kin, a friend, a professional colleague or a doctor or nurse. The norm is to expose the face and, if relevant, any easily accessible distinguishing features, e.g., tattoos or birthmarks, and confirm recognition. If there is an identification label attached, this should be inspected and confirmed as the correct one. When the body is unrecognizable then further measures such as witnesses to the event of death and/or DNA become necessary.

It is important to note that *identification only is not a sufficient process* to allow a professional member of staff to sign to say that they have examined a body after death, e.g., as on a cremation form.

External examination of the body

The external examination of a dead body has considerable legal implications, so it is important that it is done properly. It authorizes procedures such as cremation (which requires the involvement of three doctors) and the transfer of bodies between jurisdictions to occur. It should be completed with a protective apron and gloves in good light.

The objectives are as follows.

- First, to identify the body being examined. If a second independent doctor has not seen the patient before death, this will be done by the identifying name label with supporting evidence from the findings on the body (e.g., amputation, jaundice).
- To exclude or otherwise detect any surface features that might suggest abuse, violence, poison, privation or neglect before death, previously unrecorded pathology or an unnatural death. Examples of such findings are ante-mortem bruising, cigarette burns, extensive bed sores and unnatural wounds.
- To confirm that the external features of the body after death are compatible with the cause of death.

When performing an external examination of the body, the body must *always* be turned over and the back inspected. The lividity will be absent from pressure areas and the skin on the buttocks is a common site of unsuspicious tissue loss. It does, however, bring a doctor's registration into question if the stab wound in the back is only found by the undertaker!

Removal of implanted items

Implanted items are important for two reasons.

- They support the fact that the body is that of the correct person.
- If left in situ, they can explode in the cremation oven.

If there is to be a post-mortem examination, all devices, intravenous and intra-arterial lines and airway access tubes should be left as when the person died. After this, and if there will be no post-mortem, anything with a battery (e.g., pacemakers) or a gas-filled space (orthopaedic telescopic implants) *must* be removed. Usually this is done and signed for by the mortuary technician, and the certificate is required by the funeral director before he can take the body away. The current English cremation forms require the doctors signing to confirm that this has been, or will be, done.

Solid implants, such as artificial hips and knees, are safe and of no consequence.

Control of infection and other hazards

Cross-infection and reporting of infections

Procedures to prevent cross-infection and the recording of certain infections continue after death as they did in life. There are no exact rules set out as to what constitutes a hazard, but it is reasonable if the deceased had a notifiable disease to treat the body as potentially infective. Notifiable diseases are those infections that have to be reported to the local professional appointed as the 'Proper Officer'. Such people can be appointed through a variety of organizations, but are now usually employed by the Health Protection Agency. A list of notifiable diseases and statutory responsibilities is published by Public Health England.[4] The list of notifiable diseases is given in Table 32.1.

TABLE **32.1** A list of notifiable diseases

Acute encephalitis	Malaria
Acute infectious hepatitis	Measles
Acute meningitis	Meningococcal septicaemia
Acute poliomyelitis	Mumps
Anthrax	Plague
Botulism	Rabies
Brucellosis	Rubella
Cholera	Severe Acute Respiratory Syndrome (SARS)
Diphtheria	Scarlet fever
Enteric fever (typhoid or paratyphoid fever)	Smallpox
Food poisoning	Tetanus
Haemolytic uraemic syndrome (HUS)	Tuberculosis
Infectious bloody diarrhoea	Typhus
Invasive group A streptococcal disease	Viral haemorrhagic fever (VHF)
Legionnaires' disease	Whooping cough
Leprosy	Yellow fever

There are, however, other infections that can be fatal but carry no statutory obligation to report them (e.g., Legionnaire's disease), whereas others (e.g., HIV infection, AIDS) have a voluntary reporting system. Such diseases that may present significant risk to human health can be reported under the category 'other significant disease'. Guidance has been produced by the Health and Safety Executive,[5] which classifies the hazard of biological agents as follows.

Hazard group 1: A biological agent unlikely to cause human disease.

Hazard group 2: A biological agent that can cause human disease and may be a hazard to employees; it is unlikely to spread to the community and there is usually effective prophylaxis or effective treatment available, e.g., tetanus, botulism, mumps, measles and other common diseases.

Hazard group 3: A biological agent that can cause severe human disease and presents a serious hazard to employees; it may present a risk of spreading to the community, but there is usually effective prophylaxis or treatment available, e.g., anthrax, tuberculosis, typhoid, rabies, yellow fever, HIV, hepatitis B.

Hazard group 4: A biological agent that causes severe human disease and is a serious hazard to employees; it is likely to spread to the community and there is usually no effective prophylaxis or treatment, e.g., Lassa fever, Ebola, SARS. These are fortunately rare in UK practice and special isolation both in life and death is necessary.

Last offices and cleaning

Under all circumstances when a patient is alive and then dead, standard infection control procedures need to be in place. In hospital practice these are usually set and overseen by the Infection Control Department. Routine measures include:

- proper hand washing
- routine use of apron and gloves
- covering cuts and abrasions on the patient and the professional
- prevention of open puncture wounds and safe management of sharps
- avoidance of personal contamination and efficient clearing of any spillages of blood and body fluids
- disposal of contaminated waste in the appropriate containers
- disposal or laundering at the correct temperature of all sheets and clothing
- cleaning and decontamination of all rooms and equipment before reuse.

In most situations involving infections, last offices can proceed routinely with the appropriate precautions (see Chapter 35), but any infection control procedures in place prior to death must be continued afterwards. The infected washed and shrouded body needs to be put into a waterproof body bag with an occlusive zip. There should be clear labelling with a 'Danger of Infection' sticker and documentation describing the problem (including serology) firmly attached to the outside. This alerts other people (porters, pathologists, mortuary staff etc.) to the potential hazards.

After the dead patient has left the ward or room where there has been a danger of infection, all items and surfaces must be cleaned and protective clothing and mops etc. disposed of into hazard-labelled waste bags as described in the relevent hospital policy.

Mortuary practice and post-mortem examinations

It is normal practice to treat any unidentified body as if it was infected. If it is a known infected body, then the waterproof bag should only be opened sufficiently for the necessary purposes, e.g., identification.

If there is a second doctor who has to examine the body for the purposes of a cremation certificate, then this should be approached with care. In these situations, when the history of the patient is well documented before death, they can do a more limited procedure with minimal exposure of the body. The reasons for this should be documented in the notes and it is good practice for the second doctor to speak with the physician caring for the patient before death.

If a post-mortem examination has to be undertaken, the main danger is via infection transmitted through airborne spray or splashing. Most current post-mortem rooms now have a safe area with downdraft ventilation for such instances. Post-mortems on hazard group 4 pathogens must be done under the guidance set out by the Dangerous Pathogens Advisory Group. In these circumstances there is no need for a second doctor to examine the body because the Consultant for Communicacable Disease Control is able to authorize cremation.

Other hazardous substances

The management of bodies containing other hazardous substances is a specialist area. An example of such an instance is a death from radiation poisoning. The most famous of these in recent history is that of Alexander Litvinenko who died on 22 November 2006. He was a Russian granted asylum in the UK who was the first confirmed victim of lethal polonium 210-induced acute radiation syndrome.[6] His autopsy was done by a pathologist in radiation-proof clothing and he was buried in a lead-lined coffin.

Notes

1 A more detailed account of these changes can be found in Wyatt J, Squires T, Norfolk G, Payne-James J (2011): *Oxford Handbook of Forensic Medicine*, Oxford University Press, section 2, pp. 29–66.

2 This is also called post-mortem hypostasis, livor stasis or livor mortis.

3 The adenosine triphosphate concentration in the muscle cells falls and the actin and myosin bind together.

4 Public Health England (2010): 'Notifiable Diseases and Causative Organisms: How to Report'. Available at: www.gov.uk/guidance/notifiable-diseases-and-causative-organisms-how-to-report#list-of-notifiable-diseases.

5 Health and Safety Executive (2003): Safe Working and the Prevention of Infection in Clinical Laboratories and Similar Facilities', pp. 13–14. Available at: www.aber.ac.uk/en/media/departmental/healthsafetyenvironment/clinical-laboratories.pdf.

6 Crown Copyright HC695 (2016): 'The Litvinenko Inquiry: Report into the Death of Alexander Litvinenko: Chairman: Sir Robert Owen January 2016'. Available at: https://webarchive.nationalarchives.gov.uk/20160613090324/https://www.litvinenkoinquiry.org/report.

Chapter 33

Disposal of the body

Introduction

After death, the body may be disposed of in different ways depending on religious reasons, the wishes of the deceased and/or custom and practice. This chapter describes some important considerations and processes involved in different forms of disposal.

Permission to dispose of the body

When the informant registers a death, after the registration process has been completed, the Registrar issues the 'Certificate for Burial or Cremation after Registration'. Part of this certificate includes a section to be returned to the Registrar after the disposal is complete. This is usually not returned by the informant but instead by the cemetery or crematorium superintendent who requires the disposal certificate to proceed with the disposal of the body.

If, for religious reasons, a rapid disposal is required, and the case is uncomplicated, the Registrar may issue a document which permits disposal before completion of the formal registration. However, this can only be done in the case of a burial, not a cremation.

Where a death has been referred to the coroner but they are content that the death is natural, the coroner will issue a Form B, which is taken from the coroner's office to the Registrar. Registration and the issuing of permission to dispose proceeds as above from thereon. If the death is unexplained and there has to be an inquest, the body is retained for as long as is deemed necessary. If a long delay is possible, the coroner may issue an interim document confirming that the individual is dead to allow the processing of necessary documentation (e.g., closing bank accounts, reading the will etc). When the coroner has been assured by pathologists and other experts that nothing further is needed and all necessary samples have been retained, at their discretion they may issue an order for disposal. This is often permission for a burial only since cremation would exclude any further examination of the remains.

For many issues related to the management of the situation after death there is excellent advice available from the Bereavement Advice Centre.[1]

Disposal by burial

Burials currently comprise about 20% of disposals in the UK. Religions such as Islam and Judaism insist upon it, but most other religions and non-religious people have few objections to cremation. Details of the wishes of individual religions can be found in Part II of this book.

Traditionally, burials occurred in churchyards on consecrated land, and common law gives the right of a churchyard burial to every parishioner. It is also custom and practice to allow burial of cremated remains. The acceptance of unbaptized adults, the site of the grave and the nature of the headstone are at the discretion of the incumbent priest. Over time, because of the growth of the population and the limitations of space, a churchyard can be closed by an Order of Council.

The majority of burials now occur in municipal cemeteries which are under the provisions of the Church of England Provisions Orders and Local Authorities Cemetery Orders. The documents dictate standards of maintenance and protection for various denominations, and provide for chapels and other necessary features. There is, however, no requirement for local authorities to maintain churchyards indefinitely and from time to time a number are flattened or sold.

Over the past two decades what are termed 'woodland burials' have increased in popularity and there are now over 200 licensed sites in the UK. There may or may not be a funeral director involved and the family usually arrange the form of service so as to meet the wishes of themselves and the deceased. Not infrequently there is a humanist celebrant. Specialist firms provide biodegradable shrouds and coffins. Such sites also inter cremation remains. For those interested, more details can be found in *The New Natural Death Handbook*.[2]

There is clear law regarding the burial of remains in private graveyards or in the garden, most of which relates to public safety and public health. Although the requirement of coffin and grave depth are not specified, there are regulations about the distance from water supplies and the need to avoid public offence. A burial authorization order must be obtained from the Registrar and the date and place of burial is entered in the land burial register referred to below.

There is a legal duty to register burials, separate to the registration of death. It applies to church, municipal or private burials and the record is maintained by the local burial authorities, not the Registrar of births, marriages and deaths.

Disposal by cremation

Because there is no further examination of the body possible after cremation, there are safeguards in place to prevent nefarious activities. It is also necessary to remove any potentially explosive devices (e.g., pacemakers) and the crematorium will want to see a certificate to the effect that this has been done.

An application to cremate is done by a relative or executor filling in the prescribed form. This requires him/her to confirm that the deceased expressed no wish not to be cremated. Following this, under normal circumstances, signatures are required by three registered medical practitioners; all three need to identify and examine the body (see Chapter 32). The three must be:

- a doctor who attended the deceased during their last illness
- a second independent doctor with no close relationship to the first doctor
- a third doctor known as the Medical Referee of the Crematorium.

The coroner can also provide authority for cremation, but the Medical Referee still has to make a final check. If dissatisfied with any aspect of the forms, the Medical Referee can make further enquiries and his signature is required for the cremation to go ahead.

There have been several Cremation Acts, the last amendment being in 2008. Technically, cremation is only permitted in a purpose-built facility. All new crematoria are required to have emission reduction technology. As with burials, each crematorium has to keep a record (with a serial number) of every cremation carried out. The crematorium returns the 'Notification of Disposal' to the Registrar with the appropriate information.

The requirement to only cremate in a purpose licensed facility was questioned in law in 2005 (R v Wrigglesworth, Leeds Crown Court[3]), when a defendant who had burnt his mother's body on a funeral pyre in his back garden was found not guilty of a crime. The case turned on whether he had been a public nuisance, and nobody had complained. The cause of his mother's death, lung cancer, was not in doubt.

Other forms of disposal

Burial at sea

Burial at sea is tightly controlled, part of the reason being to prevent bodies being washed ashore later or becoming entangled in fishing nets. The government has issued detailed guidance.[4] This does not apply to the simple scattering of ashes at sea, which has no restrictions.

To bury a body at sea, a licence has to be applied for and granted. The process takes at least three months, and there are a number of stipulations.

- You must make sure the coffin is built to the specified design with appropriate weights and bands.
- You must also make sure that the body of the deceased:
  - isn't embalmed
  - is lightly dressed in biodegradable material
  - has a durable identification tag with the details of the funeral director.
- You must be prepared for the body and coffin to be inspected before the burial.

When you apply you must have:

- the death certificate
- a Certificate of Freedom from Fever and Infection (available from the deceased person's GP or hospital doctor)
- a Notice to a Coroner of Intention to Remove a Body out of England (available from the coroner in exchange for a Certificate of Disposal provided by the Registrar).

You might also have to provide evidence your proposed burial location is suitable. Things like water depth, currents, pipelines and fishing will be considered.

Burial at sea by military forces, e.g., the Royal Navy, is outside civil law and will not be considered here.

Donation of body for research

The Human Tissue Authority does not accept bodies as donations, but it inspects the organizations that do.[5] Information on such organizations, usually medical schools, is easily available from a web search. The basic principles are as follows.

- Under the Human Tissue Act 2004, written and witnessed consent for anatomical examination must be given prior to death. Consent cannot be given by anyone else after your death.
- A consent form can be obtained from your local medical school and a copy should be kept with your will. You should also inform your family, close friends, and GP that you wish to donate your body.
- After use, medical schools will usually arrange for donated bodies to be cremated, unless the family requests the return of the body for a private burial or cremation. Medical schools may also hold a committal, memorial or thanksgiving services.

Notes

1 www.bereavementadvice.org.
2 Albery N, Weinrich S (2000): *The New Natural Death Handbook*, Rider.
3 Green J, Green M (2006): *Dealing with Death*, Jessica Kingsley, p. 113.
4 www.gov.uk/guidance/how-to-get-a-licence-for-a-burial-at-sea-in-england.
5 www.hta.gov.uk/donating-your-body.

Chapter 34

Life support, brain death and transplantation

Introduction

As previously discussed in Chapter 26, the matter of how death is determined and some details of its diagnosis remain a matter of debate amongst various medical and non-medical groups. Although there is agreement on the science underlying the determination of death, much of the broader debate considers the reliability of its application from clinician to clinician, and also internationally, from region to region. These scientific debates can be quite specialist, confined as they are to clinical and academic groups, and so are not widely known or understood by the general public. This is an important social and ethical observation to make since, in these kinds of end-of-life circumstances, it is members the general public who are commonly expected to make final decisions about life support or organ donation for themselves or their dying family member. In this chapter then, the aim is to describe the current clinical practice of determining brain-stem death. In addition, the issues surrounding life support, organ donation, the sensitive matter of consent and the involvement of coroner are discussed.

The diagnosis of brain-stem death

When death is diagnosed clinically, it means the death of the individual as a whole. The person has irreversibly lost the capacity for consciousness and the capacity for breathing, but not all cells in their body are dead.

This concept of the definition of death has already been considered in Chapter 26. The fact that there may be continuing cellular activity when death is diagnosed is usually originally attributed to the French description of Coma Depassé[1] in 1959. However, practical observation of brain-stem death dates back much earlier and is well demonstrated in relation to the

283

biblical story of Judith.[2] Judith, a beautiful widow, is desired by Holofernes, an invading Assyrian general who will shortly attack her home town. She uses her female guile to get into his tent, render him stuporous with alcohol and then chop his head off. This story so interested the painter Johann Liss that he painted the beheading scene five times. The version in the National Gallery, London (see Figures 34.1 and 34.2), painted in 1622, clearly shows Judith holding the decapitated head whilst blood continues to spurt from arteries in the neck. Whilst Holofernes is clearly dead as an intact human, his heart is continuing to beat; i.e., he is brain-stem dead.

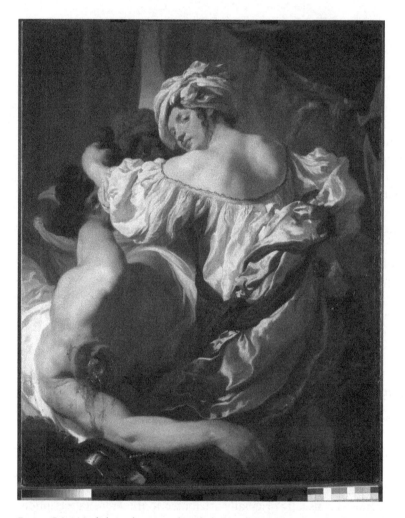

FIGURE **34.1** Judith in the tent of Holofernes. Reproduced under licence from National Gallery Picture Library, London

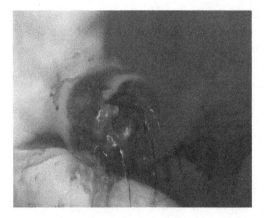

FIGURE 34.2 Detail of neck with spurting arteries

In modern clinical practice the diagnosis of death by brain-stem testing is relevant only to patients who are on an intensive-care unit, and who required ventilation of the lungs as part of overall intensive-care management of the condition for which they were admitted. In these situations, the diagnosis of brain-stem death has three main functions.

- To establish when any further treatment is futile, and to allow the diagnosis of death before further deterioration of the body.
- To allow the efficient use of scarce resources.
- To allow the possibility of transplantation to be considered.

The document 'A Code of Practice for the Diagnosis and Confirmation of Death' issued in 2008 by the Academy of Medical Royal Colleges (AoMRC) remains the reference guide to practice in this area,[3] although there have been several additional guidance documents issued to clarify and update various aspects. For clinicians involved in brain-stem death testing we would recommend a thorough reading of this guideline. The NHS has also produced information for relatives and carers,[4] and NICE has reviewed the possibilities of increasing the numbers of donor organs.[5] *It needs to be emphasized that brain-stem death testing needs to be carried out with great care to ensure maximum reliability of the outcome.*

The diagnosis of death on the basis of brain-stem tests can be difficult to comprehend by the relatives and other non-clinical members of public. Therefore, it is important that a full and detailed explanation is given to the relatives, including the rationale for the tests, what brain-stem death really means, and the implications. It is important that all involved fully understand why the tests are being done, and what the outcome of the tests mean. It should be emphasized that the clinicians involved have to be professional, experienced and meticulous to ensure that the tests are carried out and interpreted with as much correctness and precision as possible.

The principle of brain-stem death testing in the UK has two major components. These are:

- preconditions that have to be satisfied before the tests can be done.
- a series of clinical neurological tests carried out twice by two medical practitioners who have been registered for more than five years, one of whom must be a consultant. On the first occasion one does the testing and the other observes, and on the second the roles are reversed. Neither must have any interest in subsequent use of the patient's organs for transplantation. If death is confirmed, the time of death is the time at which the first set was completed.

Preconditions

In summary the preconditions are there to prevent reversible causes mimicking brain-stem death. A representative list would be as follows.

- The patient must be deeply comatose, unresponsive, apnoeic and necessarily on a mechanical ventilator to preserve oxygenation.
- There should be no doubt that the patient's condition is known to due to irremediable and untreatable brain damage.
- The exclusion on other reversible causes of unconsciousness and apnoea, e.g., absence of any sedative therapeutic drugs or relaxants, an overdose of illegal drugs, tranquillizers, poisons or other chemical agents, an abnormally low body temperature or severe under-activity of the thyroid gland.

Tests for brain-stem function

The tests to confirm death of the brain-stem are as follows.

- There must be no pupillary response to changes in light intensity. Because of trauma it may only be possible to examine one eye.
- There must be no eyelid movement when each cornea is touched.
- There must be no motor responses within the cranial nerve distribution that can be elicited by adequate stimulation of any somatic area.
- There must be no reflex activity (cough or gag) to bronchial stimulation from a catheter placed in the trachea as far as the carina.

- There must be no gag reflex from stimulation of the posterior pharyngeal wall.

- There must be no eye movements seen following the slow injection of at least 50 mls of ice-cold water over one minute into each external auditory meatus in turn. Note: the meati must be clear of wax and debris when this is done.

- The apnoea test should only be performed after all other brain-stem reflexes have been shown to be absent. This test exposes the patient to an adequate respiratory acidosis as a stimulus to breathing during a five-minute disconnection from the ventilator. Prior to the test the patient is pre-oxygenated to ensure that hypoxia does not occur during the test and the minute ventilation is adjusted to ensure that the PaCO2 is more than 6 kPA and the pH is less than 7.4. An arterial blood gas is taken to confirm this. The patient is then physically disconnected from the ventilator and observed for five minutes. During disconnection oxygenation is maintained with a non-ventilated Mapleson type C circuit or by insufflation down the ET tube. At the end of the five-minute period the arterial blood gases are repeated to confirm that the PaCO2 must have increased by at least 0.5kPA and the pH fallen still further.

- At the end of the first set of tests the patient is reconnected to the ventilator and his/her physiology returned to the starting position in preparation for the second set of tests. There is no time period specified as a minimum between the two tests except that on both occasions the patient should have stable physiology. The time between the tests is often a good point at which to speak to relatives with the likelihood of confirmed bad news to follow. Relatives are increasingly being offered the opportunity to observe the second set of tests. When this is done, they should be warned that there may be some residual reflex movement of the limbs but that this movement is independent of the brain and is controlled through the spinal cord. It is useful to emphasise that this movement is neither indicative of the ability to feel, be aware of or to respond to, any stimulus, nor to sustain respiration or allow other bodily functions to continue.

NHS Blood and Transplant, a special health authority, has produced excellent advice in a series of videos on all aspects of brain-stem death testing and the wider aspects of organ transplantation to which the reader is directed.[6]

A comprehensive form based on the AoMRC guidance to record the event of brain-stem death has been issued jointly by the Faculty of Intensive Care Medicine, the Intensive Care Society and the National Organ Donation Committee.[7] Some hospitals have their own version of such a form.

It goes without saying that in all aspects of brain death testing, it is necessary to have meticulous note-keeping.

What is life support?

Life support is a term well known within society as indicating that a patient is dependent upon machinery to stay alive. In medicine it is defined more closely.

- It can refer to the management of patients who are able and often expected to recover because of a temporary loss of consciousness or the ability to breathe (e.g., after trauma, surgery or a drug overdose)
- It can refer to patients who may not be expected to recover and whose physiological status is being maintained prior to brain-stem death testing or, after they have been declared dead, when waiting for organ retrieval to occur.

There is now a considerable literature and optimal practice guidelines on the maintenance of the dead organ donor awaiting retrieval which is out of the scope of this publication. Interested readers are directed to the review of McKeown et al.[8] This is a specialized area of clinical practice.

The non-heart-beating donor

When transplantation started, all organs were retrieved from patients immediately after cardio-respiratory arrest, i.e., from non-heart-beating donors. After the recognition that death resulted from irreversible damage to the brain-stem, organ retrieval switched to patients certified dead after brain-stem testing.

However, to take organs from a non-ventilated patient immediately after death significantly increases the pool of donor organs. For successful organ harvest, the retrieval process has to be done immediately after death has been certified. Although there are ethical issues with this, it is now being employed, usually for kidney and liver homografts and is termed 'Donation after Circulatory Death'. Related issues are discussed in Chapter 27, and interested readers are directed to the reviews of the British Transplantation Society[9] and Manara et al.[10]

Consent for organ and tissue donation

Consent for organ donation is now under the management of the Human Tissue Authority. All aspects of permission for donation etc. are covered in Chapter 27. Consent also involves powers of attorney, living wills, whether or not the person is a registered organ donor and the wishes of the relatives. At the time of writing, there is consideration at parliamentary level of changing the law and introducing an 'opt-out' rather than an 'opt-in' system of organ retrieval.

In December 2011, the National Institute for Health and Clinical Excellence (NICE) published a short clinical guideline on organ donation (CG135 (see note 5)). This guideline, which applies to practice in England, Wales and Northern Ireland, includes detailed recommendations on how to best approach the family of a potential organ donor. Key messages from this guidance are that:

- the family approach should always be planned in collaboration with the Specialist Nurse for Organ Donation
- the approach should only occur when it is clear that the family have accepted the inevitability of their loss
- organ donation should be presented as part of the care that a dying person might wish to receive
- the individual leading the family approach must be competent to do so, have the requisite knowledge to answer any family questions and have the time to take the family through what can be a lengthy process.

Despite the importance and logic of these guidelines it is vitally important to recognize two further points in considering their professional application with families.

First, always remember that one is dealing with a grieving family. Any appearance of undue haste in end-of-life decision-making runs the risk of untoward outcomes – anger, confusion, combative attitudes or even merely suspicion of motives. Patience and care are crucial in end-of-life circumstances precisely because of this emotional context. The request to take anything from families in the context of grief must be approached with great care, caution and respect. Second, a large minority of people in the UK (in fact, about one-third) do NOT desire to participate in organ donation practices.[11]

These two facts lead to a single, important social message when approaching families to discuss consent. All discussions with the family should begin as simply discussions – not about consent itself – but rather about the family's fears, concerns or questions related to the dying family member's impending death. Therefore the first clinical goal is not to directly obtain consent or counsel as a first-order approach to families, but rather, to offer support, discussion opportunities and information sharing, and that includes attentive listening for information about the dying person's or family's attitudes to *what death means to them*, or *their organ donation preferences*.

We should take care not to prejudge or to pressure the outcome simply because many surveys now show that most people are positively disposed towards organ donation. To hastily move towards obtaining consent before making time and space to discuss these matters openly, or being prepared (or more importantly *being seen to be prepared*) to accept alternative views, will be to appear insensitive and prejudiced at best, or self-interested at worst. Both outcomes will be damaging to trust in the professional relationship and to the wider national aspirations for optimizing organ donation. Consistent with the spirit of any book about the diversity of human belief systems, we recommend all due diligence and respect for those differences in the context of organ donation.

Involvement of the coroner

It is usual for organ donor deaths to be reported to the coroner, and it becomes essential if there it is an unnatural death (e.g., road traffic accident). Different coroners handle the details of transplantation in different ways, so local custom and practice should be followed.

Notes

1 Moularet P, Goudon M (1959): 'Coma Depassé et necrosis nerveuses central massives'. *Revue Neurologique*, Vol. 101, 116–139.
2 The Book of Judith is a so-called deuterocanonical biblical text because it is included in the Roman Catholic Christian Old Testament but not in the Hebrew Bible.
3 AoMRC (2008): 'A Code of Practice for the Diagnosis and Confirmation of Death'. Available at: http://aomrc.org.uk/wp-content/uploads/2016/04/Code_Practice_Confirmation_Diagnosis_Death_1008-4.pdf.
4 NHS (2016): 'Diagnosis of Brain Stem Death'. Available at: www.nhs.uk/conditions/brain-death/diagnosis/.
5 NICE (2016): 'Organ Donation for Transplantation: Improving Donor Identification and Consent Rates for Deceased Organ Donation'. Available at: www.nice.org.uk/guidance/CG135.
6 www.odt.nhs.uk/deceased-donation/best-practice-guidance/donation-after-brainstem-death/diagnosing-death-using-neurological-criteria/.
7 Faculty of Intensive Care Medicine (2014): 'Form for the Diagnosis of Death using Neurological Criteria'. Available at: https://ficm.ac.uk/sites/default/files/Form%20for%20the%20Diagnosis%20of%20Death%20using%20Neurological%20Criteria%20-%20Full%20Version%20%282014%29.pdf.
8 McKeown DW, Bonser RS, Kellum JA (2012): 'Management of the Heartbeating Brain-Dead Organ Donor'. *British Journal of Anaesthesia*, Vol. 108, No. 51, i96–i107.
9 British Transplantation Society (2013): 'Transplantation from Deceased Donors after Circulatory Death'. Available at: https://bts.org.uk/wp-content/uploads/2016/09/15_BTS_Donors_DCD-1.pdf.
10 Manara AR, Murphy PG, O'Callaghan G (2012): 'Donation after Circulatory Death'. *British Journal of Anaesthesia*, Vol. 108, No. 51, i108–i121.
11 British Medical Association (2018): 'Two Thirds of People Support a "Soft" Opt-Out Organ Donation System, Reveals New BMA Survey'. www.bma.org.uk/news/media-centre/press-releases/2017/february/two-thirds-of-people-support-an-optout-organ-donation-system.

Chapter 35

Performing last offices

Introduction

Members of hospital staff, usually nurses, are normally required to perform last offices – the laying out of a dead person. This symbolizes the termination of medical and nursing care with a final act of respect. In principle, modesty, respect and privacy need to be retained, the body washed and laid out with the limbs straight and the mouth closed. The body should be as acceptable as possible for others, e.g., relatives, to see. In the following, we will describe when not to perform last offices, and the procedure for routine deaths.

When not to perform last offices

There are some instances in which performing last offices with routine hospital staff is inappropriate. These are as follows.

- Circumstances in which the religious or ethnic status of the patient dictates that it should be done by particular appointed professionals or religious officers. These occasions are set out in Part II of this book.
- If the death is suspicious, potentially litigious or being reported to the coroner it is accepted practice to leave in place all ET tubes, cannulae and any arterial or central venous catheters. Once official enquires are complete and satisfactory, all such equipment is removed and the laying out done by the funeral director.
- Organ donors are kept on ventilation and may have inotropic infusions running until the organs have been removed. After the retrieval procedure, the body is usually taken directly to the mortuary. Often before leaving the operating theatre, the nursing staff will wash the body and put it in a shroud.

All other cases can follow the procedure below.

Procedure for 'routine deaths'

When a person dies, there is a continuing duty to both the deceased and to their relatives, and if the relatives are absent to contact them. The immediate wishes of the relatives should be accommodated whenever possible. Some may wish to sit quietly with their deceased relative for a while; some like to offer a prayer when a priest arrives.

When death happens in the community it is the norm for the funeral director to remove the body and perform the last offices in the funeral parlour. In hospital it is done in the hospital bed before transporting the body to the mortuary, in a side room if possible. There is some need to try to get on with things within two or three hours after death before rigor mortis starts to develop (Chapter 32). It is good practice to offer the option to the relatives of being able to assist in the preparation of the body (e.g., helping with washing), and if they want to be involved to continue to address the deceased with their name as the process proceeds (e.g., 'we are just going to move your arm now Mary').

Most hospitals have a prescribed procedure for the laying out of bodies and the precise details of laying out will not be described here. The principles are to make the deceased look as lifelike as possible by inserting any false teeth, closing the eyelids and supporting the chin to prevent it falling open and fixing in that position. Vaseline on the lips prevents them drying out.

The body should be laid in an anatomically neutral position with the head on a pillow, the arms and legs straight, the orifices secured and the body washed and dressed in a shroud. Particular care needs to be taken to retain any religious or cultural jewelry or icons and all rings should be left *in situ* and bound with transparent tape. The relatives may wish to remove some of these items (e.g., wedding and engagement rings), for sentimental reasons, and this should be permitted with a record made in the accompanying documentation. Finally, the body needs to be accurately labelled.

If the body has been infected, it should be placed in an occlusive zipped body bag as described in Chapter 32.

Chapter 36

Less common circumstances

Introduction

This chapter aims to cover some less common circumstances that are associated with their own unique challenges. These circumstances include missing persons, major disasters, exhumation and exporting a body overseas. It is not uncommon for some of these to become high-profile due to general public and media interest. Although few hospital and community staff may become directly involved in such issues, relatives and friends of the deceased will ask about them (the commonest being return to the birthplace for disposal), and it is best to be informed.

Missing persons

The law in England and Wales regulating missing persons is the Presumption of Death Act 2013,[1] and this has been updated with the Guardianship (Missing Persons) Act,[2] which was due to be enacted in 2018. There are similar laws, the Presumption of Death (Scotland) Act 1977 and the Presumption of Death (Northern Ireland) Act 2009, which follow similar lines in these jurisdictions.

A missing person is not automatically presumed dead. It is necessary to make a claim for a declaration of presumed death if you want to do certain things, for example, deal with their estate or claim an inheritance.

You can make a claim for a 'declaration of presumed death' from the High Court. If this is granted it cannot be appealed and the missing person is treated in law as if they were dead. In order to advance a claim, you have to be one of the following to the missing person:

- spouse or civil partner
- parent

- child
- sibling.

If none of these apply, you need to prove to the Court that you have enough of a connection to the missing person ('sufficient interest'), for example, you are a distant relative and you have a birth certificate to prove it.

In addition, one or more of the following must also apply:

- you are the missing person's spouse or civil partner and you treat England or Wales as your permanent home ('domicile') on the date you make the claim
- you are the missing person's spouse or civil partner and you've been living in England or Wales for the whole year before the date you make the claim
- the missing person treated England or Wales as their permanent home ('domicile') on the date they were last known to be alive
- the missing person was living in England or Wales for the whole year before the date they were last known to be alive.

A case can be advanced if the person normally domiciled in England and Wales has been missing for:

- seven years or more
- less than seven years and you think they have died, for example, they went missing during a natural disaster, or were killed in an aeroplane crash and there are no mortal remains.

If the claim is successful, then to all intents and purposes the survivor's relationship to the missing person is as if they had died naturally and all the legal ramifications that follow come into play.

There are similar provisions applying in the legislations of Northern Ireland and Scotland.

Exporting a body overseas

It is illegal to move a dead body overseas without the specific permission of the coroner, to whom application must be made on the prescribed form. The application must be accompanied by the Registrar's 'Permission to Dispose' certificate. If all is satisfactory, the coroner issues an 'Out of England' certificate and the removal can go ahead.

The actual export process is not without its problems and there are some specialist funeral directors who undertake it. Both air and sea carriers place strict rules on the size and construction of the coffin and demand freedom-from-infection certificates. Most insist that the body is embalmed.

The export of cremation ashes is much simpler and although detailed checks need to be made, most airlines permit them to be carried in hand luggage in a non-metal container accompanied by the cremation certificate.

Major disasters

A major disaster is probably best defined (for our purposes) as an event with multiple casualties and deaths which overwhelms the resources available to deal with it. Whenever such an event happens contentious situations automatically follow. Examples of these are as follows.

- The need to preserve those lives that can be preserved without destroying forensic evidence.
- The need to identify who is dead as soon as possible.
- The shortage of ambulances that preclude the dead being moved immediately.
- The need to protect the workers at the scene.
- The need not to prejudice a future accident investigation by destroying forensic evidence.
- The need to identify the dead and return them to their families; the longer this takes, the more protracted the bereavement.

Most jurisdictions have a 'major accident plan' with a flow diagram, but inevitably when the event occurs, flexibility is needed. It must be remembered that only certain people are able to cope psychologically with working under such circumstances. There is therefore a need to provide for their support as well as for the relatives. Often there are temporary facilities erected on the spot and it is not uncommon for pathologists to be resourced from nearby countries.

The Health and Safety Executive publishes advice on emergency planning for major accidents.[3]

Exhumation

It is still the case in law that a dead body (unlike tissues removed for study) belongs to nobody; it can have no owner. A body can however be subject to procedures that engage the law. Once buried, exhumation from a grave or vault is only permissible for six purposes:[4]

- to rebury the body elsewhere
- to clear a piece of ground required for redevelopment
- on the order of the coroner or Home Secretary to further investigate a death
- to recover items thought to be buried with it
- to confirm the identity of the deceased
- to confirm the identity of a descendent of the deceased.

Unsurprisingly, exhumations are commoner in detective novels than in practice.

Permission for exhumation can be authorized by a coroner, the Home Secretary or by the use of an arcane ecclesiastical process. An application can be made by anybody but there is an exacting application process which also takes evidence from objectors. The application must also state the proposals for the re-internment of the body or (via complex rules) for its future cremation.

When an order to disinter is granted, the process is under the control of the police. When recovered the coffin is taken unopened to a post-mortem examination room.

Notes

1 www.legislation.gov.uk/ukpga/2013/13/contents/enacted.
2 Available at: www.legislation.gov.uk/ukpga/2017/27/enacted.
3 HSE (2009): 'Emergency Planning for Major Accidents'. Available at: www.hse.gov.uk/pUbns/priced/hsg191.pdf.
4 Green J, Green M (2006): *Dealing with Death*, Jessica Kingsley, chapter 19, p. 132.

Chapter 37

Deaths in Northern Ireland and Scotland

Introduction

The objectives of death certification and registration in Northern Ireland and Scotland are essentially the same as in England and Wales. For natural deaths this means providing an accurate cause of death in a timely manner and in other cases ensuring that appropriate procedures are followed. The methodologies are similar in principle but differ in some details. As in England and Wales, natural deaths require a doctor to give an immediate cause of death with the antecedent and contributing causes supporting it on the medical certificate of the cause of death (MCCD). All the points of good practice listed in Chapter 29 (e.g., clear printing of all details, no abbreviations etc.) apply.

The differences in investigative procedures in Northern Ireland and Scotland result in a reduced number of autopsies being performed. The Luce Review[1] drew attention to the variation in deaths referred to the coroner and the number of autopsies carried out in different countries. Its findings in 2003 are shown in Table 37.1 (to the nearest whole %).

Deaths in Northern Ireland

In Northern Ireland (NI) the death certification process is in transition from hand-written to electronic MCCD forms and guidelines have been issued by the NI Department of Health, Social Services and Public Safety (DHSSPS).[2] At the time of writing, electronic reporting is done in hospitals and hand-written reporting in general practices. The electronic form is signed with the doctor's usual signature after it has been printed. If the electronic system fails, hand-written forms can still be issued in hospitals. NI has no plans to introduce Medical Examiners at present.

TABLE 37.1 International comparisons in autopsy rates

Jurisdiction	Percentage of total annual deaths referred to coroner (or equivalent)	Percentage of total annual deaths subject to an autopsy
England and Wales	38%	23%
Scotland	24%	12%
Ontario, Canada	27%	11%
New South Wales, Australia	14%	10%
British Columbia, Canada	28%	10%
New Zealand	14%	10%
Victoria, Australia	13%	10%
Republic of Ireland	27%	9%
Northern Ireland	24%	9%
Alberta, Canada	25%	7%
England and Wales (2013)+	45%	19%

+These figures given in Chapter 31 are included for comparison

Natural deaths

Doctors certifying deaths do so as a *statutory* duty under the Births and Deaths Registration (Northern Ireland) Order 1976 Section 25(2), which states:

> Where any person dies as a result of any natural illness for which he has been treated by a registered medical practitioner within *twenty-eight days* prior to the date of his death, that practitioner shall sign and give forthwith to a qualified informant a certificate in the prescribed form stating to the best of his knowledge and belief the cause of death, together with such other particulars as may be prescribed.

MCCDs can only be completed by a registered medical practitioner who saw and treated the deceased during their last illness. No other person or practitioner may sign the certificate on his/her behalf. A doctor who has not been directly involved in the patient's care at any time during the illness from which they died can determine life extinct, but cannot certify the cause of death. In hospital, there may be several doctors in a team caring for the patient who will be able to certify the cause of death. It is ultimately the responsibility of the consultant in charge of the patient's care to ensure that the death is properly certified. Foundation-level doctors should only complete MCCDs when they have received appropriate training. Discussion of a case with a senior colleague may help clarify issues about completion of an MCCD or referral to a Coroner. In general practice, more than one GP may have been involved in the patient's care and so be able to certify the cause of death. All causes of death must be written out in full. The only abbreviations a Registrar of Births, Marriages and Deaths can accept are:

- HIV for Human Immunodeficiency Virus infection
- AIDS for Acquired Immune Deficiency Syndrome
- MRSA for Methicillin Resistant Staphylococcus Aureus.

The hand-written and electronic MCCD forms are shown in Figures 37.1 and 37.2.

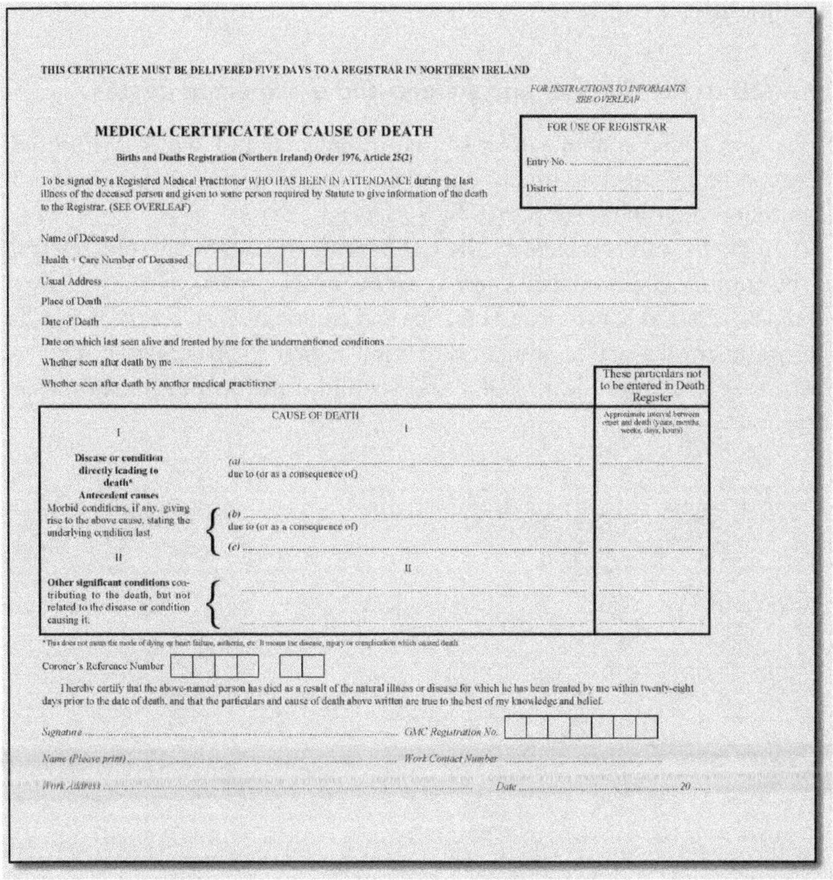

THIS CERTIFICATE MUST BE DELIVERED FIVE DAYS TO A REGISTRAR IN NORTHERN IRELAND

FOR INSTRUCTIONS TO INFORMANTS SEE OVERLEAF

MEDICAL CERTIFICATE OF CAUSE OF DEATH

Births and Deaths Registration (Northern Ireland) Order 1976, Article 25(2)

To be signed by a Registered Medical Practitioner WHO HAS BEEN IN ATTENDANCE during the last illness of the deceased person and given to some person required by Statute to give information of the death to the Registrar. (SEE OVERLEAF)

FOR USE OF REGISTRAR

Entry No. ....

District ....

Name of Deceased ....

Health + Care Number of Deceased

Usual Address ....

Place of Death ....

Date of Death ....

Date on which last seen alive and treated by me for the undermentioned conditions ....

Whether seen after death by me ....

Whether seen after death by another medical practitioner ....

CAUSE OF DEATH		These particulars not to be entered in Death Register
I	I	Approximate interval between onset and death (years, months, weeks, days, hours)
Disease or condition directly leading to death*	(a) .... due to (or as a consequence of)	....
Antecedent causes Morbid conditions, if any, giving rise to the above cause, stating the underlying condition last.	(b) .... due to (or as a consequence of)	....
	(c)	....
II	II	
Other significant conditions contributing to the death, but not related to the disease or condition causing it.	....	....

*This does not mean the mode of dying eg heart failure, asthenia, etc. It means the disease, injury or complication which caused death

Coroner's Reference Number

I hereby certify that the above-named person has died as a result of the natural illness or disease for which he has been treated by me within twenty-eight days prior to the date of death, and that the particulars and cause of death above written are true to the best of my knowledge and belief.

Signature .... *GMC Registration No.*

Name (Please print) .... *Work Contact Number* ....

Work Address .... *Date* .... 20 ....

FIGURE 37.1 A sample Northern Ireland handwritten MCCD form. Please note that each MCCD has a retained counterfoil section similar to the English MCCD shown in Figure 29.1

Once the MCCD has been completed, the MCCD is given to 'The Informant' for transmission to the Registrar. The informant is usually the next of kin, but can also be a friend or an executor. In practice it is the most appropriate person in the circumstances. The informant must state accurately to the Registrar the deceased's name, address, civil status, date and place of birth, and occupation, and show their NI Medical Card. The cause-of-death details (excluding the interval between onset of condition and death), as certified by a medical practitioner, are entered by the Registrar in the Death Register and a copy of the entry is given to the informant. Cremation legislation, and the certificates required, is essentially like that in England and Wales. In NI there is a social tradition of three days between death and disposal, so there are pressures to do things expeditiously.

Referrals to the Coroner and sudden and unexpected deaths

NI has a coronial system similar to that in England and Wales. Within NI there are three full-time legally qualified coroners appointed by the Lord Chancellor and each is supported by a Medical Adviser.

If no doctor can complete an MCCD because of the 28-day rule, referral to the coroner is automatic. There is no definitive list of what other cases should be referred. Custom and practice and common sense are the key indicators and any list will be similar to that in Chapter 31. Basically, it is when the cause of a natural death is not known, and if the death is unnatural or suspicious.

b

FOR INSTRUCTIONS TO INFORMANTS SEE OVERLEAF

MEDICAL CERTIFICATE OF CAUSE OF DEATH

Births and Deaths Registration (Northern Ireland) Order 1976, Article 25(2)

FOR USE OF REGISTRAR

ENTRY NO. ....

To be signed by a Registered Medical Practitioner WHO HAS BEEN IN ATTENDANCE during the last illness of the deceased person and given to some person required by Statute to give information of the death to the Registrar. (SEE OVERLEAF)

DISTRICT ....

Name of Deceased: Mr Joe Bloggs

The Health & Care Number of the Deceased: 1234567891

Usual Residence: 100 Any Street, Anytown, BTXX 5XX

Place of Death: BELFAST CITY HOSPITAL (123)

Date of Death: 17-July-2018 12:12

Date on which last seen alive and treated by me for 09-July-2018
the undermentioned conditions:

Whether seen after death by,
- me   Yes
- another medical practitioner   Yes

These particulars not to be entered in Death Register

CAUSE OF DEATH		Approximate interval between onset and death (years, months, weeks, days, hours)
I **Disease or condition directly leading to death**[a]	**I** (a) IMMEDIATE CAUSE OF DEATH Due to (or as a consequence of)	2d
Antecedent causes Morbid conditions, if any, giving rise to the above cause, stating the underlying condition last.	(b) ANTECEDENT CAUSE(S) Due to (or as a consequence of) (c) UNDERLYING CAUSE OF DEATH	1 yr 20 yrs
II **Other significant conditions** contributing to the death, but not related to the disease or condition causing it	**II** OTHER SIGNIFICANT CONDITION(S)	5 yrs

*This does not mean the mode of dying e.g. heart failure, asthenia, etc. It means the disease, injury or complication which caused death.

Coroner's Reference Number: [1][2][3][4]–[1][8]

I hereby certify that the above-named person has died as a result of the natural illness or disease for which he has been treated by me within twenty-eight days prior to the date of death, and that the particulars and cause of death above written are true to the best of my knowledge and belief.

Signature	*JR Johnston*	Date	*17 July 2018*
Name (Please Print)	RDE Doctor	Work Contact Number	124354y5yt4t
Work Address	123 street	GMC Registration No.	1234567

Page 1 of 2

FIGURE 37.2 A sample electronic Northern Ireland MCCD form. The doctor works through a series of screens, the first of which is shown in Figure 37.2a on p.300. After this is complete, a paper record of the necessary information for registration is printed out in hard copy as shown here (Figure 37.2b)

Referral to the coroner can be done in any manner (telephone, electronically, by post etc.); there are no statutory referral forms or procedures. On receipt of the referral the coroner will 'make inquiries'. The inquiries usually involve both professional and family members. The coroner may then:

- allow disposal of the body
- order an autopsy
- order an inquest.

In each of these cases, the coroner will determine the cause(s) of death and register the death with the Registrar on the information obtained, and if there is an autopsy he/she liaises closely with the pathologist.

Because NI is a compact province with a population of 1.8 million, all autopsies, whether hospital, coronial or forensic, are done in the State Pathologist's Department in Belfast. This office is funded and appointed through the Department of Justice for all autopsies. All cases, whether routine or forensic, are in the first instance 'single pathologist procedures'.

Deaths in Scotland

Scotland differs from the rest of the UK in two very significant ways, one longstanding and one very recent.

- The Scottish legal system is different from that of the UK, its roots being in Roman and European law, with little modification from the effects of the Norman Conquest. Scotland's most famous connection with Europe was the 1295 'Auld Alliance' with France to support Scotland and France's shared need to curtail English expansion. The legacy of this is the Procurator Fiscal system, which contrasts significantly with the coronial system.
- The system for death certification in Scotland changed on 13 May 2015. The move came in response to an extensive review of the existing arrangements. The Certification of Death (Scotland) Act 2011 introduced a 'Death Certification Review Service' (DCRS) to:
  - create a single system of independent, effective scrutiny for deaths that do not require a Procurator Fiscal (PF) investigation
  - improve the quality and accuracy of MCCDs (medical certificates of cause of death)
  - provide improved public health information
  - strengthen clinical governance in relation to deaths.

Natural deaths and the Death Certification Review Service (DCRS)

The previous system was considerably revised and advice was issued by the Chief Medical Officer of Scotland.[3] Particular revisions and advice are as follows.

- There was to be the same level of scrutiny of the cause of death regardless of whether burial, cremation or any other form of disposal is intended.
- Because of the above, Cremation Forms B and C ('Certificate of Medical Attendant' and 'Confirmatory Medical Certificate', respectively), and Cremation Medical Referees were abolished.
- There is still an application for Cremation Form A and a Permission to Cremate from the Procurator Fiscal (Form E1) as there always was.
- Independent Medical Reviewers were established to review a random sample of MCCDs (excluding those deaths reported to the the Crown and the Procurator Fiscal Service (COPFS).
- There was to be statutory provision of information and clinical records to Medical Reviewers (MRs) by certifying doctors and Health Boards to allow the MRs to undertake the scrutiny function.
- The new Form 11, medical certificate of cause of death (MCCD), now records hazards associated with implants (to include radioactive substances and cardiac pacemakers) and infection risks. The same information is required on the revised Cremation Form A (Application for Cremation), and on Form 14 (Certificate of Registration of Death), which is given to the informant by the Registrar of Births, Deaths and Marriages.
- It was intended that the MCCD should be completed electronically. At the time of writing this was happening in general practice but not in hospital practice, where paper was still being used. When electronic completion occurs, a copy is printed off and provided to the next of kin.
- The MCCD was considerably changed and enlarged to include additional information although the cause-of-death section was in the previous format with the immediate cause supported by additional underlying causes. An example of the new MCCD is shown in Figure 37.3. The MCCDs are distributed in books of 20, each with a unique serial number.

Doctors are required *not* to complete MCCDs where there is a legal impediment in doing so. That is to say, doctors can refuse to issue MCCDs where they do not believe they know the cause of death or there is a reason to believe that death is the result of unnatural causes, when such a refusal

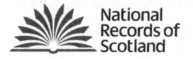

National
Records of
Scotland

Serial Numbers 0487221-0487240

MEDICAL CERTIFICATE OF CAUSE OF DEATH
(Section 24(1) of the Registration of Births, Deaths and Marriages (Scotland) Act 1965)

GUIDANCE FOR COMPLETION OF THE FORM 11 IS AVAILABLE AT
www.nrscotland.gov.uk/MCCDGuidance

MEDICAL CERTIFICATE OF CAUSE OF DEATH (Form 11)
Please print information on the Form 11 clearly and do not use abbreviations.
The Form 11 provides legal evidence that the person has died, and states the cause of death. It is essential that the information on the certificate is accurate as it is used to compile statistics about death, monitor public health, improve planning in the National Health Service and assist in medical research. Information from the certificate will be included in a register of deaths open to public scrutiny.

The Registrar of Births, Deaths and Marriages may ask you to clarify the information you have provided. Please be as helpful as you can.

Books of medical certificate of cause of death (Form 11) may be obtained from the NHS Board in which you practise. The following link contains contact details for each NHS Board:

https://www.nrscotland.gov.uk/reorder-mccd

WHERE TO TAKE THE COMPLETED FORM
A death which takes places in Scotland may be registered by an informant at any Scottish registration office. Contact details for local authority Registrars of Births, Deaths and Marriages may be found in the telephone directory or on council websites.

MEDICAL REVIEWS
Please advise the family of the deceased that when they attend the registrar's office to register the death, the death may be selected for review by a Medical Reviewer which may delay funeral arrangements. Selection of deaths for review is a random process over which the registrar has no control.

If a death is selected for a Level 1 Review, the Medical Reviewer will check the medical certificate of cause of death and speak to the certifying doctor to obtain background clinical information. This will usually be a quick process and the most common review to be carried out.

If a death is selected for a Level 2 Review this will involve a more in-depth review of the available information and may take longer.

Forms 11 are serially numbered. Ensure that you complete the Record of Issue for each form you complete. This will assist you when dealing with future enquiries about the death.

National Records of Scotland
New Register House
Edinburgh
EH1 3YT

PRINTED BY AUTHORITY OF THE REGISTRAR GENERAL FOR SCOTLAND

MEDICAL CERTIFICATE OF CAUSE OF DEATH (Form 11)   *Serial number: 04872292*
(Section 24(1) of the Registration of Births, Deaths and Marriages (Scotland) Act 1965)

The completed certificate should be taken to the Registrar of Births, Deaths and Marriages and will be retained by them.

GUIDANCE FOR COMPLETION OF THIS FORM IS AVAILABLE AT www.nrscotland.gov.uk/MCCDGuidance

PLEASE PRINT CLEARLY IN BLOCK CAPITALS AND DO NOT ABBREVIATE

PART A - DETAILS OF DECEASED

Name of deceased	
Date of death (dd/mm/yyyy)	
Time of death (24-hour clock – hh:mm)	
Place of death	
Health Board area in which death occurred	
Community Health Index (CHI) number	
Date of birth (dd/mm/yyyy)	

PART B - DETAILS OF CERTIFYING DOCTOR

Name	
GMC number	
Business address	
Business contact telephone number	
For a death in hospital Name of the consultant responsible for the deceased	

I hereby certify that to the best of my knowledge and belief the information contained in this Medical Certificate of Cause of Death is correct.

Signature of certifying doctor	
Date	

For registration office use	RD Number	Year	Entry number

08/2014

FIGURE **37.3** *(continued)*

(continued)

PART C - CAUSE OF DEATH

PLEASE PRINT CLEARLY IN BLOCK CAPITALS AND DO NOT ABBREVIATE

	Approximate interval between onset and death		
	Years	Months	Days
I Disease or condition directly leading to death * (a)			
Antecedent causes – Morbid conditions, if any, giving rise to the above cause, stating the underlying condition last			
due to (or as a consequence of) (b)			
due to (or as a consequence of) (c)			
due to (or as a consequence of) (d)			
II Other significant conditions contributing to the death, but not related to the disease or condition causing it			

* *This does not mean mode of dying, such as heart or respiratory failure; it means the disease, injury or complication that caused death.*

PART D - HAZARDS

	To the best of your knowledge and belief;	Y	N
DH1	Does the body of the deceased pose a risk to public health: for example, did the deceased have a notifiable infectious disease or was their body "contaminated", immediately before death?		
DH2	Is there a cardiac pacemaker or any other potentially explosive device currently present in the deceased?		
DH3	Is there radioactive material or other hazardous implant currently present in the deceased?		

PART E – ADDITIONAL INFORMATION

Post mortem examination by a pathologist *(tick one)*	
PM1	Post mortem has been done and information is included above	
PM2	Post mortem information may be available later	
PM3	No post mortem	

Attendance on deceased *(tick one)*	
A1	I was in attendance upon the deceased during last illness	
A2	I was not in attendance upon the deceased during last illness: the doctor who was is unable to provide the certificate	
A3	No doctor was in attendance on the deceased	

Procurator Fiscal *(tick if applicable)*	
PF	This death has been reported to the procurator fiscal	

Extra information for statistical purposes *(tick if applicable)*	
X	I may be able to supply the Registrar General with additional information	

Maternal Deaths *(tick if applicable)*	
M1	Death during pregnancy or within 42 days of the pregnancy ending	
M2	Death between 43 days and 12 months after the end of pregnancy	

08/2014

RECORD OF ISSUE (Page 4)

04872369	Name of deceased	Date of death	Certifying doctor
I (a)			
(b)			
(c)			
(d)			
II			
04872375	Name of deceased	Date of death	Certifying doctor
I (a)			
(b)			
(c)			
(d)			
II			
04872381	Name of deceased	Date of death	Certifying doctor
I (a)			
(b)			
(c)			
(d)			
II			
04872398	Name of deceased	Date of death	Certifying doctor
I (a)			
(b)			
(c)			
(d)			
II			
04872406	Name of deceased	Date of death	Certifying doctor
I (a)			
(b)			
(c)			
(d)			
II			

PRINTED BY AUTHORITY OF THE REGISTRAR GENERAL FOR SCOTLAND

FIGURE 37.3 A Scottish MCCD form: it has four pages, as shown

will make the death a matter of legal interest (i.e., it must be reported to COPFS). There is no clear legal definition of 'attended', but it is generally accepted to mean a doctor who has cared for the patient during the illness or condition that led to death and so is familiar with the patient's medical history, investigations and treatment. There is no 14- or 28-day rule. In those circumstances when it is not possible for the doctor who was in attendance to provide the certificate, another doctor in the team, with knowledge of the deceased and/or access to the relevant clinical records, can complete the MCCD. MCCDs can also be completed by a pre-registration doctor in training (FY1), with the involvement of a senior doctor. The consultant in charge of the patient's care should be made aware of all deaths that result in a report to the COPFS. The criteria for referral to the COPFS remain the same.

The date and time of death should be recorded as accurately as possible. If a person such as a nurse, relative or a carer was present when the person died, reliable information that they give about the date and time of death may be recorded. Otherwise, the best estimate is given based on all the information available. This may be different from when life was certified as extinct. The correct date of death must be recorded in the MCCD when a death is certified which occurred before midnight, but the certificate is completed the following day.

Once completed, the MCCD is taken to the Registrar by the next of kin, an executor or other suitable person within eight days of completion. The law allows a death to be registered in any registration district in Scotland and the Registrar will issue certificate of registration of death for production to the person in charge of the burial ground or crematorium and an abbreviated extract of the death entry.[4]

Medical Reviewers (MR) and Senior Medical Reviewers (SMR) are now in place to undertake level-1 and level-2 reviews. Certifying doctors (or a clinical member of the team with knowledge of the patient and/or access to the clinical records), must make themselves available to discuss a death with the MR, but it is recognized that doctors' time is often constrained and MRs should try to accommodate working patterns. Reviews of MCCDs are at random, with the randomization process starting either when the electronic MCCD is submitted or when the paper version is taken to the registrar.

It is proposed that 10 per cent of all MCCDs (approximately 5,000 per annum) will undergo a level-1 review, with a timescale for completion of one working day with the MR examining the MCCD and speaking to the certifying doctor on the phone for around five minutes. They may also speak with other members of the team if they have access to patient records and to other interested parties. Approximately 2 per cent of all MCCDs will undergo a level-2 review. This is a more comprehensive review with a target of three working days for completion. If any review finds that a case should, in their opinion, have been referred to the COPFS, then that case will be passed on to the PF's office. The status of the original MCCD is determined by the COPFS. Reviews can also be requested by 'interested persons'. These include relatives, carers, healthcare professionals and funeral directors, and informing can be done online as well as by telephone or surface mail.

Referrals to the the Crown and Procurator Fiscal Service (COPFS), and sudden and unexpected deaths

'Sudden and unexpected' deaths include unnatural (homicide, suicide and accident), as well as sudden natural deaths of no known cause (which have to be investigated to exclude unnatural causes).

The Crown and Procurator Fiscal Service (COPFS) is different from the English coronial system but performs similar functions in relation to deaths. A Procurator Fiscal (PF) is a legally qualified professional appointed through the office of the Lord Advocate. The Lord Advocate is the chief legal officer of the Scottish Government and the Crown in Scotland covering both civil and criminal matters that are under the aegis of the Scottish Parliament. The office carries the duties of chief public prosecutor for Scotland and all prosecutions are conducted by the Crown Office and Procurator Fiscal Service, nominally in the Lord Advocate's name. There are designated areas in Scotland (serving a distributed total population of 5.3 million) identified for the investigation of normal, sudden and unnatural, truly criminally suspicious deaths and health-and-safety-related incidents. The COPFS handles all unnatural and suspicious deaths and conducts Public Fatal Accident Inquiries.

A doctor who cannot complete an MCCD because they are uncertain of the cause of death has to report the death to the PF. Other causes needing reporting, as in England and Wales, are sudden and unexpected deaths, suspicious deaths, when the deceased's body is hazardous to others and when it is in the public interest to allay anxiety. The COPFS has issued guidance on this.[5] The death should be reported to the PF's team in the area in which it occurred and they investigate with their authority under statute and at common law. Medical practitioners are generally expected (but not exclusively) to report deaths by an electronic format but another mechanism (probably less preferred by COPFS in many circumstances) would be by contacting the police as a conduit to inform the PF. This referral can be done by anybody but frequently is done via the police, the Registrar of Births, Marriages and Deaths or through a medical person.

PFs handle all unexplained, sudden deaths including unnatural and suspicious deaths. Fatal Accident Inquiries (FAIs) are conducted in certain circumstances, some mandatory (deaths in legal custody and deaths as the result of an accident at work) and others discretionary (at the discretion of the Lord Advocate), to explore the facts about the nature of, and circumstances surrounding, a death; this public inquiry replaces the coroner's inquest, is much less frequently held and has a rather broader remit. There are no inquests (as such) in Scotland, that function being at least partly subsumed by the FAI.

The PF has a number of options available.

- They can accept an offered death certificate where there may be minor uncertainty but no suspicious circumstances.
- They can request a police report.
- They can instruct that an autopsy be held.

Sometimes a PF instructs a pathologist to 'take a view' after consideration of the history and external examination of the body. This so-called 'view and grant' procedure allows the pathologist to issue a death certificate and may be largely responsible for the low autopsy rate when compared with England. The PF has a responsibility to identify if any criminal action has occurred and, where appropriate, to prosecute. Where a criminal offence is suspected to have occurred the procurator fiscal will instruct the local police to investigate. If it is an accident that caused death, a public fatal accident inquiry will be held.

All sudden and unexpected deaths are investigated by an autopsy. In the case of suspicious deaths which might result in prosecution, two forensically trained pathologists complete the autopsy together (the so-called double-doctor system).

Notes

1 Secretary of State for the Home Department (2003): 'Death Certification and Investigation in England, Wales and Northern Ireland: The Report of a Fundamental Review'. Available at: https://webarchive.nationalarchives.gov. uk/20131205105739/http://www.archive2.official-documents.co.uk/document/ cm58/5831/5831.pdf.
2 www.health-ni.gov.uk/publications/guidelines-death-certification-handwritten-mccd and www.health-ni.gov.uk/publications/guidelines-death-certification-issuing-mccd-using-niecr.
3 www.sehd.scot.nhs.uk/cmo/CMO(2014)27.pdf.
4 www.nrscotland.gov.uk/registration/registering-a-death.
5 COPFS (2015): 'Reporting Deaths to the Procurator Fiscal; Information and Guidance for Medical Practitioners'. Available at: https://dokumen.tips/ documents/reporting-deaths-to-the-procurator-deaths-to-thereporting-deaths-to-the-procurator.html.

Chapter 38

Future changes in England and Wales

Introduction

The current system of death certification is undergoing change in England and Wales. In this chapter, problems with the existing arrangements are considered, followed by the new medical examiner system.

Problems with the existing arrangements

The problems with death certification came into prominence because of the activities of Dr Harold Shipman, a GP who was Britain's most prolific serial killer. Many of his victims (i.e., his patients) were cremated and the second-signature doctors on the cremation forms proved to be inadequate in detecting that the deaths were unnatural. An inquiry was set up to investigate his activities and the Department of Health accepted the conclusions of the Shipman inquiry third report:[1] that existing arrangements for death certification are confusing and provide inadequate safeguards.

Following extensive consultation, which closed in 2007,[2] and input from medical Royal Colleges and legal bodies, changes to the death registration system were included within the Coroners and Justice Act 2009.[3] This introduced the role of medical examiners (MEs), together with that of a National Medical Examiner. An ME is a senior, specially appointed doctor who is independent of the case under consideration and can apply independent scrutiny. Since then, despite professional pressure, there have been repeated delays to nation-wide introduction, although there have been pilot sites assessing the feasibility and practicality of the proposals. The government set a date of April 2019 for the commencement of the roll-out of the national implementation of MEs in hospitals, but not in the community. There is an irony in that the problems with the abuse of the death certificate

311

process were detected in the community but that it is the hospital sector that is the first to be reformed.

The Medical Examiner system

The government published its rationale and aspirations for the new system complete with the creation of MEs in 2016.[4] The remainder of this section closely follows this government publication. Readers should note that the information was correct at the time it was written but changes may still occur.

The reforms, now enabled in the Coroners and Justice Act 2009, are intended to:

- increase transparency for bereaved families
- improve the quality and accuracy of medical certificates of cause of death (MCCDs – see Chapter 29)
- introduce Medical Examiners to provide a system of effective medical scrutiny applicable to all deaths that do not require a coroner's post-mortem or inquest
- enable Medical Examiners to report matters of a clinical governance nature to support local learning and changes to practice and procedures
- provide information on public health surveillance requested by a Director of Public Health.

The new Medical Examiner system aims to provide a common approach as follows

- All deaths will be scrutinized in a robust and proportionate way, regardless of whether they are followed by burial or cremation, making the system fairer (this is similar to the new Scottish system – see Chapter 37).
- Medical certification and the registration of all deaths not requiring a coroner's post-mortem or inquest will be examined in the same way, including:
  - unified arrangements for burial and cremation
  - a simpler process for arranging funerals
  - removal of any inequalities.

- All medical certificates of cause of death (MCCDs) will be confirmed by local medical examiners. There will also be an out-of-hours scrutiny service where it is needed, for example, for organ donation or to comply with religious practices.
- There will be strengthening of safeguards for the public and to ensure that the right deaths are referred to a coroner.

It is intended that the certified cause of death will be explained to all relatives, either face-to-face or over the telephone. Relatives will also be given an opportunity to discuss any concerns they might have about the care provided to the person who has died and report the death to a coroner. Any unnecessary distress for those who are bereaved, resulting from unanswered questions about the certified cause of death or from unexpected delays when registering a death, will be avoided. It is expected that rejections of MCCDs by the Registrar will be all but eliminated.

Other perceived advantages

- Information will be more complete on MCCDs, including contributory conditions and factors leading to cause of death and spotting of unusual trends in deaths for local public health surveillance. This will improve the quality of the cause-of-death information for local clinical governance and public health surveillance to help the NHS learn and save more lives in the future.
- Malpractice will be easier to detect. The new system will also confirm to the registrar that the death has been discussed and that no concerns were raised that might require the death to be investigated by a coroner.
- Medical Examiners will have powers to report matters of patient safety to the local clinical governance team for prompt action. This will improve safety in the NHS, allowing easier identification of trends and unusual patterns, and enable local learning and changes to practice and procedures.

The new process

- Doctors who are unsure of the cause of death on the MCCD will be able to discuss it with a Medical Examiner for guidance. This will increase the quality and accuracy of the MCCDs and reduce the number of deaths that are unnecessarily reported to a coroner.
- Where a death does not need to be investigated by a coroner, the attending doctor will prepare the MCCD with the guidance of the ME.
- When a death that has been notified to a coroner is found not to require a post-mortem or inquest, the doctor, with the ME, will prepare an MCCD in the same way as for a non-reportable death. If there is no attending doctor or none available, then the MCCD can be prepared and signed by the Medical Examiner.
- During scrutiny, a Medical Examiner may determine that the death is reportable and will refer the death to a coroner. This activity is currently

undertaken by the Registrar and can be difficult if it requires medical knowledge or if it causes distress for bereaved families.

- The Medical Examiner scrutinizes the MCCD and the medical records of the deceased.
- The Medical Examiner may determine that the MCCD appears to be incorrect. This would be discussed with the attending doctor, to agree any changes that may need to be made.
- The Medical Examiner may identify clinical governance issues and will advise colleagues who are responsible for taking appropriate local action.
- The Medical Examiner or a Medical Examiner's officer will discuss the cause of death with a member or representative of the family of the deceased – 'The Informant'. This is an opportunity for any questions or concerns about the cause of death to be raised. If there are no concerns to be addressed then the Medical Examiner will prepare and sign a notification stating the confirmed cause of death.
- The notification includes the name of the informant – the person with whom the cause of death has been discussed – their relationship to the deceased and the date and time of the discussion. The notification must be signed by the informant, to confirm that the discussion has taken place, before registration of the death can be completed.
- The notification will be given to the attending doctor and the Registrar that the MCCD is confirmed and can be issued to the informant.
- The Registrar compares the MCCD and the notification, ensures the notification is signed by the informant, and registers the death.
- Once the confirmed MCCD has been issued, the funeral director will be able to prepare the body for burial, cremation or other chosen legal action. Removal of implants and medical devices will need to be confirmed prior to cremation. The informant is expected to give information about any infection hazards to a funeral director or funeral arranger so that appropriate action is taken to meet health and safety requirements.
- A death is usually registered before burial, cremation or other chosen legal action. However, where a funeral needs to take place very quickly after a death, possibly to comply with religious or cultural practices, the Registrar may be able to issue authority to proceed prior to registration, provided that the scrutiny is completed, and the MCCD and notification form are confirmed.
- Burials are authorized by the Registrar – they issue the Green Form to the informant once they are satisfied all the safeguards have been completed. The Green Form must be handed to the funeral director or arranger.

Professional standards and training and medical examiner recruitment

The Academy of Medical Royal Colleges has developed a curriculum and training materials for medical examiners.[5]

The curriculum developed for medical examiners will help them:

- navigate the system of death certification and develop strong relationships with their partners.
- understand the issues when discussing the cause of death with the recently bereaved.
- identify and overcome death certification problems.
- Local authorities will have responsibility for appointing medical examiners in England; Local Health Boards will be responsible for appointing medical examiners in Wales.
- It is expected that around 385 experienced doctors will be recruited to work as medical examiners, mostly on a part-time basis.
- Medical examiners must be registered medical practitioners with at least five years' experience and have been practising within the previous five years.

The future

Given the delays that have dogged the introduction of MEs, readers should ascertain just what the situation is for themselves in their locality at the time of reading.

Notes

1 Secretary of State for the Home Department (2013): 'The Shipman Inquiry Third Report: Death Certification and the Investigation of Deaths by Coroners'. Available at: www.gov.uk/government/publications/the-shipman-inquiry-third-report-death-certification-and-the-investigation-of-deaths-by-coroners.
2 Department of Health (2007): 'Consultation on Improving the Process of Death Certification'. Available at: http://webarchive.nationalarchives.gov.uk/+/http://www.dh.gov.uk/en/Consultations/Closedconsultations/DH_076971.
3 Available at: www.legislation.gov.uk/ukpga/2009/25/contents.
4 Department of Health and Social Care (2016): 'An Overview of the Death Certification Reforms'. Available at: www.gov.uk/government/publications/changes-to-the-death-certification-process/an-overview-of-the-death-certification-reforms.
5 Royal College of Pathologists and E-Learning for Healthcare (2017): 'The Medical Examiner'. Available at: www.e-lfh.org.uk/programmes/medical-examiner/.

Index

Locators in *italics* refer to figures and those in **bold** to tables.

Abraham (Bible) 163
Abrahamic religions 92, 94; *see also* Baha'i faith; Christianity; Islam; Judaism; Rastafarianism
accidents as cause of death 295–296, 309–310
adolescence, rites and societal interventions 71–72
advance directives 223–224
African heritage 171–172; *see also* Rastafarianism
Afro-Caribbean community: Christianity 133, 134; Rastafarianism 171–172
afterlife: belief in 42–46; exploitation 41–42; near-death experiences and deathbed visions 65–67; scepticism 39–41; what happens when we die? 32, 33–34, 39–46
agnosticism: current practice 177; global distribution 100; historic emergence and trends 93–94, *95*; meaning of 176; UK distribution 101–102; *see also* secularism
ahimsa 156
Ahura Mazda 201–202
Allah 46, 145, 151
allegory 20–21
Alston, W. P. 16
alternative facts 10
amoebas 207, *208*, 210–211
anatomical examination 222, 282; *see also* autopsies
Anglicanism 128–129

Angra Mainyu 201–202
animism 26–28
Antyesti 141
Arab Spring 9
Aristotle 52, 53
Armstrong, Karen 83
Arnold, Matthew 33
Asimov, Isaac 58
assisted dying 225–226
assisted suicide 225–226
Assyrians 33
atheism: current practice 177; global distribution 100; historic emergence and trends 93–94, *95*; meaning of 176; UK distribution 101–102; *see also* secularism
atman 34, 137
Aurelius, Marcus 32, 33, 50–51
autolysis 212–213
autopsies: Baha'i faith 105; Buddhism 114; Chinese beliefs 122; Christianity 134; consent 222, 228–235; coroners 259, 263, 264–266, 268–269; forensic 268–269; Hinduism 141; infection control 276; international comparisons 297, **298**; Islam 152; Jainism 159; Judaism 169, 266; Rastafarianism 173; secularism 183; Shintoism 190; Sikhism 198; Zoroastrianism 203
Avicenna 53
Ayatollahs 77, 84, 148
Ayer, A. J. 66–67
Ayurveda 140

Babylonians 33
Baha'i faith 92, *94*; autopsy and organ transplantation 105; care of the dying 105; description of the religion 103–105; management of death 105
baptism 132
belief paradigms 26–31; animism 26–28; deism 29–30; dualism 30; monotheism 28; pantheism 26, 28–29; polytheism 26
beliefs: in an afterlife 42–46; justifications 7–8; need for tolerance 6–12; why people believe 5–6, 7–12; *see also* religion; *individually named religions e.g. Christianity, Islam*
bereavement: Confucianism 121; family members' roles around death 239–240; and grief 240–243; Islam 152; Roman Catholicism 133
Bible: allegory and metaphor 20–21; Judaism 162–163
Biblical Christianity 127
bikur cholim 167
biological understanding: the body after death 211–213, 271–272; death 210–211; decay 208–209; life 207–208
Bland, Tony 227
the body after death 271; biological understanding 211–213, 271–272; control of infection and other hazards 274–276; diagnosis of death 213–219; identification and external examination 272–273; last offices 275–276, 291–292; removal of implanted items 273–274; *see also* autopsies; disposal of the body; management of death
brain death: diagnosis of 283–288; Judaism 169; meaning of 36, 211; persistent vegetative state 227; reversibility 61–62; Shintoism 190; the soul 57
brain-stem testing 285–288
Broks, P. 59
Buddha 42, 52, 107, 108
Buddhism: autopsy and organ transplantation 114; care of the dying 113, 120–121; in China 117–118; description of the religion 107–113; global followers 97; management of death 113–114, 121–122; perfect peace 43–44
Buddhology 110

Bunkotsu 190
burial: Christianity 133; funeral director's role 243; Islam 151; Judaism 168; at sea 281; in the UK 279–280
Bush, George W. 75

Calvin, Susan 58
care of the dying: Baha'i faith 105; Buddhism 113; Chinese beliefs 120–121; Christianity 131–132; healthcare professionals' roles 237–239; Hinduism 140; Islam 150–151; Jainism 157–158; Judaism 167–168; Rastafarianism 173; secularism 183; Shintoism 188–189; Sikhism 197; Zoroastrianism 202–203
Caribbean community: Christianity 133, 134; Rastafarianism 171–172
Cartesian dualism 54–55
caste systems: Hinduism 138–139; Sikhism 196
certification *see* medical certification of the cause of death
Charismatic Christianity 129
charities, religious basis **81**, 81–82
Chief Coroners 262, 265, 268
Chief Coroner's Guide (CCG) 261–262
childhood, rites and societal interventions 71
Chinese beliefs 91, 92, **95**; autopsy and organ transplantation 122; care of the dying 120–121; description of the religions/philosophies 117–120; management of death 121–122; *see also* Confucianism; Shintoism; Taoism
Christ 124–125
Christian Scientists 131; autopsy 134; interventions 132; management of death 133
Christianity: abuses of 83–84; allegory and metaphor 20–21; autopsy and organ transplantation 134; care of the dying 131–132; denominations today *126*, 128–131; description of the religion 124–131; dualism 30; global followers 97, 98, 124; historic emergence *94*, 125–127; management of death 133; the soul 52–53; and spirituality 179; what happens when we die? 34, 40, 44, 45
church Christianity 127

Church of Jesus Christ of Latter-Day Saints 130
circulatory criteria for death 217
cleaning procedures 275–276
Cold War 73
comatose *see* brain death
Conan Doyle, Arthur 55–56
confidentiality 221
Confucianism: autopsy and organ transplantation 122; care of the dying 120–121; in China and Japan 91; description of the religion 117–119; management of death 121–122
Confucius 44
consciousness 56
consent: autopsies 222, 228–235; disposal of the body 278–279; donation of body for research 282; organ transplantation 288–290
conservative Judaism 166
conversion 73–75
coroners: autopsy request 263, 264–266; Chief Coroners 262, 265, 268; exhumation 296; forensic autopsy 268–269; inquests and 'verdicts' or 'findings' 266–268; Judaism 169; medical certification of the cause of death 246–247, 250, 263–264; Northern Ireland 300–302; organ donors 290; referral of a death to 263–264; registration of death 254; retained tissues 269; what is a coroner and what does the coroner do? 260–262; when a coroner is needed 258–259
Coroners and Justice Act (2009) 260–262
cosmological argument for God 22
cremation: Christianity 133; exporting ashes overseas 295; Harold Shipman case 311; Hinduism 141; Islam 151; Jainism 158; Judaism 168; removal of implanted items 273–274; Sikhism 198; in the UK 280
Crick, Francis 41
cross-infection 274–276
Crown and Procurator Fiscal Service (COPFS), Scotland 309–310
cultural entanglements 69–71

Dante's *Inferno* 34
Darius, King of Persia 7
Darwin, Charles 30, 80

death: approaches from literature 37–39; biological understanding 208–209; the body after death 211–213; brain-stem testing 285–288; concepts surrounding 32–34, 206; declaration of 213–214; definition 210–211, 214; diagnosis of 213–219, **218**; different religions 7; discussions about 2–3; how does death happen? 211; meaning of 34–37, 210–212; registration of 253–259; reversibility 61–62; what happens when we die? 32, 33–34, 39–46; *see also* care of the dying; management of death; medical certification of the cause of death; medico-legal issues at end of life
death certificates 247, 256, 258, 311–312; *see also* medical certification of the cause of death
Death Certification Review Service (DCRS) 302, 303
deathbed visions (DBVs) 65–67
decay, biological 208–209
deism 29–30
dementia 35, 63
demographics: distribution of religions across the world 97–100; national health service 102; population projections 100, **101**; religion in the UK **101**, 101–102
Descartes, Rene 49, 54–55
Dhamma 108, 111
Dharma 109, 137
Dharmic religions 91
diet *see* fasting; food requirements
disease: infection control 274–276; Sikhism 197
disposal of the body 279–282; *see also* burial; cremation
doctrinal dimension of religion 17
donation of body for research 281–282
donation of organs/tissues 288–290
Donne, John 38–39
double effect 222–223
Drummond, Edward 57
dualism 30, 49, 54–55
Dylan, Bob 23–24

Eagleman, David 34–35
Eddy, Mary Baker 131
Egyptian religion 33
Eistein, Albert 30

elective ventilation of potential organ
donors 226–227
emotion: and beliefs 10; bereavement
and grief 240–243; healthcare
professionals 239; *see also* mourning
emotional dimension of religion 17
end of life *see* care of the dying; death;
management of death; medico-legal
issues at end of life
England and Wales: autopsies in
264–265; future changes 311–315;
missing persons 293–294; registration
of death 253–259
entanglements: cultural 69–71; religion,
politics and the law 75–78; rites and
societal interventions 71–75
ethical dimension of religion 17–18
euthanasia: Christianity 131–132;
Judaism 167; types of and the law
224–225
Evangelical Christianity 129
evil, religious understanding of 23–25
exhumation 295–296
experiential dimension of religion 17, 23
exploitation, of religion 41–42
exporting a body overseas 294–295

faith *see* religion
family members: bereavement 240–243;
discussions about death 2–3; grief
240–243; last offices 292; organ
donation 288–290; registration of
death 255–259; tasks around death
239–240; what does death mean?
61–63; *see also* mourning
fasting: Baha'i faith 105; Hinduism
140; Islam 151; Jainism 157–158;
Orthodox Christians 129; *see also*
food requirements
Fatal Accident Inquiries (FAIs)
309–310
fear, of the afterlife 41–42
Flying Man thought experiment 53
folk religions: global followers 97,
98–100; meaning of 16
food requirements: Islam 150–151;
Judaism 167–168; Rastafarianism
172; Sikhism 197; Zoroastrianism
202; *see also* fasting
forensic autopsy 268–269
'free' churches 129–130
free will 23, 58, 158, 202
freedom of speech 84–85

freedom of thought, conscience and
religion 77–78, 169
Fricker, M. 8–9
funeral director's role 243
funerals *see* management of death
future changes, medical examiner
system 311–315

Gage, Phineas 57
Galton, Francis 80
Gardiner, Gerald 182
Garvey, Marcus 171–172
Gautama, Siddhartha *see* Buddha
Glaucon 51
global distribution of religion 97–100,
99, 101
God: characteristics of a supreme being
21–23; distinctive features of religion
16; evil and unpleasant events 23–24;
existence of 22–23, 54; monotheism
28; *see also individually named
religions*
gods: Greek and Roman 21–22;
polytheism 26; *see also individually
named religions*
Graves, Robert 73
Greek philosophy 51–52
Greek religion 21–22, 34
grief 240–243; *see also* mourning
Guru Granth Sahib 195–196
Guruship in Sikhism 195

Hadiths 145
Haldane, J. B. S. 58, 59
hazardous substances 276; *see also*
infection control
Health and Safety Executive, major
accidents 295
healthcare professionals: declaration
of death 213–214; discussions about
death 2–3; last offices 291–292;
medical certification of the cause
of death 245–252; medical
examiners 311–315; registration
of death 253–259; roles around
death 237–239; *see also*
management of death
Heaven 46, 128; *see also* afterlife
Hebrew Bible 162–163
Hell 34, 46; *see also* afterlife
Herodotus 7
Herzl, Theodore 164
Hindu Trinity 137

Hinduism: autopsy and organ
transplantation 141; care of the
dying 140; description of the
religion 136–140; dualism 30; global
followers 97, 98; management
of death 141; rebirth 43, 44; and
Sikhism 193, 194; what happens
when we die? 34
Holocaust 164–165
Holy Piby 171
homicide: autopsy 269; Harold
Shipman case 311; *see also*
suspicious deaths
Human Rights 77–78, 86, 158, 169, 266
Human Tissue Act (2004) 235, 269, 282
Human Tissue Authority (HTA) 222,
228–235, 269, 281–282
humanism 177–178
Hume, David 7–9, 40–41
Huxley, T. H. 176

identification of a dead body 272–273
implanted items, the body after death
273–274
independent, everlasting soul 44
Indian subcontinent 91–92, *93*, **95**; *see
also* Buddhism; Hinduism; Jainism;
Sikhism
infection control 274–276
the informant, registration of death
255–257
inquests 266–268
institutional dimension of religion 18
international consensus on the diagnosis
of death 216–218, *217*, **218**
involuntary euthanasia 225
Islam: abuses of 84–85; autopsy and
organ transplantation 152; care of
the dying 150–151; description of the
religion 144–150; divisions within
147–149; global followers 97, 98,
144, 144; historic emergence *94*, *149*;
management of death 151–152; rites
and societal interventions 72; and
Sikhism 193, 194; what happens
when we die? 34, 44, 46
Israel 164–165
Israelites 33–34

Jainism: autopsy and organ
transplantation 159; care of the dying
157–158; description of the religion
155–157; management of death 158
Jamaica 171; *see also* Rastafarianism

James, William 179
Japanese beliefs: brain death 36;
historic emergence and trends
91, *92*, **95**; Shintoism as lifestyle
religion 186; *see also* Confucianism;
Shintoism; Taoism
Jehovah's Witnesses 131, 134
Jesus 124–125
Jihad 147
Judaism 44; autopsy and organ
transplantation 169, 266; branches
of 161–162, 165–167, *166*; care of
the dying 167–168; description of the
religion 161–167; global followers
97, 98, 161; historic emergence 94;
management of death 168; Passover
85–86; what happens when we die?
44–45
Judith (Bible) 284

kami 187–188, 189
karma 109, 139–140
Keats, John 37, 38
Khalsa 195
Koran *see* Qur'an
Kosher food 167–168

language, accurate meaning of written
texts 19
last offices 275–276, 291–292
latter-day saints 133, 134
law: advance directives 224; capacity
223–224; confidentiality 221; consent
222; coroners 260–262; cremation
280; defining the Hindu religion
136–137; diagnosis of death 213–219,
218; elective ventilation of potential
organ donors 226–227; euthanasia
224–225; exhumation 295–296;
'Freedom of thought, conscience and
religion' 77–78; Hindu caste system
139; Human Rights 77–78, 86, 158,
169, 266; Islamic beliefs on scriptures
and the law 145–147; Judaism 162,
169; medico-legal considerations
at end of life 221; missing persons
293–294; powers of attorney 224;
registration of death 253–259;
relationship with religion and politics
75–78; retained tissues 222, 269,
281–282; Scottish system 302; suicide
225–226; unnatural death 227–228;
see also medical certification of the
cause of death

legal death 36–37, 213
legal dimension of religion 17–18
Liberal Christianity 129
liberal Judaism 166
liberalism, rites and societal
    interventions 72–73
life: complex forms of 209, *210*; as
    concept 206; definition 206–207;
    humans 209–210; simple forms of
    207–209, *208*
life expectancy **80**, 80–81
life support 288
Lindsell, Annie 223
lividity 271–272
living wills 224
lobbying 76
Lodge, Oliver 55, 56
Lucretius 40
Luther, Martin 42, 127, 164

Machiavelli, N. 32
Mahāyāna (East Asian) Buddhism
    111, *111*
Maimonides 53–54
major disasters 295–296, 309–310
mammalian life 209–210, *210*
management of death: Baha'i faith
    105; Buddhism 113–114; Chinese
    beliefs 121–122; Christianity 133;
    family members' role 239–243;
    funeral director's role 243; healthcare
    professionals' roles 237–239;
    Hinduism 141; humanism 178; Islam
    151–152; Jainism 158; Judaism 168;
    Rastafarianism 173; secularism 183;
    Shintoism 189–190; Sikhism 198;
    Zoroastrianism 203; *see also* burial;
    cremation
marriage: Hinduism 139;
    Rastafarianism 172; Sikhism
    196–197
Marx, Karl 41–42
material dimension of religion 18
McNaughton, Denis 57
medical certification of the cause of
    death (MCCD): coroners' role
    246–247, 250, 263–264; doctor's
    role 214, 245; filling in 250–252;
    funeral director's role 243; future
    changes 311–312; importance of
    245–246; new Medical Examiner
    system 312–314; Northern Ireland
    297, 298–300, *299*, *301*; procedure
    and description of the forms

246–250, *248–249*; registration of
    death 254–255; Scotland 302–309,
    304–307
medical examiners (MEs) 311–315
medico-legal issues at end of life 221;
    advance directives 244; capacity
    223–224; confidentiality 221;
    consent 222, 228–229; elective
    ventilation of potential organ donors
    226–227; euthanasia 224–225;
    powers of attorney 224; unnatural
    death 227–228
Mental Capacity Act 2005 223
Mental Health Act 2007 223
metaphors 20–21
Michener, James 70
Middle East 92–93, **95**
middle way (Buddhism) 110
Midgley, Mary 58
missing persons 293–294
monastic Christianity 127
monotheism 28
Moor, David 223
moral argument for God 22
moral dimension of religion 17–18
moral norms 12
Mormon Church 130
mortuary practice 276
Moses 162
mourning: bereavement and grief
    240–243; Confucianism 121;
    Islam 152; Judaism 168; Roman
    Catholicism 133; Sikhism 198
Muhammad 145–146
multi-cultural society: discussions about
    death 2–3; tolerance of belief 10–12
mystical Christianity 127
mythic dimension of religion 17

naming conventions: secularism 178;
    Sikhism 196, 197
Nanak (first Guru of Sikhism)
    193–195, *194*
narrative dimension of religion 17
National Confidential Enquiry
    into Patient Outcome and Death
    (NCEPOD) 265
national health service (NHS) 102
National Institute for Health and
    Clinical Excellence (NICE) 289
National Medical Examiners 311–314
natural disasters 295
near-death experiences (NDEs) 65–67
neo-paganism 182

neurological criteria for death 218
neuroscience, the soul 56, 57–59
New Age beliefs 94, *95*, 180–181
Nicene Creed 126
Nirvana 108–109
Noble Eightfold Path (Buddhism) 110
non-conformist churches 127, 129–130
non-heart-beating donors 288
non-therapeutic elective ventilation
    (NTEV) 226–227
Northern Ireland, certification and
    registration processes 297–302

Oedipus the King 21
Office of the Area Coroner 260–262
ontological argument for God 22
opioids, double effect 222–223
organ examination 231; *see also*
    autopsies
organ transplantation: Baha'i faith 105;
    Buddhism 114; Chinese beliefs 122;
    Christianity 134; consent 288–290;
    elective ventilation of potential organ
    donors 226–227; Hinduism 141; Islam
    152; Jainism 159; Judaism 169; last
    offices 291; non-heart-beating donors
    288; Rastafarianism 173; secularism
    183; Shintoism 190; Sikhism 198;
    Zoroastrianism 203
Orthodox Churches 129
orthodox Judaism 165–166, 168, 169

paganism 181–182
pain killers, double effect 222–223
Paine, Thomas 29–30, 76
Palestine 164–165
Pali Canon 108
palliative care: Baha'i faith 105; care of
    the dying 238; Christianity 131–132;
    Jainism 157; Judaism 167
pantheism 26, 28–29, 137
Parsee *see* Zoroastrianism
Passover 85–86
patients, what does death mean?
    61–63
Pentecostal Christianity 129, 133
perfect peace 43–44
persistent vegetative state 227; *see also*
    brain death
personality, death of 35–36
philosophical dimension of religion 17
physiological death 36
Plato 51
police involvement 227–228, 263

politics, relationship with religion and
    the law 75–78
polytheism 26
the Pope (Catholic Church) 45, 77,
    84, 128
population projections 100, **101**
post-mortem examination *see* autopsies
post-truth 10
powers of attorney 223–224
practitioners *see* healthcare
    professionals
prayer, and life expectancy 80–81
Presumption of Death Act 2013
    293–294
primary flaccidity 272
professionals *see* healthcare
    professionals
Protestantism 127, 128–130
Purgatory 45
putrefaction 212–213

Qur'an: accurate meaning of written
    texts 19–20; care of the dying 151;
    freedom of speech 84–85; Islamic
    beliefs on scriptures and the law
    145–147; as word of God 83

Rabbis 163, 168
Ramadan 151
Rastafarianism: autopsy and organ
    transplantation 173; care of the
    dying 173; description of the religion
    171–173; historic emergence 94;
    management of death 173
rebirth 43, 109
reconstructionist Judaism 167
reform Judaism 166
Reformation 128, 164
Register Offices 253–254
registration of death: England and
    Wales 253–259; Northern Ireland
    297–302; Scotland 302–310
reincarnation: Hinduism 34; Jainism 156;
    meaning of 43; Rastafarianism 172
relatives *see* family members
relativism 8–10
religion: abuses of 82–86; belief
    paradigms 26–31; beliefs about death
    3–4; characteristics of a supreme
    being 21–23; as comfort at death
    243; cultural entanglements 69–71;
    definition 15–16; distinctive features
    16–18; evil and unpleasant events
    23–25; interpretation of religious

texts 18–21; need for tolerance 6–12; relationship with politics and the law 75–78; rites and societal interventions 71–75; uses of 80–82; what happens when we die? 33–34, 39–46; why people believe 5–6, 7–12
religious experience argument for God 23
religious systems: categorization 90–91, 94; Chinese and Japanese beliefs 91, 92; distribution of religions across the world 97–100, **99**, **101**; distribution of religions in the UK **101**, 101–102; historic timeline 95, 96; Indian subcontinent 91–92, 93; Middle East 92–93; secular ethics and new faiths 93–94, 95; *see also individually named religions e.g. Christianity, Islam*
research, donation of body for 281–282
retained tissues 222, 231, 269
'revelation' 5, 92–93
rigor mortis 217, 272, 292
rites 71–75
ritual dimension of religion 17; Baha'i faith 104; cultural entanglements 69–71; Hinduism 138; Islam 151; Jainism 157; rites and societal interventions 71–75; Shintoism 188, 190; Sikhism 194; Taoism 122; Zoroastrianism 202, 203
Robinson, J., Bishop 179
robots, and the soul 58
Roman Catholicism: death rites 132; description of the religion 128; the soul 56–57; Spanish Inquisition 83–84; the 'wake' 133; what happens when we die? 45
Roman religion 21–22, 34
Rorty, Richard 9
Rushdie, Salman 84–85
Russell, Bertrand 11, 41, 42

sacraments, Christianity 132
Sallekhana 157–158
Salmon, George 73
samsara 6, 34, 43–44, 109
Sanatana Dharma 137
Sangha 108
Santayana, George 33
Sargant, William 73–74
Saudi Arabia 77
scepticism, to the afterlife 39–41
Schrödinger, Erwin 214
scientology 182–183

Scotland, certification and registration processes 297, 302–310
Scruton, Roger 9
secular Judaism 162, 167
secularism: autopsy and organ transplantation 183; care of the dying 183; description of philosophies and belief systems 175–183; ethics and new faiths 93–94, 95; historic emergence 93–94, 95; management of death 183; near-death experiences 66–67; religion, politics and the law 76–77; religious wars 83; rites and societal interventions 72–73
sedatives, double effect 222–223
Selassie, Haile 172
Shari'a law 146–147
Shelley, Percy Bysshe 28–29
Shi'ite Islam 147–148
Shintoism: autopsy and organ transplantation 190; care of the dying 188–189; in China and Japan 91; description of the religion 186–188; management of death 189–190
Shipman, Harold 311
shraddha 141
shrutis 138
Sikhism: autopsy and organ transplantation 198; care of the dying 197; description of the religion 193–197; management of death 198; names 196, 197
Smart, Ninian 6, 12, 16–17
smritis 138
social class: Hinduism 138–139; life expectancy 80
social death 36
social dimension of religion 18
social media 9
social relationships: reciprocity 63; what does death mean? 61–63
societal interventions 71–75
society: cultural entanglements 69–71; religion, politics and the law 75–78; rites and societal interventions 71–75
Socrates 51, 52
Solomon (Bible) 163
somatic criteria for death 216–217
the soul: arguments for and against the existence of 51–59; meaning of 49–51; near-death experiences and deathbed visions 67; what happens when we die? 44–45

Spanish Inquisition 83–84
Spencer, Herbert 10–11, 206–207
Spinoza, B. 28, 30
spiritualism 55–56, 181
spirituality 178–180
sudden deaths 309–310; *see also* suspicious deaths
Sufism 148
suicide: Christianity 131–132; Jainism 158; law 225–226; Shintoism 189; Sikhism 197
Sunna 145
Sunni Islam 147–148
survival of the fittest 10–11
suspicious deaths: forensic autopsy 268–269; Harold Shipman case 311; last offices 291; police involvement 227–228; Scotland 309–310

Tanakh 162
Taoism: autopsy and organ transplantation 122; care of the dying 120–121; in China and Japan 91; description of the religion 117–118, 119–120; management of death 122
teleological argument for God 22
Tengoku 190
terrorism: abuses of religions 82–86; War on Terror 75
theocracy 77
theodicy 6
Theravāda (Southern) Buddhism 112, *112*
thermodynamics 208, 212–213, 214, 215
Thetan 183
Thomas, Dylan 37–38
Tibetan (Northern) Buddhism 112
tissue donation 288–290
tolerance: Buddhism 111; different religions 6–12; universality 11–12
Torah 162
training needs 2

transplantation *see* organ transplantation
tribalism 3
Trimurti 137
the Trinity 126–127
truth, and relativism 9
turbans 195

unexpected deaths 309–310; *see also* major disasters; suicide; suspicious deaths
universal tolerance 11–12
unnatural death *see* suspicious deaths
Uthmanic Codex 145

Vatican City 77
vegetative state 227; *see also* brain death
visions of the bereaved (VBs) 65–67
voluntary euthanasia 225

War on Terror 75
wars: abuses of religions 82–84; Jewish mistreatment 164–165
Weber, Max 5–6
Wesley, John 74
Wicca 182
wills 223–224
'witchcraft' 182
Wong, David 12
woodland burials 279–280
Wordsworth, William 180

yin and *yang* 119–120, *120*

Zoroastrianism: autopsy and organ transplantation 203; care of the dying 202–203; description of the religion 201–202; dualism 30; evil and unpleasant events 23; historic context 92, *93*; management of death 203